Gastrointestinal Malignancies:
Screening, Diagnosis, and Treatment

Gastrointestinal Malignancies: Screening, Diagnosis, and Treatment

Editor

Ugo Grossi

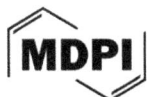

Basel • Beijing • Wuhan • Barcelona • Belgrade • Novi Sad • Cluj • Manchester

Editor
Ugo Grossi
University of Padua
Treviso, Italy

Editorial Office
MDPI
St. Alban-Anlage 66
4052 Basel, Switzerland

This is a reprint of articles from the Special Issue published online in the open access journal *Journal of Clinical Medicine* (ISSN 2077-0383) (available at: https://www.mdpi.com/journal/jcm/special_issues/Gastrointestinal_Malignancies_Screening_Diagnosis_Treatment).

For citation purposes, cite each article independently as indicated on the article page online and as indicated below:

Lastname, A.A.; Lastname, B.B. Article Title. *Journal Name* **Year**, *Volume Number*, Page Range.

ISBN 978-3-0365-9386-9 (Hbk)
ISBN 978-3-0365-9387-6 (PDF)
doi.org/10.3390/books978-3-0365-9387-6

© 2023 by the authors. Articles in this book are Open Access and distributed under the Creative Commons Attribution (CC BY) license. The book as a whole is distributed by MDPI under the terms and conditions of the Creative Commons Attribution-NonCommercial-NoDerivs (CC BY-NC-ND) license.

Contents

About the Editor vii

**Marina Nogueira Silveira, Lara Pozzuto, Maria Carolina Santos Mendes,
Lorena Pires da Cunha, Felipe Osório Costa, Lígia Traldi Macedo, et al.**
Association of Albumin-Corrected Serum Calcium Levels with Colorectal Cancer Survival
Outcomes
Reprinted from: *J. Clin. Med.* **2022**, *11*, 2928, doi:10.3390/jcm11102928 1

**Monika Zajkowska, Maciej Dulewicz, Agnieszka Kulczyńska-Przybik, Kamil Safiejko,
Marcin Juchimiuk, Marzena Konopko, et al.**
The Significance of Selected C-C Motif Chemokine Ligands in Colorectal Cancer Patients
Reprinted from: *J. Clin. Med.* **2022**, *11*, 1794, doi:10.3390/jcm11071794 11

Yu-Min Huang, Po-Li Wei, Chung-Han Ho and Chih-Ching Yeh
Cigarette Smoking Associated with Colorectal Cancer Survival: A Nationwide,
Population-Based Cohort Study
Reprinted from: *J. Clin. Med.* **2022**, *11*, 913, doi:10.3390/jcm11040913 23

**Noriyuki Arakawa, Atsushi Irisawa, Kazuyuki Ishida, Takuya Tsunoda, Yoshiko Yamaguchi,
Goro Shibukawa, et al.**
Clinical Differences in c-Myc Expression in Early-Stage Gastric Neoplasia: A Retrospective
Study Based on the WHO Classification
Reprinted from: *J. Clin. Med.* **2022**, *11*, 544, doi:10.3390/jcm11030544 37

**Choong-Kyun Noh, Eunyoung Lee, Gil Ho Lee, Sun Gyo Lim, Bumhee Park, Sung Jae Shin,
et al.**
Association of Regular Endoscopic Screening with Interval Gastric Cancer Incidence in the
National Cancer Screening Program
Reprinted from: *J. Clin. Med.* **2022**, *11*, 230, doi:10.3390/jcm11010230 47

**Masashi Fukushima, Hirokazu Fukui, Jiro Watari, Chiyomi Ito, Ken Hara, Hirotsugu Eda,
et al.**
Gastric Xanthelasma, Microsatellite Instability and Methylation of Tumor Suppressor Genes in
the Gastric Mucosa: Correlation and Comparison as a Predictive Marker for the Development
of Synchronous/Metachronous Gastric Cancer
Reprinted from: *J. Clin. Med.* **2022**, *11*, 9, doi:10.3390/jcm11010009 57

**Sung Yong Han, Sung Hee Park, Hyun Suk Ko, Aelee Jang, Hyung Il Seo, So Jeong Lee,
et al.**
Vimentin-Positive Circulating Tumor Cells as Diagnostic and Prognostic Biomarkers in Patients
with Biliary Tract Cancer
Reprinted from: *J. Clin. Med.* **2021**, *10*, 4435, doi:10.3390/jcm10194435 69

Shu-Wei Huang, Yen-Chin Chen, Yang-Hsiang Lin and Chau-Ting Yeh
Clinical Limitations of Tissue Annexin A2 Level as a Predictor of Postoperative Overall Survival
in Patients with Hepatocellular Carcinoma
Reprinted from: *J. Clin. Med.* **2021**, *10*, 4158, doi:10.3390/jcm10184158 85

**Young Ki Lee, Eun Kyung Lee, You Jin Lee, Bang Wool Eom, Hong Man Yoon, Young-Il Kim,
et al.**
Metabolic Effects of Gastrectomy and Duodenal Bypass in Early Gastric Cancer Patients with
T2DM: A Prospective Single-Center Cohort Study
Reprinted from: *J. Clin. Med.* **2021**, *10*, 4008, doi:10.3390/jcm10174008 99

Ju-Hee Lee, Sung-Joon Kwon, Mimi Kim and Bo-Kyeong Kang
Prevalence and Clinical Implications of Ascites in Gastric Cancer Patients after Curative Surgery
Reprinted from: *J. Clin. Med.* **2021**, *10*, 3557, doi:10.3390/jcm10163557 . . . . **113**

Szu-Chia Liao, Hong-Zen Yeh, Chi-Sen Chang, Wei-Chih Chen, Chih-Hsin Muo and Fung-Chang Sung
Colorectal Cancer Risk in Women with Gynecologic Cancers—A Population Retrospective Cohort Study
Reprinted from: *J. Clin. Med.* **2021**, *10*, 3127, doi:10.3390/jcm10143127 . . . . **123**

Yin-Yi Chu, Jur-Shan Cheng, Ting-Shu Wu, Chun-Wei Chen, Ming-Yu Chang, Hsin-Ping Ku, et al.
Association between Hepatitis C Virus Infection and Esophageal Cancer: An Asian Nationwide Population-Based Cohort Study
Reprinted from: *J. Clin. Med.* **2021**, *10*, 2395, doi:10.3390/jcm10112395 . . . . **133**

About the Editor

Ugo Grossi

Dr. Ugo Grossi is an accomplished medical professional with a distinguished educational background and a wealth of experience in the field of gastrointestinal surgery. He earned his Medical Degree from the Catholic University of Rome in 2007, followed by a Postgraduate Degree in Surgery from the same institution at A. Gemelli University Hospital IRCCS in 2015. Dr. Grossi furthered his academic journey by completing a PhD in Digestive Diseases at Queen Mary University of London, UK, in 2021. Dr. Grossi has been an Assistant Professor at the University of Padua since 2022, and his research interests are primarily centered around the surgical management of benign coloproctological conditions, including functional and inflammatory bowel disorders, as well as pelvic floor disorders. His extensive contributions to this field are evident through his numerous publications. Notably, he has been recognized for his outstanding work with awards from esteemed organizations such as the Italian Society of Surgery (Ettore Ruggieri Award), the European Crohn's and Colitis Organisation (ECCO Travel Award), and the Italian Society of Colorectal Surgery (John Nicholls Prize). His dedication to advancing the field is further underscored by his recent appointment to the Anorectal Disorders Committee for the V Revision of the Rome Criteria for the Rome Foundation.

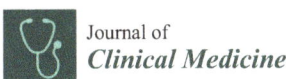

Article

Association of Albumin-Corrected Serum Calcium Levels with Colorectal Cancer Survival Outcomes

Marina Nogueira Silveira, Lara Pozzuto, Maria Carolina Santos Mendes, Lorena Pires da Cunha, Felipe Osório Costa, Lígia Traldi Macedo, Sandra Regina Brambilla and José Barreto Campello Carvalheira *

Division of Oncology, Department of Anesthesiology, Oncology and Radiology, School of Medical Sciences, State University of Campinas (UNICAMP), Campinas, SP 13083-888, Brazil; marina.nogueira2@gmail.com (M.N.S.); larapozzuto.nutri@gmail.com (L.P.); mariacarol.op@gmail.com (M.C.S.M.); lorenapcunha@yahoo.com (L.P.d.C.); felipeoc@unicamp.br (F.O.C.); ligiamed@gmail.com (L.T.M.); sandraunicamp2@gmail.com (S.R.B.)
* Correspondence: jbcc@unicamp.br; Tel.: +55-19-3521-7496

Abstract: In epidemiological studies, higher calcium intake has been associated with decreased colorectal cancer (CRC) incidence. However, whether circulating calcium concentrations are associated with CRC prognosis is largely unknown. In this retrospective cohort analysis, we identified 498 patients diagnosed with stage I–IV CRC between the years of 2000 and 2018 in whom calcium and albumin level measurements within 3 months of diagnosis had been taken. We used the Kaplan–Meier method for survival analysis. We used multivariate Cox proportional hazards regression to identify associations between corrected calcium levels and CRC survival outcomes. Corrected calcium levels in the highest tertile were associated with significantly lower progression-free survival rates (hazard ratio (HR) 1.85; 95% confidence interval (CI) 1.28–2.69; $p = 0.001$) and overall survival (HR 1.86; 95% CI 1.26–2.74, $p = 0.002$) in patients with stage IV or recurrent CRC, and significantly lower disease-free survival rates (HR 1.44; 95% confidence interval (CI) 1.02–2.03; $p = 0.040$) and overall survival rates (HR 1.72; 95% CI 1.18–2.50; $p = 0.004$) in patients with stage I–III disease. In conclusion, higher corrected calcium levels after the diagnosis of CRC were significantly associated with decreased survival rates. Prospective trials are necessary to confirm this association.

Keywords: gastrointestinal malignancies; cancer survivorship; calcium carbonate; hypercalcemia; cancer outcomes

1. Introduction

Every year, it is expected that approximately 1.88 million people will be diagnosed with colorectal cancer (CRC) worldwide, while 915,880 deaths are attributed to the disease [1]. Although current changes in risk factors such as decreased smoking and red meat consumption may have contributed to the decline in overall incidence of CRC in some countries, it is still the third most common type of cancer [2]. For this reason, research that considers possible predictive as well as prognostic factors is needed.

Higher calcium intake has been associated with a decreased risk of CRC [3–5]. Results from a meta-analysis of 21 publications showed that for each 300 mg of calcium consumed, there was a reduction of 8–9% in the risk of acquiring CRC [6]. Consistently, a pooled analysis of 534,536 individuals also revealed a reduction in CRC with higher calcium intake [7]. In contrast, a recently published, large prospective trial found that calcium and calcitriol supplementation was associated with an increased risk of the development of serrated polyps, a CRC precursor lesion [8]. Although calcium signaling is a key player in the fundamental stages of cancer development, the complexities of calcium intersections with oncogenic pathways are context dependent (i.e., the alignment of calcium channels in cancer cells, extracellular calcium concentrations, and calcium interactions with the microenvironment are factors that determine calcium influence in cancer cell fate) [9]. Moreover, increased levels of extracellular calcium are insufficient to modulate cancer cell proliferation. Rather, cytosolic calcium levels, which are mainly determined by the activity of calcium channels, pumps, and exchangers, are key to the control of intracellular calcium levels in a context-dependent manner [9]. Thus, it is simple to delineate a plausible biological framework of how the modulation of extracellular calcium levels by calcium intake influences carcinogenesis.

Much less is known about the effects of serum calcium on the risk of developing CRC. In striking opposition to the association between calcium intake and a reduced risk of CRC, a retrospective analysis of a Swedish databank (Apolipoprotein Mortality Risk (AMORIS)) showed a modest increase in the risk of developing CRC in the highest quartiles of albumin-corrected serum calcium [10]. Calcium homeostasis is regulated not only by calcium intake but also by bidirectional fluxes of this ion at the level of the kidneys and bones [11]. Importantly, calcium homeostasis is disrupted in 20–30% of patients during the course of cancer development [12], making it biologically plausible that the association between higher calcium levels and CRC observed in the AMORIS study may be related to calcium homeostasis disturbances mediated by the initial stages of tumor development.

In normal physiology, extracellular calcium levels are mainly regulated by parathyroid hormone (PTH), calcitonin, and calcitriol [11]. On the other hand, in cancer pathology, the vast majority of hypercalcemia of malignancy is associated with increased PTH-related peptide (PTHrP) levels [12]. Interestingly, PTHrP has a limited role during cartilage embryogenesis through the activation of the hedgehog signaling pathway in cartilage cells [13,14]. In cancer cells, this dormant pathway is reactivated, increasing circulating levels of PTHrP [15], which leads to the elevation of the extracellular calcium concentration in a tumor-burden- and aggressiveness-dependent manner [16,17]. Thus, bearing in mind the hypothesis that the corrected calcium level is a biomarker of cancer progression, we sought to examine the impact of corrected calcium levels in the outcomes of patients with CRC, using both calcium and albumin levels routinely measured during clinic visits reported in medical records.

2. Materials and Methods

2.1. Study Population

This study was a single-center, retrospective, and analytical study conducted at the State University of Campinas Hospital (HC-UNICAMP) in Campinas, Brazil. The study population was composed of patients diagnosed with stage I–IV CRC between the years of 2000 and 2018, admitted to the HC-UNICAMP. Patients that met the following inclusion criteria were selected: histologically confirmed CRC between 2000 and 2018; CRC stage I–IV according to the 8th edition of the American Joint Committee on Cancer (AJCC) cancer staging manual [18]; the availability of calcium and albumin measurements within 3 months of the diagnosis for stage IV or recurrent CRC; the availability of calcium and albumin measurements before surgery in patients with stage I–III CRC; and complete medical record information regarding age, date of diagnosis, topography, histological type, and tumor staging. Patients with concomitant malignancies, CRC that was not adenocarcinoma, in situ CRC, or unreported data regarding treatment were excluded (Figure 1).

The study was approved by the local Institutional Review Board (CAAE number: 15505419.1.0000.5404) with a consent form waiver. The principles recommended by the Declaration of Helsinki were adhered to.

2.2. Body Composition

Two consecutive computed tomography (CT) images of the third lumbar vertebra were evaluated; the images were obtained from routine examinations of the patients. Baseline imaging was performed within 3 months of diagnosis for patients with stage I–III CRC and 3 months before diagnosis or chemotherapy initiation for patients with stage IV or recurrent CRC. Skeletal muscle (SM) values of the psoas, abdominal, rectus abdominis, and paravertebral muscles were measured [19,20]. The visceral adipose tissue (VAT), intramuscular adipose tissue (IMAT), and subcutaneous adipose tissue (SAT) were also measured; from these values, we determined the SM index (SMI), the SAT index (SFI), and the VAT index (VFI), measured in units of square centimeters (cm^2) and normalized by height in square meters (m^2). The software used was SliceOmatic V. 5.0. (Tomovision, Canada); standard Hounsfield units (HUs) established for tissues were −150 to −50 for VAT, −190 to −30 for IMAT and SAT, and −29 to 150 for SM. The images were analyzed by two evaluators (M.N.S. and L.P.) blinded to the outcomes, and the coefficients of variation for the cross-sectional areas analyzed were 1.07%, 1.05%, 1.61%, and 3.57% for SM, SAT, VAT, and IMAT, respectively, and 1.60% for SM density.

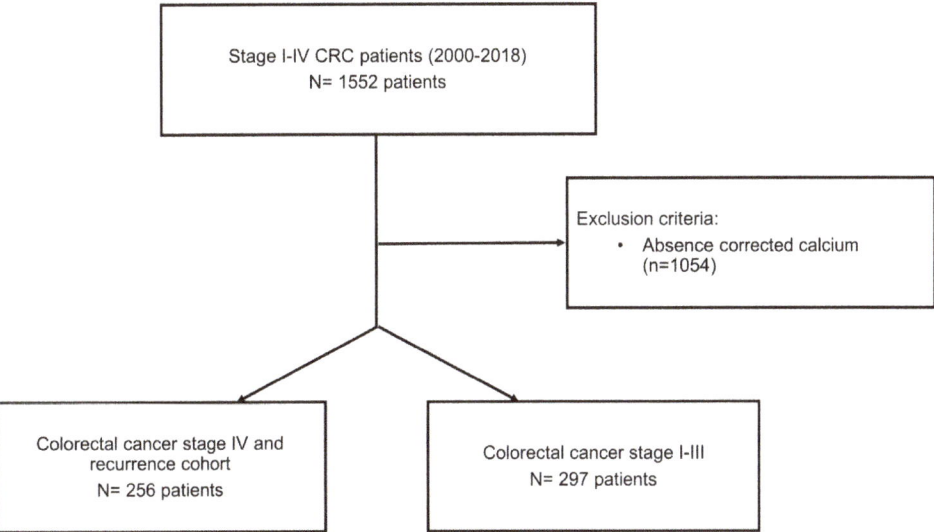

Figure 1. Study flowchart.

2.3. Data Collection

Data were collected from medical records, specifically from the time of CRC diagnosis until the date of death or last follow-up. Research Electronic Data Capture (REDCap) software was used for the construction of case report forms (CRFs) and database management [21].

2.3.1. Clinical Variables

The variables collected comprised sociodemographic characteristics (age, sex, ethnicity, smoking status, and alcohol use status) and anthropometric characteristics (weight, weight loss (WL), height, and body mass index (BMI) at diagnosis). Additionally, disease-related covariates were obtained regarding the date of CRC diagnosis, the Eastern Cooperative Oncology Group Performance Status Scale (ECOG) status, chemotherapy regimens, the primary tumor location, the Charlson Comorbidity Index [22], carcinoembryonic antigen (CEA), the number of metastases, emergency surgery, and the clinical and pathological stage according to the AJCC cancer staging manual (tumor, node, and metastasis (TNM)) [23].

2.3.2. Biochemical Exam Data

Serum albumin and calcium levels were measured using calorimetric assays according to the HC-UNICAMP clinical pathology protocol. Calcium (mg/dL; reference range: 8.8–10.2 mg/dL for adults aged 21–50 years and 8.4–9.7 mg/dL for adults > 50 years old), albumin (mg/dL; reference range: 3.4–4.8 g/dL), baseline CEA levels (ng/mL; cut-off value: 5 ng/mL), and complete blood count levels were collected within 3 months of diagnosis for patients with stage IV or recurrent CRC, and before surgery for patients with stage I–III CRC.

2.3.3. Corrected Calcium Measurement

Given that ionized calcium is not measured routinely in clinics, we used corrected calcium to estimate the free calcium concentration, which was calculated using the following formula: corrected calcium = serum calcium + [(4.0 − serum albumin) × 0.8] [24]. The corrected calcium levels were categorized into tertiles.

2.3.4. Systemic Inflammatory Indexes

The neutrophil-to-lymphocyte ratio (NLR) was calculated by dividing the absolute count of neutrophils by the absolute count of lymphocytes [25]. The platelet-to-lymphocyte ratio (PLR) was calculated by dividing the absolute count of platelets by the absolute count of lymphocytes [26]. The lymphocyte-to-tomonocyte ratio (LMR) was calculated by dividing the absolute count of lymphocytes by the absolute count of monocytes. The NLR and PLR were analyzed as continuous variables.

2.3.5. Endpoints

The co-primary endpoints were progression-free survival and overall survival, which were calculated using the time between disease diagnosis or recurrence and the first event (disease progression or death) and death from any cause, respectively. Data regarding mortality were obtained from medical records. To evaluate the outcomes, the last date of follow-up recorded in the medical record or the date of death of the patient was considered.

2.4. Statistical Analysis

After summarizing the baseline characteristics based on the corrected calcium levels using descriptive statistics, the characteristics were compared by using chi-square and Kruskal–Wallis tests. Multivariate-adjusted Cox proportional hazards regression models were used to investigate associations between corrected calcium and progression-free and overall survival. Time was calculated in months from the diagnosis to the time of the event or the last follow-up visit (through August 2018).

To minimize the effects of potential confounders in our regression model, we included variables related to CRC-specific mortality outcomes established in previous studies. We also included variables that were associated ($p < 0.10$ in the unadjusted Cox analysis) with CRC mortality. We used the Kaplan–Meier method for survival analysis.

Analyses stratified by stage, cancer site, age, and gender were performed. Two-sided p values < 0.05 were considered to be statistically significant. The STATA 12 software was used for statistical analysis.

3. Results

3.1. Patient Disposition and Baseline Characteristics

A total of 256 patients with stage IV or recurrent CRC were included in our study; 207 died of any cause, with a median follow-up of 15.7 months (interquartile range (IQR) 5.8–32.6 months) at the time of the analysis.

Baseline characteristics according to corrected calcium levels are shown in Table 1. Generally, subjects with high levels of corrected calcium ($\geq$9.46 mg/dL) were younger, had more metastases, the highest CEA levels, were less often submitted to prior neoadjuvant or adjuvant treatment, and were less often submitted to a backbone chemotherapy regimen with oxaliplatin. The other characteristics evaluated were similar among the calcium levels.

We also evaluated 243 patients with CRC stage I–III for calcium levels < 9.44 mg/dL and $\geq$9.44 mg/dL; only sex correlated with higher calcium levels ($p = 0.002$) (Table S1).

Table 1. Selected demographic and clinical characteristics and laboratory findings according to calcium tertiles of patients with metastatic colorectal cancer.

Characteristic	All Patients, n = 256	Corrected Calcium, mg/dL			p
		Low Tertile, n = 85 7.18–8.98	Middle Tertile, n = 81 9.00–9.44	High Tertile, n = 90 9.46–14.24	
Age (years), number (%)					
<55	93 (36.3)	26 (30.6)	24 (29.6)	43 (47.8)	0.039 [a]
55–70	112 (43.8)	37 (43.5)	39 (48.2)	36 (40.0)	
>70	51 (19.9)	22 (25.9)	18 (22.2)	11 (12.2)	
Sex, number (%)					
Male	150 (58.6)	56 (65.9)	45 (55.6)	49 (54.4)	0.246 [a]
Female	106 (41.4)	29 (34.1)	36 (44.4)	41 (45.6)	
BMI (kg/m^2), number (%)					
<18.5	24 (9.4)	7 (8.3)	5 (6.2)	12 (13.3)	0.682 [a]
18.5–24.9	135 (52.7)	45 (52.9)	41 (50.6)	49 (54.4)	
25–29.9	63 (24.6)	22 (25.9)	22 (27.2)	19 (21.1)	
≥30	34 (13.3)	11 (12.9)	13 (16.0)	10 (11.1)	
Weight loss, number (%)					
<5%	69 (27)	30 (35.3)	21 (25.9)	18 (20.0)	0.233 [a]
5–10%	39 (15.2)	10 (11.8)	13 (16.1)	16 (17.8)	
>10%	148 (57.8)	45 (52.9)	47 (58.0)	56 (62.2)	
Active smoker, number (%)	116 (45.9)	40 (47.6)	38 (47.5)	38 (42.7)	0.760 [a]
Active alcohol user, number (%)	81 (31.9)	31 (36.5)	28 (34.6)	22 (25.0)	0.222 [a]
Topography, number (%)					
Left	208 (81.2)	70 (82.3)	68 (84)	70 (77.8)	0.558 [a]
Right	48 (18.8)	15 (17.7)	13 (16.0)	20 (22.2)	
ECOG, number (%)					
0	209 (90.5)	71 (94.7)	67 (93.1)	71 (84.5)	0.070 [b]
I	22 (9.5)	4 (5.3)	5 (6.9)	13 (15.5)	
II					
Stage, number (%)					
I–II	33 (12.9)	15 (17.7)	12 (14.8)	6 (6.7)	0.026 [b]
III	21 (8.2)	8 (9.4)	10 (12.3)	3 (3.3)	
IV	202 (78.9)	62 (72.9)	59 (72.8)	81 (90.0)	
Metastasis, number (%)					
1	143 (55.9)	54 (63.5)	44 (54.3)	45 (50.0)	0.017 [b]
2 or more	104 (40.6)	26 (30.6)	33 (40.7)	45 (50.0)	
Local recurrence	9 (3.5)	5 (5.9)	4 (4.9)	0 (0.0)	
CEA (ng/mL), median (IQR)	30.9 (6.37–157.3)	20.1 (4.6–74.4)	26.9 (4.4–122.9)	87.6 (11.2–406.0)	<0.001 [c]
Prior neoadjuvant or adjuvant treatment, number (%)	81 (31.6)	34 (40.0)	31 (38.3)	16 (17.8)	0.002 [a]
Bevacizumab containing regimen, number (%)	53 (27.0)	14 (21.9)	20 (33.9)	19 (26.0)	0.315 [a]
Backbone chemotherapy regimen, number (%)					
Oxaliplatin	62 (32.8)	25 (40.3)	21 (36.2)	16 (23.2)	0.016 [a]
Irinotecan	105 (55.6)	33 (53.2)	34 (58.6)	38 (55.1)	
5-Fluorouracil	22 (11.6)	4 (6.5)	3 (5.2)	15 (21.7)	

Abbreviations: BMI: body mass index; CEA: carcinoembryonic antigen; ECOG: Eastern Cooperative Oncology Group Performance Scale; IQR: interquartile range. [a] Chi-square test, [b] Fisher's exact test, [c] Kruskal–Wallis test.

3.2. Body Composition and Inflammatory Indexes

The serum calcium levels of patients with stage IV or recurrent CRC showed no correlation with body composition variables; however, when evaluating inflammatory markers, there were higher levels of the NLR and the PLR (Table S2).

In non-metastatic patients, serum calcium levels ≥ 9.44 mg/dL correlated with lower IMAT ($p = 0.016$), lower NLR ($p = 0.005$), and higher LMR ($p = 0.025$) (Table S3).

3.3. Survival Analysis

As shown in Table 2, unadjusted Cox regression revealed that higher levels of corrected calcium were associated with reduced median progression-free survival ($p < 0.001$) and overall survival ($p < 0.001$) rates in patients with stage IV or recurrent CRC. The significant association persisted after adjusting the model for age, BMI, ECOG, baseline CEA levels, the number of metastases, chemotherapy use, and WL. High levels of calcium were associated with decreased median progression-free survival (hazard ratio (HR) 1.85; 95% confidence interval (CI) 1.27–2.69, $p = 0.001$) (Figure 2a) and overall survival rates (HR 1.86; 95% CI 1.26–2.74, $p = 0.002$) (Figure 2b).

Table 2. Corrected calcium and survival for patients with metastatic colorectal cancer.

	Corrected Calcium, mg/dL [HR (95% CI)]			
	Low Calcium	Middle Calcium	High Calcium	p
	(7.18–8.98)	(9.00–9.44)	(9.46–14.24)	
Progression-free survival				
Number of events/at risk	68/85	74/81	84/90	
Unadjusted	Referent	1.27 (0.91–1.76)	1.94 (1.41–2.69)	<0.001
Adjusted [a]	Referent	1.17 (0.80–1.71)	1.85 (1.27–2.69)	0.001
Overall survival				
Number of events/at risk	63/85	67/81	77/90	
Unadjusted	Referent	1.44 (1.02–2.04)	1.98 (1.41–2.79)	<0.001
Adjusted [a]	Referent	1.16 (0.78–1.74)	1.86 (1.26–2.74)	0.002

Abbreviations: CI, confidence interval; HR, hazard ratio. [a] Cox model adjusted for age, body mass index, Eastern Cooperative Oncology Group Performance Scale, number of metastases, chemotherapy use, and weight loss.

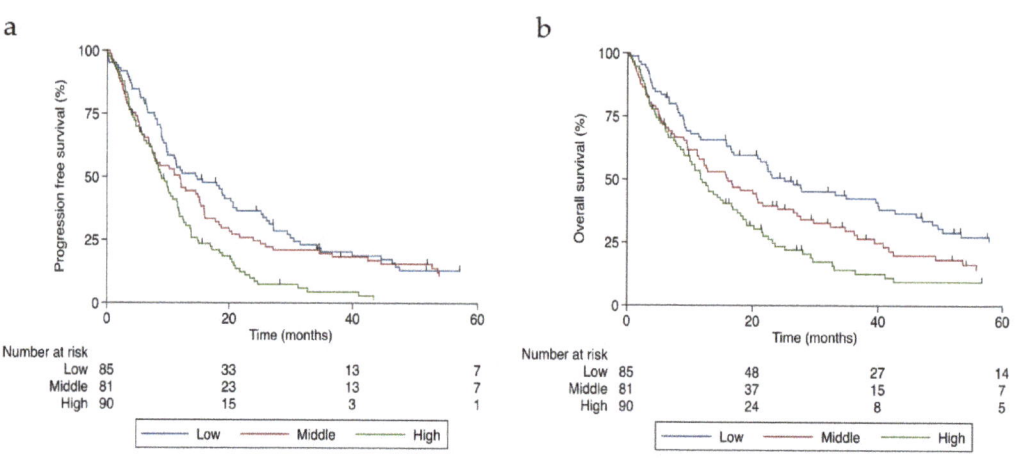

Figure 2. Survival curves of patients with stage IV or recurrent colorectal cancer divided by corrected calcium tertiles (in mg/dL): (**a**) progression-free survival and (**b**) overall survival.

Likewise, higher levels of calcium were associated with decreased progression-free survival (HR 1.44; 95% CI 1.02–2.03, $p = 0.040$) (Figure 3a) and overall survival rates (HR 1.72; 95% CI 1.18–2.50, $p = 0.004$) (Figure 3b) in patients with stage I–III CRC, even after adjusting the model for age, BMI, WL, smoking, the Charlson Comorbidity Index, cancer stage, and emergency surgery.

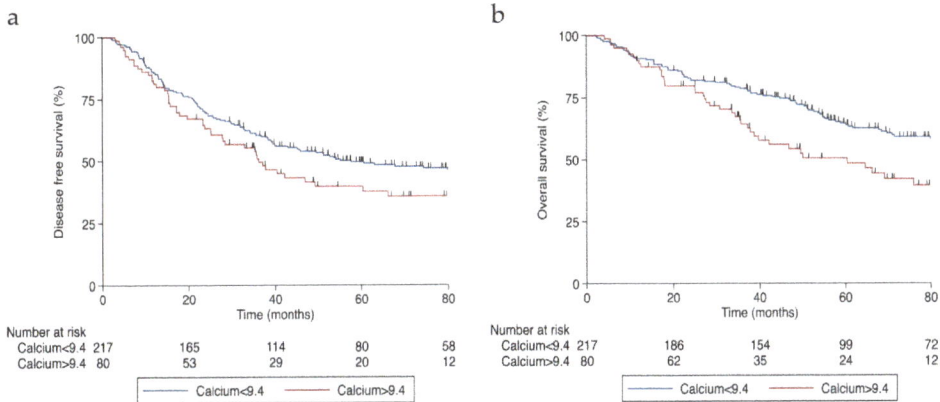

Figure 3. Survival curves of patients with stage I–III colorectal cancer divided by corrected calcium levels (in mg/dL): (**a**) disease-free survival and (**b**) overall survival.

4. Discussion

In this retrospective cohort, patients with metastatic disease presented with significantly decreased progression-free and overall survival rates in a corrected-calcium-dependent manner. Importantly, this association appeared to be independent of age, BMI, ECOG, CEA levels, the number of metastases, chemotherapy regimen, and WL. Moreover, patients with non-metastatic disease had increased risk of progression and mortality even after adjusting the model for age, BMI, WL, smoking, the Charlson Comorbidity Index, and emergency surgery. However, our analysis with body composition was not associated with corrected calcium levels.

Previous studies have evaluated the effects of hypercalcemia of malignancy (calcium greater than upper limit of normal (ULN)) on disease outcomes but not the influence of calcium as a biomarker of CRC progression. These reports consistently associate hypercalcemia with a poor prognosis [27,28]. Thus, a key question is that beyond corrected calcium directly influencing cancer outcomes, is it also a biomarker of cancer progression?

Interestingly, a few reports have investigated the role of corrected calcium as a marker of cancer progression without categorizing it in the ULN. For example, in the setting of metastatic kidney cancer, the set level of corrected calcium commonly used in prognostic models of survival (a tool used routinely in clinics) is lower than the ULN [29,30]. Interestingly, extracellular calcium levels per se have an established CRC chemoprotective effect [31–33]. Extracellular calcium levels may be considered a marker for increased PTH and vitamin D levels. Like extracellular calcium levels, serum vitamin D level is associated with reduced cancer mortality [34]; thus, a possible biological explanation for the association of corrected calcium levels with cancer progression is that corrected calcium may reflect the spectrum of PTHrP secreted by the tumor. PTHrP is expressed in >90% of CRC cases, and the grade of its expression was previously correlated with poor differentiation and aggressiveness [17]. We also found an association between higher levels of corrected calcium and a greater number of metastases and higher levels of CEA, which are important prognostic biomarkers for metastatic CRC. Consistent with this finding, PTHrP was recently linked to the increased proliferation of colon cancer cells [35]. Moreover, elevated PTHrP levels have been associated with cancer cachexia [16]. However, in our analysis, body composition, excluding IMAT in nonmetastatic patients, was not associated with corrected calcium, corroborating the findings of a recent study where the serum PTHrP level was not correlated with WL, uncoupling protein (UCP)-1, and other white adipose tissue browning markers [36]. Thus, additional prospective studies are needed to elucidate the role of PTHrP in determining body composition in humans.

Interestingly, in a cohort of patients with gastroesophageal cancer, the levels of PTHrP were associated with poor prognosis independently of overt hypercalcemia. Hence, one could assume that PTHrP interferes with calcium levels within the normal range [37]. In accordance, the antibody neutralization of PTHrP in mice bearing tumors improved survival [38]. In another animal model, PTHrP showed great influence on tumorigenesis, progression, and metastasis formation in breast cancer xenografts [39]. Moreover, Carriere et al. [40] recently suggested the involvement of PTHrP, secreted protein acidic and rich in cysteine (SPARC), and epithelial–mesenchymal transition (EMT) in CRC, favoring a more aggressive phenotype of the disease. Consistent with the idea of an unmediated effect of calcium levels on survival outcomes, our assessment of inflammatory indexes revealed the opposite results. While patients with stage IV or recurrent CRC with higher calcium levels had greater inflammation, in patients with local and locoregional disease, higher calcium levels were associated with lower inflammatory rates. This suggests that calcium levels do not modulate the inflammatory milieu of the host; rather, the higher calcium levels observed in metastatic patients may be a consequence of the greater tumor burden.

The strength of our study is that it is the first to separately report this association in patients with both locoregional and advanced CRC. Nonetheless, our study has limitations. First, the retrospective nature of this study impeded any further analysis of the mechanisms involved in the association of corrected calcium with prognosis, such as the measurement of PTHrP. Second, the generalizability of our study is limited. We conducted our study in a single institution, and patients attended HC-UNICAMP; these patients represent a population in São Paulo that does not have private insurance and thus does not represent the higher socioeconomic spectra. Third, although the calcium and albumin measurements were obtained in a manner that was dependent on the assistant physician's choice, the notable number of missing data points in our cohort (of the 1552 patients in this cohort, only 498 had calcium and albumin measurements at the given time) may have potentiated unrecognized changes in clinical practice during the study timeframe. Finally, our findings need to be tested in future studies that examine other populations, which must include information regarding PTHrP, calcium, PTH, and vitamin D levels.

In summary, we demonstrated that higher corrected calcium levels might be associated with worse CRC survival outcomes. Although reverse causality may have contributed to our findings, the use of corrected calcium levels as a biomarker of CRC prognosis holds promise for better understanding the mechanisms of CRC aggressiveness and deserves further evaluation in prospective trials to be implemented as a prognostic predictor in clinical practice.

Supplementary Materials: The following supporting information can be downloaded at: https://www.mdpi.com/article/10.3390/jcm11102928/s1, Table S1: Selected demographic and disease characteristics according to calcium levels of stage I–III colorectal cancer patients; Table S2: Body composition and inflammatory indexes according to calcium tertiles of metastatic colorectal cancer patients; Table S3: Body composition and inflammatory indexes according to calcium tertiles of stage I–III colorectal cancer patients

Author Contributions: Conceptualization, M.N.S., M.C.S.M., L.P.d.C. and J.B.C.C.; methodology, M.N.S., L.P., M.C.S.M., L.P.d.C., L.T.M. and J.B.C.C.; software, M.N.S., L.P., M.C.S.M., L.P.d.C. and J.B.C.C.; validation, M.N.S., L.P., M.C.S.M., L.P.d.C. and J.B.C.C.; formal analysis, M.N.S., M.C.S.M. and J.B.C.C.; investigation, M.N.S., L.P., M.C.S.M., L.P.d.C. and J.B.C.C.; resources, M.N.S., L.P., M.C.S.M., L.P.d.C. and J.B.C.C.; data curation, M.N.S., L.P., M.C.S.M., L.T.M. and J.B.C.C.; writing—original draft preparation, M.N.S., M.C.S.M.,L.P.d.C. and J.B.C.C.; writing—review and editing, M.N.S., L.P., M.C.S.M., L.P.d.C., F.O.C., L.T.M., S.R.B. and J.B.C.C.; visualization, M.N.S., M.C.S.M. and J.B.C.C.; supervision, M.N.S., M.C.S.M. and J.B.C.C.; project administration, M.N.S., M.C.S.M. and J.B.C.C. All authors have read and agreed to the published version of the manuscript.

Funding: The MNS was funded by Conselho nacional de desenvolvimento científico e tecnológico (CNPq), grant number 140596/2019-4; The JBCC was funded by CNPq, grant number 303429/2021-6, and funded by Fundação de Amparo à Pesquisa do Estado de São Paulo (FAPESP), grant number 2018/23428-0.

Institutional Review Board Statement: The study was conducted in accordance with the Declaration of Helsinki, and approved by the Ethics Committee of State University of Campinas (CAAE number: 15505419.1.0000.5404, approved in 5 July 2019).

Informed Consent Statement: Patient consent was waived due to this is a retrospective work and the research method used guaranteed the anonymity of the participants, as the search was carried out using the identification number generated in HC-UNICAMP for the records hospital. The collected data were stored in a restricted location, and accessed only by the work researchers.

Data Availability Statement: Not applicable.

Conflicts of Interest: The authors declare no conflict of interest.

References

1. Sung, H.; Ferlay, J.; Siegel, R.L.; Laversanne, M.; Soerjomataram, I.; Jemal, A.; Bray, F. Global Cancer Statistics 2020: GLOBOCAN Estimates of Incidence and Mortality Worldwide for 36 Cancers in 185 Countries. *CA Cancer J. Clin.* **2021**, *71*, 209–249. [CrossRef] [PubMed]
2. Siegel, R.L.; Miller, K.D.; Fedewa, S.A.; Ahnen, D.J.; Meester, R.G.S.; Barzi, A.; Jemal, A. Colorectal cancer statistics, 2017. *CA Cancer J. Clin.* **2017**, *67*, 177–193. [CrossRef] [PubMed]
3. McCullough, M.L.; Robertson, A.S.; Rodriguez, C.; Jacobs, E.J.; Chao, A.; Carolyn, J.; Calle, E.E.; Willett, W.C.; Thun, M.J. Calcium, vitamin D, dairy products, and risk of colorectal cancer in the Cancer Prevention Study II Nutrition Cohort (United States). *Cancer Causes Control* **2003**, *14*, 1–12. [CrossRef] [PubMed]
4. Wu, K.; Willett, W.C.; Fuchs, C.S.; Colditz, G.A.; Giovannucci, E.L. Calcium intake and risk of colon cancer in women and men. *J. Natl. Cancer Inst.* **2002**, *94*, 437–446. [CrossRef] [PubMed]
5. Han, C.; Shin, A.; Lee, J.; Lee, J.; Park, J.W.; Oh, J.H.; Kim, J. Dietary calcium intake and the risk of colorectal cancer: A case control study. *BMC Cancer* **2015**, *15*, 966. [CrossRef]
6. Keum, N.; Aune, D.; Greenwood, D.C.; Ju, W.; Giovannucci, E.L. Calcium intake and colorectal cancer risk: Dose-response meta-analysis of prospective observational studies. *Int. J. Cancer* **2014**, *135*, 1940–1948. [CrossRef]
7. Cho, E.; Smith-Warner, S.A.; Spiegelman, D.; Beeson, W.L.; van den Brandt, P.A.; Colditz, G.A.; Folsom, A.R.; Fraser, G.E.; Freudenheim, J.L.; Giovannucci, E.; et al. Dairy foods, calcium, and colorectal cancer: A pooled analysis of 10 cohort studies. *J. Natl. Cancer Inst.* **2004**, *96*, 1015–1022. [CrossRef]
8. Crockett, S.D.; Barry, E.L.; Mott, L.A.; Ahnen, D.J.; Robertson, D.J.; Anderson, J.C.; Wallace, K.; Burke, C.A.; Bresalier, R.S.; Figueiredo, J.C.; et al. Calcium and vitamin D supplementation and increased risk of serrated polyps: Results from a randomised clinical trial. *Gut* **2018**, *68*, 475–486. [CrossRef]
9. Monteith, G.R.; Prevarskaya, N.; Roberts-Thomson, S.J. The calcium-cancer signalling nexus. *Nat. Rev. Cancer* **2017**, *17*, 367–380. [CrossRef]
10. Wulaningsih, W.; Michaelsson, K.; Garmo, H.; Hammar, N.; Jungner, I.; Walldius, G.; Lambe, M.; Holmberg, L.; Van Hemelrijck, M. Serum calcium and risk of gastrointestinal cancer in the Swedish AMORIS study. *BMC Public Health* **2013**, *13*, 663. [CrossRef]
11. Blaine, J.; Chonchol, M.; Levi, M. Renal control of calcium, phosphate, and magnesium homeostasis. *Clin. J. Am. Soc. Nephrol.* **2015**, *10*, 1257–1272. [CrossRef] [PubMed]
12. Stewart, A.F. Clinical practice. Hypercalcemia associated with cancer. *N. Engl. J. Med.* **2005**, *352*, 373–379. [CrossRef] [PubMed]
13. Karaplis, A.C.; Luz, A.; Glowacki, J.; Bronson, R.T.; Tybulewicz, V.L.; Kronenberg, H.M.; Mulligan, R.C. Lethal skeletal dysplasia from targeted disruption of the parathyroid hormone-related peptide gene. *Genes Dev.* **1994**, *8*, 277–289. [CrossRef] [PubMed]
14. Lanske, B.; Karaplis, A.C.; Lee, K.; Luz, A.; Vortkamp, A.; Pirro, A.; Karperien, M.; Defize, L.H.; Ho, C.; Mulligan, R.C.; et al. PTH/PTHrP receptor in early development and Indian hedgehog-regulated bone growth. *Science* **1996**, *273*, 663–666. [CrossRef] [PubMed]
15. Mundy, G.R.; Edwards, J.R. PTH-related peptide (PTHrP) in hypercalcemia. *J. Am. Soc. Nephrol.* **2008**, *19*, 672–675. [CrossRef] [PubMed]
16. Hong, N.; Yoon, H.-j.; Lee, Y.-h.; Kim, H.R.; Lee, B.W.; Rhee, Y.; Kang, E.S.; Cha, B.-S.; Lee, H.C. Serum PTHrP Predicts Weight Loss in Cancer Patients Independent of Hypercalcemia, Inflammation, and Tumor Burden. *J. Clin. Endocrinol. Metab.* **2016**, *101*, 1207–1214. [CrossRef]
17. Nishihara, M.; Ito, M.; Tomioka, T.; Ohtsuru, A.; Taguchi, T.; Kanematsu, T. Clinicopathological implications of parathyroid hormone-related protein in human colorectal tumours. *J. Pathol.* **1999**, *187*, 217–222. [CrossRef]
18. Amin, M.B.; Greene, F.L.; Edge, S.B.; Compton, C.C.; Gershenwald, J.E.; Brookland, R.K.; Meyer, L.; Gress, D.M.; Byrd, D.R.; Winchester, D.P. The Eighth Edition AJCC Cancer Staging Manual: Continuing to build a bridge from a population-based to a more "personalized" approach to cancer staging. *CA Cancer J. Clin.* **2017**, *67*, 93–99. [CrossRef]

19. Mourtzakis, M.; Prado, C.M.; Lieffers, J.R.; Reiman, T.; McCargar, L.J.; Baracos, V.E. A practical and precise approach to quantification of body composition in cancer patients using computed tomography images acquired during routine care. *Appl. Physiol. Nutr. Metab.* **2008**, *33*, 997–1006. [CrossRef]
20. Mitsiopoulos, N.; Baumgartner, R.N.; Heymsfield, S.B.; Lyons, W.; Gallagher, D.; Ross, R. Cadaver validation of skeletal muscle measurement by magnetic resonance imaging and computerized tomography. *J. Appl. Physiol.* **1998**, *85*, 115–122. [CrossRef]
21. Harris, P.A.; Taylor, R.; Thielke, R.; Payne, J.; Gonzalez, N.; Conde, J.G. Research electronic data capture (REDCap)—A metadata-driven methodology and workflow process for providing translational research informatics support. *J. Biomed. Inform.* **2009**, *42*, 377–381. [CrossRef] [PubMed]
22. Quan, H.; Li, B.; Couris, C.M.; Fushimi, K.; Graham, P.; Hider, P.; Januel, J.M.; Sundararajan, V. Updating and validating the Charlson comorbidity index and score for risk adjustment in hospital discharge abstracts using data from 6 countries. *Am. J. Epidemiol.* **2011**, *173*, 676–682. [CrossRef] [PubMed]
23. Edge, S.B.; Compton, C.C. The American Joint Committee on Cancer: The 7th edition of the AJCC cancer staging manual and the future of TNM. *Ann. Surg. Oncol.* **2010**, *17*, 1471–1474. [CrossRef] [PubMed]
24. Payne, R.B.; Little, A.J.; Williams, R.B.; Milner, J.R. Interpretation of serum calcium in patients with abnormal serum proteins. *Br. Med. J.* **1973**, *4*, 643–646. [CrossRef]
25. Templeton, A.J.; McNamara, M.G.; Šeruga, B.; Vera-Badillo, F.E.; Aneja, P.; Ocaña, A.; Leibowitz-Amit, R.; Sonpavde, G.; Knox, J.J.; Tran, B.; et al. Prognostic role of neutrophil-to-lymphocyte ratio in solid tumors: A systematic review and meta-analysis. *J. Natl. Cancer Inst.* **2014**, *106*, dju124. [CrossRef]
26. Templeton, A.J.; Ace, O.; McNamara, M.G.; Al-Mubarak, M.; Vera-Badillo, F.E.; Hermanns, T.; Seruga, B.; Ocaña, A.; Tannock, I.F.; Amir, E. Prognostic role of platelet to lymphocyte ratio in solid tumors: A systematic review and meta-analysis. *Cancer Epidemiol. Biomarkers Prev.* **2014**, *23*, 1204–1212. [CrossRef]
27. Ralston, S.H.; Gallacher, S.J.; Patel, U.; Campbell, J.; Boyle, I.T. Cancer-associated hypercalcemia: Morbidity and mortality. Clinical experience in 126 treated patients. *Ann. Intern. Med.* **1990**, *112*, 499–504. [CrossRef]
28. Ramos, R.E.O.; Perez Mak, M.; Alves, M.F.S.; Piotto, G.H.M.; Takahashi, T.K.; Gomes da Fonseca, L.; Silvino, M.C.M.; Hoff, P.M.; de Castro, G., Jr. Malignancy-Related Hypercalcemia in Advanced Solid Tumors: Survival Outcomes. *J. Glob. Oncol.* **2017**, *3*, 728–733. [CrossRef]
29. Motzer, R.J.; Mazumdar, M.; Bacik, J.; Berg, W.; Amsterdam, A.; Ferrara, J. Survival and prognostic stratification of 670 patients with advanced renal cell carcinoma. *J. Clin. Oncol.* **1999**, *17*, 2530–2540. [CrossRef]
30. Manola, J.; Royston, P.; Elson, P.; McCormack, J.B.; Mazumdar, M.; Negrier, S.; Escudier, B.; Eisen, T.; Dutcher, J.; Atkins, M.; et al. Prognostic model for survival in patients with metastatic renal cell carcinoma: Results from the international kidney cancer working group. *Clin. Cancer Res.* **2011**, *17*, 5443–5450. [CrossRef]
31. Lipkin, M. Preclinical and early human studies of calcium and colon cancer prevention. *Ann. N. Y. Acad. Sci.* **1999**, *889*, 120–127. [CrossRef] [PubMed]
32. Wargovich, M.J.; Jimenez, A.; McKee, K.; Steele, V.E.; Velasco, M.; Woods, J.; Price, R.; Gray, K.; Kelloff, G.J. Efficacy of potential chemopreventive agents on rat colon aberrant crypt formation and progression. *Carcinogenesis* **2000**, *21*, 1149–1155. [CrossRef] [PubMed]
33. Chakrabarty, S.; Radjendirane, V.; Appelman, H.; Varani, J. Extracellular calcium and calcium sensing receptor function in human colon carcinomas: Promotion of E-cadherin expression and suppression of beta-catenin/TCF activation. *Cancer Res.* **2003**, *63*, 67–71. [PubMed]
34. Kim, H.; Giovannucci, E. Vitamin D Status and Cancer Incidence, Survival, and Mortality. *Adv. Exp. Med. Biol.* **2020**, *1268*, 39–52. [CrossRef]
35. Martin, M.J.; Calvo, N.; de Boland, A.R.; Gentili, C. Molecular mechanisms associated with PTHrP-induced proliferation of colon cancer cells. *J. Cell Biochem.* **2014**, *115*, 2133–2145. [CrossRef]
36. Anderson, L.J.; Lee, J.; Anderson, B.; Lee, B.; Migula, D.; Sauer, A.; Chong, N.; Liu, H.; Wu, P.C.; Dash, A.; et al. Whole-body and adipose tissue metabolic phenotype in cancer patients. *J. Cachexia Sarcopenia Muscle* **2022**, *13*, 1124–1133. [CrossRef]
37. Deans, C.; Wigmore, S.; Paterson-Brown, S.; Black, J.; Ross, J.; Fearon, K.C. Serum parathyroid hormone-related peptide is associated with systemic inflammation and adverse prognosis in gastroesophageal carcinoma. *Cancer* **2005**, *103*, 1810–1818. [CrossRef]
38. Sato, K.; Yamakawa, Y.; Shizume, K.; Satoh, T.; Nohtomi, K.; Demura, H.; Akatsu, T.; Nagata, N.; Kasahara, T.; Ohkawa, H.; et al. Passive immunization with anti-parathyroid hormone-related protein monoclonal antibody markedly prolongs survival time of hypercalcemic nude mice bearing transplanted human PTHrP-producing tumors. *J. Bone Miner. Res.* **1993**, *8*, 849–860. [CrossRef]
39. Li, J.; Karaplis, A.C.; Huang, D.C.; Siegel, P.M.; Camirand, A.; Yang, X.F.; Muller, W.J.; Kremer, R. PTHrP drives breast tumor initiation, progression, and metastasis in mice and is a potential therapy target. *J. Clin. Investig.* **2011**, *121*, 4655–4669. [CrossRef]
40. Carriere, P.; Calvo, N.; Novoa Díaz, M.B.; Lopez-Moncada, F.; Herrera, A.; Torres, M.J.; Alonso, E.; Gandini, N.A.; Gigola, G.; Contreras, H.R.; et al. Role of SPARC in the epithelial-mesenchymal transition induced by PTHrP in human colon cancer cells. *Mol. Cell Endocrinol.* **2021**, *530*, 111253. [CrossRef]

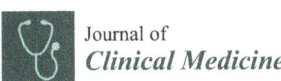

Article

The Significance of Selected C-C Motif Chemokine Ligands in Colorectal Cancer Patients

Monika Zajkowska [1,*], Maciej Dulewicz [1], Agnieszka Kulczyńska-Przybik [1], Kamil Safiejko [2], Marcin Juchimiuk [2], Marzena Konopko [2], Leszek Kozłowski [2] and Barbara Mroczko [1,3]

[1] Department of Neurodegeneration Diagnostics, Medical University of Bialystok, 15-269 Bialystok, Poland; maciejdulewicz@gmail.com (M.D.); agnieszka.kulczynska-przybik@umb.edu.pl (A.K.-P.); barbara.mroczko@umb.edu.pl (B.M.)
[2] Department of Oncological Surgery with Specialized Cancer Treatment Units, Maria Sklodowska-Curie Oncology Center, 15-027 Bialystok, Poland; kamil.safiejko@gmail.com (K.S.); jumedica.onkologia@gmail.com (M.J.); marzeniedoc@yahoo.com (M.K.); leszek@kozlowski.pl (L.K.)
[3] Department of Biochemical Diagnostics, Medical University of Bialystok, 15-269 Bialystok, Poland
* Correspondence: monika.zajkowska@umb.edu.pl; Tel.: +48-686-5168; Fax: +48-686-5169

Abstract: Colorectal cancer (CRC) is one of the most frequently diagnosed neoplasms. Despite the advances in diagnostic tools and treatments, the number of CRC cases is increasing. Therefore, it is vital to search for new parameters that could be useful in its diagnosis. Thus, we wanted to assess the usefulness of selected CC chemokines (CCL2, CCL4, and CCL15) in CRC. The study included 115 subjects (75 CRC patients and 40 healthy volunteers). The serum concentrations of all parameters were measured using a multiplexing method (Luminex). The CRP levels were determined by immunoturbidimetry, and the classical tumor markers (CEA and CA 19-9) were measured using CMIA (chemiluminescent microparticle immunoassay). The concentrations of all parameters were higher in the CRC group when compared to the healthy controls. The diagnostic sensitivity, specificity, positive and negative predictive value, and area under the ROC curve (AUC) of all estimated CC chemokines were higher than those of CA 19-9. Interestingly, the obtained results also suggest CCL2's significance in the determination of local metastases and CCL4's significance in the determination of distant metastases. However, further studies concerning the role of selected CC chemokines in the course of colorectal cancer are necessary to confirm and to fully clarify their diagnostic utility and their clinical application as markers of CRC development.

Keywords: CRC; CCL2; CCL4; CCL15; diagnostic utility

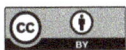

1. Introduction

Colorectal cancer (CRC) is one of the most frequent malignancies worldwide, being the second most common malignancy in men and third in women, and accounting for almost 11% and over 9% of all cancer cases, respectively. According to the World Health Organization (WHO), the global incidence of CRC is almost 2 million new cases per year, with approximately 920,000 deaths annually. Importantly, there is an observed increase in both the incidence and the mortality of colorectal cancer, as estimated year-to-year. It was predicted by WHO that the number of new CRC cases may exceed 3,000,000 in 2040, with the number of fatalities reaching 1.5 million per year [1,2]. What should be stressed is CRC is a preventable disease—even in up to 50% of cases—by some modifications of lifestyle, such as a high-fiber and a balanced diet, moderate physical activity, or avoidance of alcohol or smoking [3,4].

Diagnosis of colorectal cancer as early as possible, particularly in the asymptomatic stages, when the tumor is still non-malignant, and initiation of appropriate treatment is of principal importance for patients' survival. The currently used methods of CRC detection include colonoscopy and sigmoidoscopy, as well as imaging diagnostics with the use of computed tomographic colonography and the magnetic resonance method. Although substantial progress has been made in this field in recent years, in the case of small lesions, with a mass not exceeding 1 g, these techniques may be ineffective. Another diagnostic tool useful in the detection of colorectal cancer are tumor markers, mainly glycoproteins or enzymes, which are synthesized by tumor cells. Tumor markers have a particular utility not only in detecting of malignancies and determining tumor advancement, but also in monitoring of treatment and early detection of recurrence [5,6]. The example of tumor markers employed in the diagnosis of CRC are CEA and CA 19-9. Unfortunately, the diagnostic usefulness of these biomarkers is relatively low and they are not specific to the colorectal cancer only [7]. Taking into account the above premises, there is an urgent need to find new diagnostic markers, the use of which will allow for detection of a developing cancer even earlier than before.

Increasing evidence suggests that small (8–12 kDa) inflammatory proteins known as chemokines are key regulators of angiogenesis, including pathological angiogenesis. They are a large family composed of 50 members. The main role of these cytokines is to direct the recruitment and the relocation of cells to locations of inflammation or injury. They are divided into four classes according to the location and the number of cysteine residues at the amino terminus. The CC-chemokine group has two adjacent cysteine residues, and the CXC chemokine group has two cysteine residues detached by an amino acid. The chemokine CX3C group has 3 amino acids between 2 cysteine residues and the C-chemokine group has only1 cysteine residue at the amino terminus. Of the four chemokine groups, the largest group is the CC chemokine group which includes a total of 28 members across all species. This is followed by the chemokine CXC group (17 members), with chemokines CX3C and XC having 1 and 2 members, respectively. All of these proteins exert their biological properties by interacting with G-protein-coupled transmembrane chemokine receptors found on the cell membrane of specific effector cells. The nomenclature of chemokines and their receptors results directly from their classification. At present, there are 19 receptors corresponding to specific groups of chemokines. Despite their large number, these receptors are structurally similar and they are activated in an analogous manner to the chemokines themselves [8].

The current state of knowledge allows us to suspect that chemokines and their receptors play a significant role in cancer development [9]. In tumor growth and metastasis, chemokines and their receptors exert a multifaceted effect on regulating angiogenesis, tumor cell proliferation, and apoptosis, mediating tumor cell metastasis in an organ-specific manner [10]. It is postulated that the CC and CXC chemokines could be the most active in the regulation of angiogenesis [11,12]. That is why the aim of our study was an attempt to clarify and to assess the usefulness of selected CC-chemokine measurement (CCL2, CCL4 and CCL15) in patients with colorectal cancer compared to the healthy volunteer group. We have also compared the obtained results to comparative, routinely used tumor markers (CA 19-9, CEA) and CRP (C-reactive protein), which is an inflammatory parameter.

2. Materials and Methods
2.1. Patients

The study included 75 colorectal cancer (CRC) patients diagnosed by the oncology group (Table 1). The patients were treated in the Department of Oncological Surgery with Specialized Cancer Treatment Units, Maria Sklodowska-Curie Oncology Center, Bialystok, Poland. Tumor classification and staging were conducted in agreement with the International Union Against Cancer Tumor–Node–Metastasis (UICC-TNM) classification. The histopathology of colorectal cancer was based on the examination of tissue samples with the use of a microscope. Moreover, all patients were grouped according to not only tumor stage (TNM), but also depth of tumor invasion (T factor), the presence of lymph node (N factor), and distant metastases (M factor), as well as the histological grade (G factor) of the tumor. The pretreatment staging procedures included physical and blood examinations, computed tomography (CT) and—in case of patients with rectal cancer—magnetic resonance imaging

(MRI) of the small pelvis. Additionally, all patients were assessed according to the Eastern Cooperative Oncology Group (ECOG) score. The control group comprised 40 healthy volunteers. For each patient qualified for the control group, the following exclusion criteria was applied: active infections and symptoms of an infection (both bacterial and viral); other comorbidities which can affect cytokine concentrations (respiratory diseases, digestive tract diseases); or systemic diseases such as lupus, rheumatoid arthritis, or collagenosis.

Table 1. Characteristics of colorectal cancer and healthy patient groups.

Study Group		No. of Patients
Colorectal Cancer		75
	Gender:	
	Female	26
	Male	49
	Type:	
	Colon Cancer	25
	Rectal Cancer	41
	Sigmoid Cancer	9
	TNM Stage:	
	0	1
	I	15
	II	13
	III	25
	IV	21
	Depth of tumor invasion:	
	In situ	1
	T1	2
	T2	19
	T3	41
	T4	12
	Nodal involvement:	
	N0	34
	N1	25
	N2	16
	Distant metastasis:	
	M0	54
	M1	21
	Age:	33–89
Control Group		40
	Gender:	
	Female	12
	Male	28
	Age:	34–80

2.2. Biochemical Analyses

Venous blood samples were collected from each patient into a tube with a clot activator (S-Monovette, SARSTEDT, Numbrecht, Germany), centrifuged to obtain serum samples, and stored at −80 °C until assayed. The tested chemokines were measured with the use of a Luminex 200 analyzer (Thermo Fisher Scientific, Waltham, MA, USA) (multiplexing, multiparametric, fluorescence laser reading system on microspheres for the simultaneous determination of multiple parameters) and Luminex Human Discovery assay plates, provided by R&D systems, Abingdon, UK. According to the manufacturer's protocols, duplicate samples were assessed for each standard, control, and sample. The serum levels of classical tumor markers were measured with chemiluminescent microparticle immunoassay (CMIA) (Abbott, Chicago, IL, USA); and, for the analysis of the CRP concentration, the immunoturbidymetric method (Abbott, Chicago, IL, USA) was used according to the manufacturer's protocols.

2.3. Statistical Analysis

Statistical analysis was performed by RStudio. The introductory statistical analysis (using the Shapiro–Wilk test) exposed that the tested parameters and tumor marker levels did not follow normal distribution. Therefore, statistical analysis between the groups was performed with the use of the U Mann–Whitney test, the Kruskal–Wallis test, and a multivariate analysis of various data by the post-hoc Dwass–Steele–Critchlow–Flinger test. The data were presented as a median and a range. Diagnostic sensitivity, specificity, and the predictive values of positive and negative test results (SE, SP, PPV, and NPV, respectively) were calculated by using the cut-off values which were calculated by the Youden's index (as a criterion for selecting the optimum cut-off point) and for each of the tested parameters they were as follows: CCL2—426.13 pg/mL, CCL4—274.45 pg/mL, CCL15—2607.49 pg/mL, CA 19-9—5.30 U/mL, CEA—1.70 ng/mL, and CRP—2.50 mg/L. We also defined the receiver operating characteristics (ROC) curve for all of the tested parameters, tumor markers, and for the CRP to estimate diagnostic accuracy, and we performed a Spearman's rank correlation test. Statistically significant differences were defined as comparisons resulting in $p < 0.05$.

3. Results

Table 2 shows the serum levels of the CCL2, CCL4, CCL15, CA 19-9, CEA, and CRP in patients with colorectal cancer and in the control group. After performing the non-parametric U Mann–Whitney test comparing the concentrations obtained in both groups, we observed that the levels of CCL2, CCL4, CEA, and CRP in the entire cancer group were significantly higher (in all cases $p < 0.05$).

Table 2. Serum levels of tested parameters in cancer and control groups.

Parameter		Colorectal Cancer	Control Group	p *
CCL2 [pg/mL]	Me	485.68	371.81	**0.02**
	Min–Max	181.12–2033.23	72.80–1117.74	
CCL4 [pg/mL]	Me	378.81	272.03	**0.02**
	Min–Max	142.60–655.50	83.58–933.72	
CCL15 [pg/mL]	Me	2853.88	2547.22	0.55
	Min–Max	204.17–12,750.00	132.63–14,677.81	
CA 19-9 [U/mL]	Me	5.30	5.39	0.82
	Min–Max	2.06–8199.90	2.06–33.34	
CEA [ng/mL]	Me	3.87	1.02	**<0.001**
	Min–Max	0.50–3688.00	0.50–15.64	
CRP [mg/L]	Me	6.00	1.36	**<0.001**
	Min–Max	1.00–248.50	0.20–5.80	

* U Mann–Whitney test; CCL—chemoattractant cytokine ligand; CA 19-9—cancer antigen 19-9; CEA—carcinoembryonic antigen; CRP—C-reactive protein. The statistically significant results are presented in bold.

In addition, we performed a more thorough analysis with use of Kruskal–Wallis and Dwass–Steel–Critchlow–Fligner tests after the division of the total CRC group into advancement groups (TNM I-IV). As a result of this analysis, we obtained significant results for almost all parameters (Table 3). Interpreting the obtained results, it can be suggested that the concentration of CCL4, CEA, and CA 19-9 increases significantly with the advancement of neoplastic changes, and it may be related not only to the number of neoplastic cells, but also to their spread—as TNM stage III is associated with the presence of metastases to nearby lymph nodes and stage IV with distant metastases. Interestingly, the CRP analysis confirms the inflammatory theory of neoplasm, as statistically significant differences were obtained only in the case of comparisons between the control group and individual stages of cancer.

Table 3. Kruskal–Wallis and Dwass–Steel–Critchlow–Fligner tests analysis results.

	Parameter	CCL2	CCL4	CCL15	CA 19-9	CEA	CRP
	Kruskal–Wallis p-value	**0.05**	**<0.001**	0.22	**0.003**	**<0.001**	**<0.001**
Dwass–Steel–Critchlow–Fligner p-value	Control vs. I	0.35	0.99	0.70	0.19	0.34	**<0.001**
	Control vs. II	1.00	0.98	1.00	0.83	0.08	**<0.001**
	Control vs. III	**0.05**	0.58	0.99	0.50	**0.002**	**<0.001**
	Control vs. IV	0.52	**<0.001**	0.41	0.25	**<0.001**	**<0.001**
	I vs. II	0.54	0.92	0.65	0.98	1.00	0.99
	I vs. III	0.99	0.53	0.63	**0.033**	0.77	1.00
	I vs. IV	0.99	**<0.001**	0.99	**0.013**	**<0.001**	0.99
	II vs. III	0.31	0.19	0.99	0.17	0.68	0.95
	II vs. IV	0.93	**<0.001**	0.67	0.15	**<0.001**	0.99
	III vs. IV	0.91	**<0.001**	0.28	0.99	**0.005**	0.97

The statistically significant results are presented in bold.

Considering the fact that in the subgroups of TNM stages I and II, the number of patients did not exceed 20, which may affect the accuracy of the obtained results, we decided to confirm them using the U Mann–Whitney test. We divided the group of all CRC patients into the group of less-advanced neoplasms (TNM I + II) and the group of advanced neoplasms (TNM III + IV). In addition, we divided the group of advanced neoplasms into separate TNM stages (III and IV) due to the sufficient number of patients in each subgroup to perform a precise analysis in different subgroups and in comparison to the control group. The results obtained were similar to those in previous analyses. Interestingly, we observed significant differences between controls and III stage TNM in the case of CCL2, which may suggest its participation in local lymph node metastasis processes. In the case of CCL4, we observed differences between the control and the most advanced stage of CRC, and what is of utmost importance, significant differences between all advancement CRC stages (similarly to CA 19-9). In comparison between the control group and all advancement stages, CEA and CRP revealed significance; but, in case of differences between TNM stages, significant results were obtained only in case of CEA between less-advanced stages and distant stage metastases (Table 4).

Table 4. U Mann–Whitney test analysis results between control group and TNM subgroups.

	Parameter	CCL2	CCL4	CCL15	CA 19-9	CEA	CRP
U Mann–Whitney test p-value	Control vs. I + II	0.44	0.99	0.91	**0.05**	**0.04**	**<0.001**
	Control vs. III + IV	**0.02**	**0.002**	0.82	0.10	**<0.001**	**<0.001**
	Control vs. III	**0.02**	0.32	0.87	0.30	**<0.001**	**<0.001**
	Control vs. IV	0.27	**<0.001**	0.24	0.14	**<0.001**	**<0.001**
	I + II vs. III + IV	0.32	**<0.001**	0.89	**<0.001**	**<0.001**	1.00
	I+II vs. III	0.17	**0.03**	0.39	**<0.001**	0.10	0.70
	I+II vs. IV	0.82	**<0.001**	0.48	**<0.001**	**<0.001**	0.67

The statistically significant results are presented in bold.

Table 5 shows the sensitivity, specificity, positive and negative predictive values (SE; SP; PPV; NPV, respectively), and the relationship between them with the use of the area under the ROC curve (AUC) of all newly tested parameters. We indicated that the highest SE from all parameters revealed CCL4 (76%). The observed value is higher than SE of commonly used tumor markers such as CEA (75%), CA 19-9 (51%) and C-reactive protein (73%). In the case of SP, the highest value was observed for CCL2 (60%) and it was higher than SP of CA 19-9 (48%), but the highest specificity from all parameters was observed in case of CRP (78%) and CEA (70%). Positive and negative predictive values were highest in case of CCL2 and CCL4 (72%/47% and 74%/53%, respectively). These values were slightly lower than PPV and NPV of CEA and CRP. What is more, the SE, SP, PPV, and NPV values of all newly tested parameters (CCL2, CCL4, CCL15) were higher than CA 19-9, which confirms their higher usefulness in case of patients with CRC than the routinely used marker.

Table 5. Diagnostic criteria of tested parameters in patients with colorectal cancer.

Tested Parameters	Diagnostic Criteria	Colorectal Cancer
CCL2	SE	64%
	SP	60%
	PPV	75%
	NPV	47%
	AUC	0.634
CCL4	SE	76%
	SP	50%
	PPV	74%
	NPV	53%
	AUC	0.630
CCL15	SE	57%
	SP	53%
	PPV	69%
	NPV	40%
	AUC	0.534
CA 19-9	SE	51%
	SP	48%
	PPV	64%
	NPV	34%
	AUC	0.513
CEA	SE	75%
	SP	70%
	PPV	82%
	NPV	60%
	AUC	0.787
CRP	SE	73%
	SP	78%
	PPV	86%
	NPV	61%
	AUC	0.836

SE—sensitivity; SP—specificity; PPV—positive predictive value; NPV—negative predictive value.

We noticed that the CCL2 and CCL4 areas under the ROC curve (0.634; 0.630, respectively) in the entire group of colorectal cancer were highest from all newly tested parameters, but lower than AUC for CEA and CRP. Additionally, similar to previously mentioned statistical parameters, in the case of all tested CC chemokines, AUC was higher than AUC for CA 19-9. A graphical version of all of the significant ROC analysis results is shown in Figure 1. The AUCs for the tested parameters, as for generally used tumor markers and combined analysis, were significantly larger in comparison to AUC = 0.5 (borderline of the diagnostic usefulness of the test) ($p < 0.05$ in all cases).

In order to complete the statistical analysis, we checked the Spearman's rank correlation coefficient to measure and to show the strength and the direction of monotonic association between variables in the CRC group. Obtained results are shown in Table 6. We observed a strong positive correlation for one of the tested parameters (CCL4) and the tumor TNM stage. This may confirm that the increasing concentration of this parameter is related to the number of neoplastic cells. This fact was also observed during the Kruskal–Wallis and Dwass–Steel–Critchlow–Fligner tests. In the case of the remaining parameters (CEA and CA 19-9), we also observed a similar correlation but of moderate strength. Moderate, positive correlation was also observed between the CEA and the CCL4 concentrations, and concentrations of both markers (CEA and CA 19-9). The rest of the observed correlations revealed weak strength (coefficient < 0.40). Interestingly, we observed also one negative but weak correlation between the CCL2 and the CCL15 concentrations.

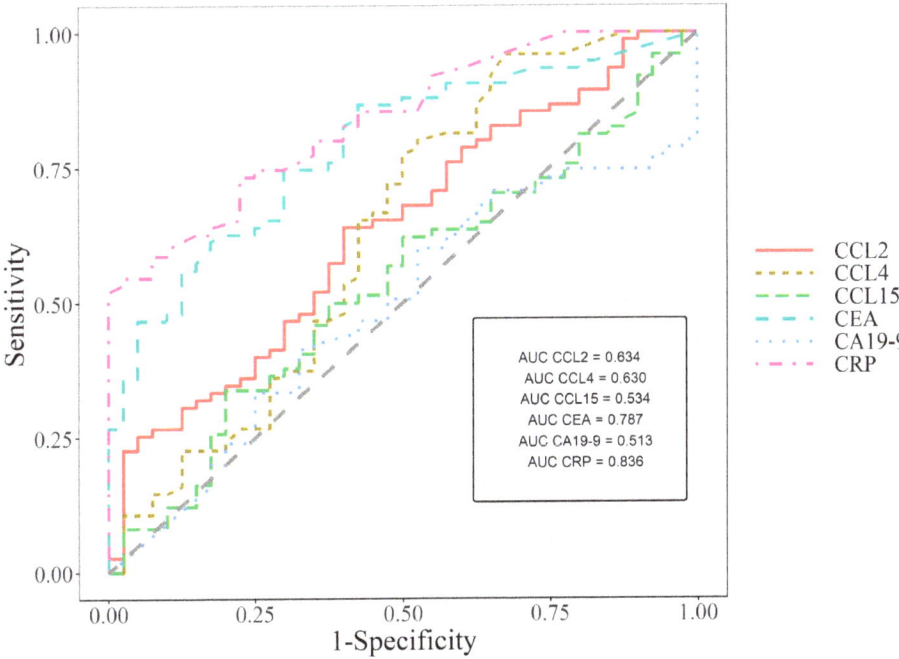

AUC CCL2 = 0.634
AUC CCL4 = 0.630
AUC CCL15 = 0.534
AUC CEA = 0.787
AUC CA19-9 = 0.513
AUC CRP = 0.836

Figure 1. Receiver operating characteristics for all significant ROC analysis results.

Table 6. Spearman's rank correlation coefficient for tested variables.

Tested Variables	CCL2	CCL4	CCL15	CA 19-9	CEA	CRP	Age
CCL4	**0.34** $p < 0.001$	-					
CCL15	**−0.24** $p = 0.04$	−0.06 $p = 0.60$	-				
CA 19-9	−0.01 $p = 0.96$	**0.39** $p < 0.001$	−0.04 $p = 0.73$	-			
CEA	0.07 $p = 0.56$	**0.56** $p < 0.001$	0.09 $p = 0.46$	**0.51** $p < 0.001$	-		
CRP	0.18 $p = 0.13$	**0.32** $p = 0.01$	0.04 $p = 0.74$	−0.01 $p = 0.90$	0.17 $p = 0.16$	-	
Age	0.18 $p = 0.11$	**0.39** $p < 0.001$	−0.00 $p = 0.98$	0.18 $p = 0.13$	**0.36** $p < 0.001$	−0.07 $p = 0.55$	-
TNM stage	0.02 $p = 0.84$	**0.62** $p < 0.001$	0.06 $p = 0.60$	**0.43** $p < 0.001$	**0.57** $p < 0.001$	0.05 $p = 0.67$	**0.34** $p < 0.001$

The statistically significant results are presented in bold.

4. Discussion

At present, in case of patients with colorectal cancer it is clinically important to search for new prognostic or predictive markers, as they might influence postoperative decisions. Generally, the guidelines for CRC are mainly based on the basis of, e.g., the TNM stage or the molecular characteristics of the tumor. In some cases, the decision whether to use or not to use adjuvant chemotherapy requires additional tests such as for a serum CEA level or an expression of p53/Ki67 [13]. In accordance with that, researchers are searching for different, new parameters to find markers for the highly accurate and non-invasive tests for colorectal cancer.

We indicated that the serum concentration for CCL2 was statistically higher in the group of colorectal cancer patients when compared to healthy controls (p = 0.02). Similar results were obtained in the work of De la Fuente López et al. [14]. These authors revealed that not only plasma levels, but also the concentration of this parameter in CRC tissue lysates is significantly higher when compared to healthy mucosa. Nevertheless, as the number of samples in these investigations were low (25 tissues; 32 CRC patients and 15 healthy patient plasma samples), these results needed a verification. Another work confirmed that a higher expression of CCL2 can be found in cancer tissue, and it is connected with a negative prognosis in CRC patients [15]. Interestingly, some researchers have indicated that an overexpression of CCL2 is associated with increased metastatic potential [16]. A different study by Nardelli et al. [17] also established that circulating CCL2 levels were associated with the presence of CRC, but the number of patients in this study was also insufficient (20 CRC patients and 20 healthy volunteers). A different research group also suggested that higher CCL2 levels may be considered as a prognostic factor in CRC, but this study was performed with the use of serum from 45 patients, and peculiarly, the control group was not included [13]. Therefore, our research carried out on a much larger group of patients with the use of a sufficiently large group of healthy volunteers, finally confirms the previously mentioned fragmentary reports.

Some studies also assessed the changes of CCL2 concentration after surgery or perioperatively. Hua et al. [18] discovered that elevated levels of this parameter are associated with a high risk of overall mortality. On the contrary, a study by Watanabe et al. [19] revealed that a decrease in the CCL2 ratio between tumoral and normal adjacent tissues is associated with lymph node involvement, and it could predict a poor prognosis. This discrepancy may be related not only to the difference in the material used for research, but also to the calculated ratio. Its reduction may be caused not only by lower expression in neoplastic tissues, but also by increased expression in healthy tissues. Interestingly, when analyzing the concentration of CCL2 in the control group and the study group by TNM stage, we showed a significant relationship between stage III and the control group, which may be a confirmation of the Watanabe et al. [19] investigation, which pointed out the relationship between CCL2 and the appearance of local lymph node metastases. In addition, the work of Johdi et al. [20] showed that there were no differences in the serum concentration of CCL2 and CRC, polyp, and healthy subjects. However, these results were performed on a basis of only 20 samples from each group. In the work of Tonouchi et al. [21], CCL2 levels were significantly raised 1 h after surgery, which suggests that this parameter can have a different role than as a marker of surgical insults, especially, as these differences did not correlate with IL-6 changes. However, a few days after surgery, the levels of this parameter were comparable to those before surgery. Due to discrepancies in the previously obtained studies, all previously mentioned results require further confirmation, which indicates a further plan for the continuation of our research.

We also found studies concerning the CCL2 concentration and expression in murine models [22,23]. These authors concluded that this cytokine may activate macrophages to become tumoricidal, resulting in the suppression of metastasis; and, they could be useful as biomarkers of colon cancer progression, which fully coincides with our discoveries.

On the other hand, one of the publications indicated that CCL2 did not show any differences between the adenoma group compared to the control group. This inconsistency may be related to a too-early period of changes leading to cancer progression. However, the serum samples used in the study were stored for many years and they were transported several times, which may have a significant impact on the results obtained by those researchers [24]. These results also suggest the need for further confirmation.

In the work of De la Fuente López et al. [14], CCL4 concentration was also found (similar to our study) to be significantly increased in CRC patients when compared to healthy controls. The previously mentioned work by Johdi et al. [20] also included the CCL4 determinations. Interestingly, in case of this parameter, significantly higher concentrations in the blood serum of patients with CRC compared to the control group were observed, as well as in the serum of patients with colorectal polyps.

Remarkably, in the work of Krzystek-Korpacka et al. [25], it was shown that CCL4 concentrations in the case of CRC are significantly higher when compared to the control group. However, after division by tumor location (rectum and colon), it turned out that in the case of rectal cancer, these concentrations are the highest and the difference is statistically significant. This can be important information when attempting to personalize therapy, and it is indicative of the heterogeneity of CRC. Surprisingly, in the work of Pervaiz et al. [26], completely contradictory results were presented. In IV stage of the tumor's advancement, statistically lower concentrations of CCL4 were demonstrated compared to the control group. These differences may be related to the number of patients, as the studies of Pervaiz et al. [26] were carried out on a group of 24 patients diagnosed with CRC, of which only 3 were at stage IV of CRC advancement.

In the case of CCL15, for which we did not observe any statistical differences, we found only one study that assessed the concentration of this parameter in the course of CRC. Inamoto et al. [27] showed that the concentrations of CCL15 in patients with CRC are statistically significantly higher than in healthy subjects, not only in the entire study group, but also at various stages of CRC advancement. These differences are extremely difficult to explain, as both experiments involved a properly large group of patients. However, the results obtained by Inamoto et al. [27] were several times higher (median for the control group 9.4 ng/mL; for the tested group 17.8 ng/mL). Possibly these differences could be influenced by the method of determination (ELISA vs. Luminex) or the ethnicity of the patients (Asian vs. European).

Unfortunately, we have not found any other papers that would focus on demonstrating the dependence and statistical significance based on the division of the study group into stages of advancement. Therefore, we believe that our work is innovative in this matter, which significantly increases its value. A more accurate demonstration of the relationships between the control group and the study group may significantly affect the understanding of changes in the course of CRC. Interestingly, our results showed a significant relationship between CCL2 and III TNM stage of CRC, which may be associated with the formation of local lymph nodes metastases, and significant differences between the concentration of CCL4 in stage IV of CRC and the control group, which may indicate its involvement in the development of distant metastasis. Due to the fact that these are the first reports on these dependencies, it is advisable to confirm them in further analyses.

According to our knowledge, the present study is also the first that assesses diagnostic criteria such as SE, SP, PPV, NPV, and ROC. However, parameters such as CCL2 and CCL4 showed high values (especially diagnostic sensitivity) compared to markers routinely used in diagnostics, and even higher than CA 19-9. This is significant evidence that these cytokines can contribute to the development of diagnostics and constitute an additional diagnostic parameter, e.g., in the case of detecting local and distant metastases. Perhaps a simultaneous analysis of the classical tumor markers and the tested cytokines would increase their diagnostic utility, which is an important task for the continuation of our research in the future. The only work assessing merely the SE and the SP of the CCL15 chemokine was the previously mentioned work of Inamoto et al. [27], whose results were significantly higher than ours (78.8%; 70% vs. 57%; 53%, respectively). These discrepancies may be due to the same reasons as for the concentrations of CCL15 described above.

We also tried to determine the correlations between the examined parameters, which showed that the concentration of CCL2 positively correlates with the concentration of CCL4 and negatively correlates with the concentration of CCL15. In contrast, CCL4 positively correlated with routine markers (CEA, CA 19-9), CRP protein, age (similar to CEA), and tumor stage (similar to CEA and CA 19-9). The study by De la Fuente López et al. [14] showed a significant correlation between CCL4 and the CD163 marker on pro-tumor macrophages and inflammatory mediators (VEGF, TNF-α). This indicates the high potential of CCL4 to induce infiltration of tumor-associated macrophages which may be related to tumor progression or metastases associated with high levels of CCL4, which was found in our study.

5. Conclusions

According to our knowledge, the current study is the first that links the diagnostic characteristics of CCL2, CCL4, and CCL15 with the well-established, classical tumor markers (CEA and CA 19-9) and CRP—which is the marker of inflammation—in CRC patients, and not only in the entire study group, but also in subjects divided according to TNM stage. The results obtained suggest the significant importance of CCL2 in the determination of local metastases and CCL4 in the case of distant metastases. However, after a careful analysis of our results and the results of other authors, it is certain that further studies concerning the concentrations of selected CC chemokines in the course of colorectal cancer are necessary to confirm and to clarify their diagnostic utility and their clinical application as potential non-invasive markers of CRC development.

Author Contributions: Conceptualization, M.Z. and B.M.; methodology, M.Z. and A.K.-P.; formal analysis, M.Z., A.K.-P. and M.D.; investigation, M.Z., M.D., K.S., M.J., L.K., M.K. and A.K.-P.; resources, M.Z.; data curation, M.Z. and M.D.; writing—original draft preparation, M.Z.; writing—review and editing, M.Z. and B.M.; supervision, B.M.; project administration, M.Z. and B.M.; funding acquisition, M.Z. All authors have read and agreed to the published version of the manuscript.

Funding: This research was funded by the Medical University of Bialystok, Poland (grant numbers: SUB/1/DN/21/004/1198 and SUB/1/DN/22/004/1198).

Institutional Review Board Statement: The study was conducted according to the guidelines of the Declaration of Helsinki, and it was approved by the Ethics Committee of the Medical University of Bialystok (R-I-002/564/2019; 28 November 2019).

Informed Consent Statement: Informed consent was obtained from all subjects involved in the study.

Data Availability Statement: The data presented in this study are available on request from the corresponding author. Key data are stated in the text.

Acknowledgments: This study was conducted with the use of equipment purchased by the Medical University of Bialystok as part of RPOWP 2007-2013 funding, Priority I, Axis 1.1, contract No. UDA-RPPD.01.01.00-20-001/15-00 dated 26.06.2015. B.M. received consultation and/or lecture honoraria from Abbott, Wiener, Roche, Cormay, and Biameditek. M.Z. received lecture honoraria from Roche.

Conflicts of Interest: The authors declare no conflict of interest.

References

1. Ferlay, J.; Colombet, M.; Soerjomataram, I.; Mathers, C.; Parkin, D.M.; Piñeros, M.; Znaor, A.; Bray, F. Estimating the global cancer incidence and mortality in 2018: GLOBOCAN sources and methods. *Int. J. Cancer* **2019**, *144*, 1941–1953. [CrossRef] [PubMed]
2. Sung, H.; Ferlay, J.; Siegel, R.L.; Laversanne, M.; Soerjomataram, I.; Jemal, A.; Bray, F. Global Cancer Statistics 2020: GLOBOCAN Estimates of Incidence and Mortality Worldwide for 36 Cancers in 185 Countries. *CA Cancer J. Clin.* **2021**, *71*, 209–249. [CrossRef] [PubMed]
3. Toma, M.; Beluşică, L.; Stavarachi, M.; Apostol, P.; Spandole, S.; Radu, I.; Cimponeriu, D. Rating the environmental and genetic risk factors for colorectal cancer. *J. Med. Life* **2012**, *5*, 152–159. [PubMed]
4. Holvoet, L.T.; Schrijvers, D. Chapter 17—Colorectal Cancer. In *Handbook of Cancer Prevention*, 1st ed.; Informa UK Ltd.: London, UK, 2008; pp. 127–136.
5. Łukaszewicz-Zając, M.; Pączek, S.; Muszyński, P.; Kozłowski, M.; Mroczko, B. Comparison between clinical significance of serum CXCL-8 and classical tumor markers in oesophageal cancer (OC) patients. *Clin. Exp. Med.* **2019**, *19*, 191–199. [CrossRef] [PubMed]

6. Pączek, S.; Łukaszewicz-Zając, M.; Gryko, M.; Mroczko, P.; Kulczyńska-Przybik, A.; Mroczko, B. CXCL-8 in Preoperative Colorectal Cancer Patients: Significance for Diagnosis and Cancer Progression. *Int. J. Mol. Sci.* **2020**, *21*, 2040. [CrossRef]
7. Das, V.; Kalita, J.; Pal, M. Predictive and prognostic biomarkers in colorectal cancer: A systematic review of recent advances and challenges. *Biomed. Pharmacother.* **2017**, *87*, 8–19. [CrossRef]
8. Zajkowska, M.; Mroczko, B. Eotaxins and Their Receptor in Colorectal Cancer—A Literature Review. *Cancers* **2020**, *12*, 1383. [CrossRef]
9. Gudowska-Sawczuk, M.; Kudelski, J.; Mroczko, B. The Role of Chemokine Receptor CXCR3 and Its Ligands in Renal Cell Carcinoma. *Int. J. Mol. Sci.* **2020**, *21*, 8582. [CrossRef]
10. Pączek, S.; Łukaszewicz-Zając, M.; Mroczko, B. Chemokines-What Is Their Role in Colorectal Cancer? *Cancer Control* **2020**, *27*, 1073274820903384. [CrossRef]
11. Zlotnik, A.; Yoshie, O. Chemokines: A new classification system and their role in immunity. *Immunity* **2000**, *12*, 121–127. [CrossRef]
12. Ridiandries, A.; Tan, J.T.; Bursill, C.A. The Role of CC-Chemokines in the Regulation of Angiogenesis. *Int. J. Mol. Sci.* **2016**, *17*, 1856. [CrossRef]
13. Szczepanik, A.M.; Siedlar, M.; Szura, M.; Kibil, W.; Brzuszkiewicz, K.; Brandt, P.; Kulig, J. Preoperative serum chemokine (C-C motif) ligand 2 levels and prognosis in colorectal cancer. *Pol. Arch. Med. Wewn.* **2015**, *125*, 443–451. [CrossRef] [PubMed]
14. De la Fuente López, M.; Landskron, G.; Parada, D.; Dubois-Camacho, K.; Simian, D.; Martinez, M.; Romero, D.; Roa, J.C.; Chahuán, I.; Gutiérrez, R.; et al. The relationship between chemokines CCL2, CCL3, and CCL4 with the tumor microenvironment and tumor-associated macrophage markers in colorectal cancer. *Tumor Biol.* **2018**, *40*, 1010428318810059. [CrossRef]
15. Bailey, C.; Negus, R.; Morris, A.; Ziprin, P.; Goldin, R.; Allavena, P.; Peck, D.; Darzi, A. Chemokine expression is associated with the accumulation of tumour associated macrophages (TAMs) and progression in human colorectal cancer. *Clin. Exp. Metastasis* **2007**, *24*, 121–130. [CrossRef]
16. Hu, H.; Sun, L.; Guo, C.; Liu, Q.; Zhou, Z.; Peng, L.; Pan, J.; Yu, L.; Lou, J.; Yang, Z.; et al. Tumor cell-microenvironment interaction models coupled with clinical validation reveal CCL2 and SNCG as two predictors of colorectal cancer hepatic metastasis. *Clin. Cancer Res.* **2009**, *15*, 5485–5493. [CrossRef]
17. Nardelli, C.; Granata, I.; Nunziato, M.; Setaro, M.; Carbone, F.; Zulli, C.; Pilone, V.; Capoluongo, E.D.; De Palma, G.D.; Corcione, F.; et al. 16S rRNA of Mucosal Colon Microbiome and CCL2 Circulating Levels Are Potential Biomarkers in Colorectal Cancer. *Int. J. Mol. Sci.* **2021**, *22*, 10747. [CrossRef]
18. Hua, X.; Kratz, M.; Malen, R.C.; Dai, J.Y.; Lindström, S.; Zheng, Y.; Newcomb, P.A. Association between post-treatment circulating biomarkers of inflammation and survival among stage II-III colorectal cancer patients. *Br. J. Cancer* **2021**, *125*, 806–815. [CrossRef]
19. Watanabe, H.; Miki, C.; Okugawa, Y.; Toiyama, Y.; Inoue, Y.; Kusunoki, M. Decreased expression of monocyte chemoattractant protein-1 predicts poor prognosis following curative resection of colorectal cancer. *Dis. Colon Rectum* **2008**, *51*, 1800–1805. [CrossRef]
20. Johdi, N.A.; Mazlan, L.; Sagap, I.; Jamal, R. Profiling of cytokines, chemokines and other soluble proteins as a potential biomarker in colorectal cancer and polyps. *Cytokine* **2017**, *99*, 35–42. [CrossRef]
21. Tonouchi, H.; Miki, C.; Ohmori, Y.; Kobayashi, M.; Mohri, Y.; Tanaka, K.; Konishi, N.; Kusunoki, M. Serum monocyte chemoattractant protein-1 in patients with postoperative infectious complications from gastrointestinal surgery for cancer. *World J. Surg.* **2004**, *28*, 130–136. [CrossRef]
22. Huang, S.; Singh, R.K.; Xie, K.; Gutman, M.; Berry, K.K.; Bucana, C.D.; Fidler, I.J.; Bar-Eli, M. Expression of the JE/MCP-1 gene suppresses metastatic potential in murine colon carcinoma cells. *Cancer Immunol. Immunother.* **1994**, *39*, 231–238. [CrossRef] [PubMed]
23. McClellan, J.L.; Davis, J.M.; Steiner, J.L.; Day, S.D.; Steck, S.E.; Carmichael, M.D.; Murphy, E.A. Intestinal inflammatory cytokine response in relation to tumorigenesis in the Apc(Min/+) mouse. *Cytokine* **2012**, *57*, 113–119. [CrossRef] [PubMed]
24. Henry, C.J.; Sedjo, R.L.; Rozhok, A.; Salstrom, J.; Ahnen, D.; Levin, T.R.; D'Agostino, R., Jr.; Haffner, S.; DeGregori, J.; Byers, T. Lack of significant association between serum inflammatory cytokine profiles and the presence of colorectal adenoma. *BMC Cancer* **2015**, *15*, 123. [CrossRef]
25. Krzystek-Korpacka, M.; Zawadzki, M.; Kapturkiewicz, B.; Lewandowska, P.; Bednarz-Misa, I.; Gorska, S.; Witkiewicz, W.; Gamian, A. Subsite heterogeneity in the profiles of circulating cytokines in colorectal cancer. *Cytokine* **2018**, *110*, 435–441. [CrossRef] [PubMed]
26. Pervaiz, A.; Zepp, M.; Georges, R.; Bergmann, F.; Mahmood, S.; Faiza, S.; Berger, M.R.; Adwan, H. Antineoplastic effects of targeting CCR5 and its therapeutic potential for colorectal cancer liver metastasis. *J. Cancer Res. Clin. Oncol.* **2021**, *147*, 73–91. [CrossRef]
27. Inamoto, S.; Itatani, Y.; Yamamoto, T.; Minamiguchi, S.; Hirai, H.; Iwamoto, M.; Hasegawa, S.; Taketo, M.M.; Sakai, Y.; Kawada, K. Loss of SMAD4 Promotes Colorectal Cancer Progression by Accumulation of Myeloid-Derived Suppressor Cells through the CCL15-CCR1 Chemokine Axis. *Clin. Cancer Res.* **2016**, *22*, 492–501. [CrossRef]

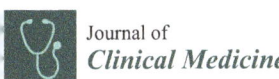

Article

Cigarette Smoking Associated with Colorectal Cancer Survival: A Nationwide, Population-Based Cohort Study

Yu-Min Huang [1,2], Po-Li Wei [1,3], Chung-Han Ho [4,5,†] and Chih-Ching Yeh [6,7,8,9,*,†]

1. Department of Surgery, School of Medicine, College of Medicine, Taipei Medical University, Taipei 11031, Taiwan; yuminhuang26@gmail.com (Y.-M.H.); poliwei@tmu.edu.tw (P.-L.W.)
2. Division of General Surgery, Department of Surgery, Taipei Medical University Hospital, Taipei 11031, Taiwan
3. Division of Colorectal Surgery, Department of Surgery, Taipei Medical University Hospital, Taipei Medical University, Taipei 11031, Taiwan
4. Department of Medical Research, Chi-Mei Medical Center, Tainan 71004, Taiwan; ho.c.hank@gmail.com
5. Department of Information Management, Southern Taiwan University of Science and Technology, Tainan 71005, Taiwan
6. Master Program in Applied Epidemiology, College of Public Health, Taipei Medical University, Taipei 11031, Taiwan
7. Cancer Center, Wan Fang Hospital, Taipei Medical University, Taipei 11696, Taiwan
8. School of Public Health, College of Public Health, Taipei Medical University, Taipei 11031, Taiwan
9. Department of Public Health, College of Public Health, China Medical University, Taichung 40402, Taiwan
* Correspondence: ccyeh@tmu.edu.tw; Tel.: +886-27361661 (ext. 6534)
† These authors contributed equally to this work.

Abstract: We investigate whether cigarette smoking is associated with survival in patients with colorectal cancer (CRC) through a nationwide population-based cohort study in Taiwan. The Taiwan Cancer Registry and National Health Insurance Research Database were used to identify data from patients with CRC from 2011 to 2017. Tobacco use was evaluated based on the smoking status, intensity, and duration before cancer diagnosis. A total of 18,816 patients was included. A Kaplan–Meier survival analysis indicated smoking to be significantly associated with the CRC mortality risk (log-rank p = 0.0001). A multivariable Cox model indicated that smoking patients had a 1.11-fold higher mortality risk (HR = 1.11, 95% CI = 1.05–1.19) than nonsmoking patients did. This increased risk was also present in patients with CRC who smoked 11–20 cigarettes per day (HR = 1.16; 95% CI = 1.07–1.26) or smoked for >30 years (HR = 1.14; 95% CI = 1.04–1.25). Stratified analyses of sex and cancer subsites indicated that the effects of smoking were higher in male patients and in those with colon cancer. Our results indicate that cigarette smoking is significantly associated with poor survival in patients with CRC. An integrated smoking cessation campaign is warranted to prevent CRC mortality.

Keywords: colorectal cancer; cigarette smoking; survival

Citation: Huang, Y.-M.; Wei, P.-L.; Ho, C.-H.; Yeh, C.-C. Cigarette Smoking Associated with Colorectal Cancer Survival: A Nationwide, Population-Based Cohort Study. *J. Clin. Med.* **2022**, *11*, 913. https://doi.org/10.3390/jcm11040913

Academic Editor: Ugo Grossi

Received: 11 December 2021
Accepted: 7 February 2022
Published: 9 February 2022

Publisher's Note: MDPI stays neutral with regard to jurisdictional claims in published maps and institutional affiliations.

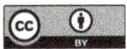

Copyright: © 2022 by the authors. Licensee MDPI, Basel, Switzerland. This article is an open access article distributed under the terms and conditions of the Creative Commons Attribution (CC BY) license (https://creativecommons.org/licenses/by/4.0/).

1. Introduction

Colorectal cancer (CRC) is among the most common cancers and among the leading causes of cancer deaths worldwide [1–4]. Although it has historically been more prevalent in the West, the incidence rates of CRC have been increasing in East Asian countries [5]. In Taiwan, CRC is one of the most commonly diagnosed cancers [6]. Despite the progress that has been achieved in its diagnosis and treatment, approximately half of patients with CRC die within 5 years of diagnosis [4]. Therefore, further efforts to identify and obviate the risk factors of CRC mortality are required to improve the prognosis of this cancer.

Cigarette smoking is a serious public health concern; it is annually responsible for millions of deaths around the world [7]. Smoking is estimated to be responsible for more than 30% of cancer deaths in the United States each year. Smoking has also been observed to increase the risk of mortality in CRC [8]. The association between smoking and CRC has been demonstrated in many studies [9–13]. Long-term smokers have been reported to have a significantly increased risk of developing CRC than nonsmokers [13–16]. Studies have reported a 15% to 60% higher risk estimate associated with active smoking [1,17,18]. Although data were insufficient for the association between smoking and CRC to be defined as casual, recent studies have suggested cigarette smoking to be a risk factor for CRC [1,4,13,19–21]. Consequently, the American College of Gastroenterology colorectal cancer screening guidelines have highlighted smokers as being at an increased risk [22].

Cigarette smoking may worsen the prognosis of CRC [23,24]. Long-term cigarette smoking has been reported to increase the risk of both overall and disease-specific CRC mortality in men and women [4,9,13,19]. However, findings regarding the influence of smoking on CRC survival have been inconsistent; several studies have also reported no significant association between smoking and CRC mortality [25,26].

Moreover, many of the aforementioned studies on the association between smoking and the risk and prognosis of CRC were conducted in Western countries [5,27]. In the 16 studies included in one meta-analysis, only 1 was conducted in East Asia [28]. Therefore, because of factors such as ethnicity, culture, and lifestyle, the reported findings of this meta-analysis may not be directly applicable to other demographic groups. Another meta-analysis reported that the relative risks (RRs) of CRC among current smokers were significantly different in different geographic areas [1]. In addition, the results of studies from Asian countries have generally been heterogeneous, which further complicates the matter [5]. Evidence regarding the effects of cigarette smoking on the prognosis of CRC remains limited. Therefore, we perform a nationwide population-based cohort study to investigate whether cigarette smoking adversely affects the survival outcomes of Asian patients with CRC.

2. Materials and Methods

2.1. Data Sources

Data in this study were collected from the Taiwan Cancer Registry (TCR) and Taiwan's National Health Insurance Research Database (NHIRD). Both of these databases are managed by the Health and Welfare Data Science Center (HWDC) of the Ministry of Health and Welfare. The TCR was established to gather information on individual demographics, cancer stages (AJCC 7th edition), primary sites, histology, and treatment types in patients with cancer to understand the incidence and mortality rates of cancer in Taiwan. The NHIRD was established for research purposes; it contains data from Taiwan's single-payer insurance system, in which more than 99% of Taiwan's 23 million citizens are registered. The NHIRD contains registration files and original inpatient and outpatient reimbursement claim data from 1996 to 2017. The datasets of the HWDC are all de-identified forms. This study was conducted in compliance with the Declaration of Helsinki of 1964 and was approved by the Research Ethics Committee of Chi Mei Hospital (IRB no. 10702-E04). The requirement for informed consent was waived by the Research Ethics Committee of Chi Mei Hospital.

2.2. Study Population

The TCR was used to identify patients with CRC based on the International Classification of Diseases for Oncology, third edition (ICD-O-3); in this study, colon (ICD-O-3: C18), rectosigmoid junction (ICD-O-3: C19), and rectum (ICD-O-3: C20) cancers were included. Because the TCR began recording smoking and drinking behavioral information in 2011, patient data from 2011 to 2017 were selected. Patients with a history of CRC before 2011 were excluded to reduce omitted variable bias. In addition, because the aim of this study was to estimate the association between cigarette smoking and risk of mortality in patients with CRC, included patients were categorized as those with and without a history of prediagnostic smoking. Those with a smoking history included both current and ever smokers, for whom the duration of smoking in years and smoking count per day were included in the analysis. To reduce the potential confounding factors of mortality, including age, gender, clinical stage, grade, and cancer subsite, between patients with smoking and those without, we randomly selected two patients without smoking to match each patient with smoking using propensity score approach. A propensity score matching approach with the nearest-neighbor matching algorithm was used in this study according to SAS macro "%OneToManyMTCH". The flowchart of the study population selection is presented in Figure 1.

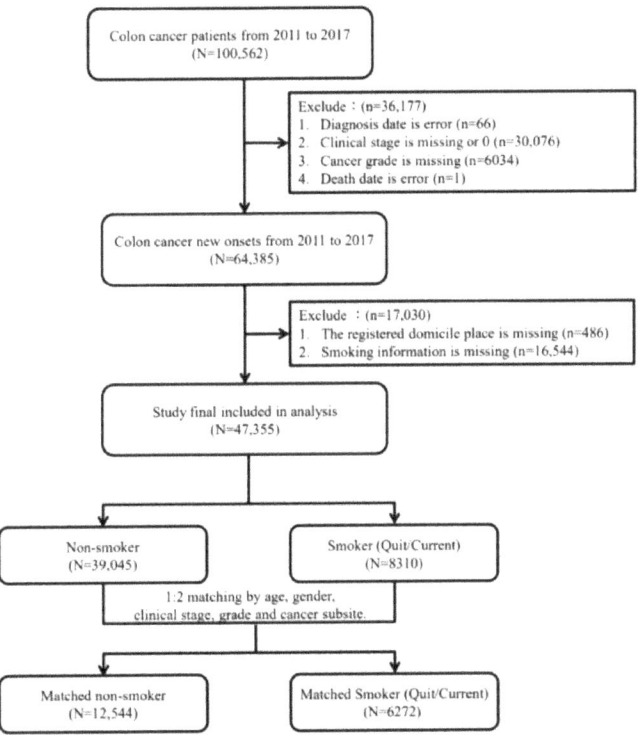

Figure 1. Flowchart of study population selection.

2.3. Measurements

The major outcome of this study was overall mortality. Mortality was defined using Taiwan's cause-of-death data. All patients were right censored to date of death or 31 December 2017, whichever came first. The study variables, namely, age at diagnosis, sex, clinical stage, histological grade, and alcohol drinking habit, were all collected from the TCR. Age was divided into groups of <40, 40–49, 50–59, 60–69, and ≥70 years. Charlson comorbidity index (CCI) scores were calculated using patients' diagnosis records from the NHIRD to represent patients' comorbidities, which were defined before the date of diagnosis of CRC. To generate the index score, each of the 19 identified medical conditions was scored from 1 to 6.

2.4. Statistical Analysis

The frequency was presented as a percentage for categorical variables among the study population. The distribution difference between smoking and nonsmoking groups was compared using Pearson's chi-square test. The trend of mortality during the study period was plotted using the Kaplan–Meier approach, with a log-rank test for estimating the statistical difference between smoking and nonsmoking patients with CRC. Multivariable Cox proportional regression was constructed to estimate the mortality risk and control for potential confounders by adjusting for age, sex, drinking habit, residence in a remote area, cancer site, cancer clinical stage, cancer grade, and CCI group. Stratified analyses of age, sex, and CRC subsites were also presented. To observe the progress of mortality risk on smoking counts per day and smoking years, the linear trend test was used to estimate the potential trends. All analyses were conducted using SAS statistical software version 9.4 (SAS Institute, Cary, NC, USA). Significance was set at $p < 0.05$. Kaplan–Meier curves were plotted using STATA (version 12; Stata, College Station, TX, USA).

3. Results

3.1. Characteristics of Study Population

The baseline characteristics of the matched cohort are presented in Table 1. Of the 18,816 patients with CRC included in this study, 6272 were smokers and 12,544 were not. The smoking group comprised more patients with drinking habits (52.1% vs. 13.8%, $p < 0.0001$). In addition, the mortality rate was significantly higher in the smoking group (30.1% vs. 27.9%, $p = 0.0012$). Otherwise, the two groups were balanced with regard to age, sex, residence in remote area, cancer subsite, clinical stage, tumor grade, and CCI grouping.

Table 1. Demographic analysis of smoking and nonsmoking patients with colorectal cancer.

	Total	Nonsmoking	Smoking	
	N = 18,816	N = 12,544	N = 6272	p
Age group, n (%), years				
<40	554 (2.94)	377 (3.01)	177 (2.82)	0.8870
40–50	1298 (6.90)	859 (6.85)	439 (7.00)	
50–60	3642 (19.36)	2421 (19.30)	1221 (19.47)	
60–70	6213 (33.02)	4163 (33.19)	2050 (32.68)	
≥70	7109 (37.78)	4724 (37.66)	2385 (38.03)	
Sex, n (%)				
Male	17,019 (90.45)	11,346 (90.45)	5673 (90.45)	1.0000
Female	1797 (9.55)	1198 (9.55)	599 (9.55)	
Drinking, n (%)				
No	13,821 (73.45)	10,817 (86.23)	3004 (47.90)	<0.0001
Yes	4995 (26.55)	1727 (13.77)	3268 (52.10)	
Remote area, n (%)				
No	18,477 (98.20)	12,334 (98.33)	6143 (97.94)	0.0628
Yes	339 (1.80)	210 (1.67)	129 (2.06)	
Cancer subsite, n (%)				
Colon	12,006 (63.81)	7999 (63.77)	4007 (63.89)	0.8722
Rectum	6810 (36.19)	4545 (36.23)	2265 (36.11)	
Clinical stage, n (%)				
I	4472 (23.77)	2986 (23.80)	1486 (23.69)	0.9532
II	3610 (19.19)	2398 (19.12)	1212 (19.32)	
III	7125 (37.87)	4742 (37.80)	2383 (37.99)	
IV	3609 (19.18)	2418 (19.28)	1191 (18.99)	
Grade, n (%)				
Well-differentiated	1221 (6.49)	794 (6.33)	427 (6.81)	0.1276
Moderately differentiated	15,877 (84.38)	10,638 (84.81)	5239 (83.53)	
Poorly differentiated	1562 (8.30)	1015 (8.09)	547 (8.72)	
Undifferentiated	156 (0.83)	97 (0.77)	59 (0.94)	
CCI group, n (%)				
0–1	14,453 (76.81)	9644 (76.88)	4809 (76.67)	0.4946
2–4	3863 (20.53)	2579 (20.56)	1284 (20.47)	
≥5	500 (2.66)	321 (2.56)	179 (2.85)	
Death, n (%)	5384 (28.61)	3495 (27.86)	1889 (30.12)	0.0012

3.2. Cigarette Smoking and Mortality Risk

As illustrated in Figure 2, a significant difference was found in the mortality risk of CRC between the smoking and nonsmoking groups (log-rank test $p = 0.0001$). The crude data, presented in Table 2, revealed that smoking patients had a 1.11-fold higher mortality risk (95% CI = 1.05–1.19; p = 0.0009) than nonsmoking patients did. Regarding the effects of smoking intensity, patients who smoked 11–20 cigarettes per day (HR = 1.17; 95% CI = 1.08–1.27; p = 0.0001) and who smoked for more than 10 years (HR = 1.12; 95% CI = 1.02–1.23; p = 0.0184 for patients smoking for 11–30 years; HR = 1.15; 95% CI = 1.06–1.26; p = 0.0014 for those smoking for >30 years) had a significantly higher mortality risk than nonsmoking patients did. After adjustment for age, sex, alcohol-drinking habit, residence in remote areas, cancer subsites, cancer clinical stage, cancer tumor grade, and CCI score grouping, smoking patients had a 1.10-fold higher mortality risk (95% CI = 1.03–1.18; p = 0.0056) than nonsmoking patients did. Patients who smoked 11–20 cigarettes (HR = 1.16; 95% CI = 1.07–1.26; p = 0.0006) per day and who smoked for more than 10 years (HR = 1.11; 95% CI = 1.01–1.23; p = 0.0356 for patients smoking for 11–30 years; HR = 1.14; 95% CI = 1.04–1.25; p = 0.0044 for those smoking for >30 years) had a significantly higher mortality risk than nonsmoking patients did. A significant trend was identified for increased mortality risk due to smoking duration (p = 0.0474).

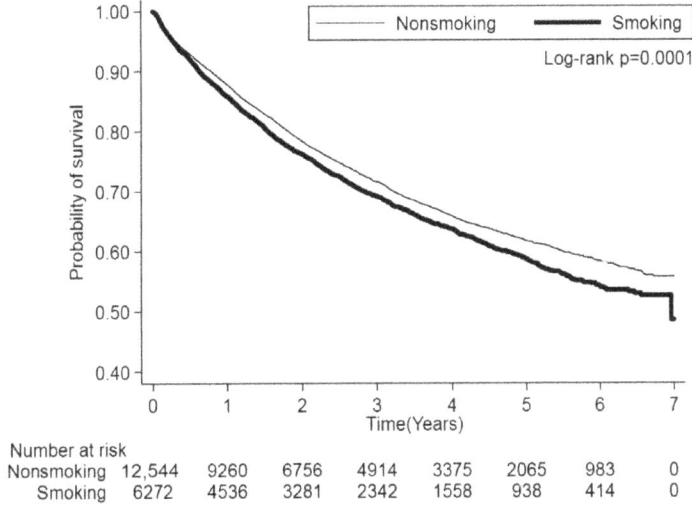

Figure 2. Association of cigarette smoking with mortality risk of colorectal cancer.

Table 2. Cigarette smoking associated with mortality risk of colorectal cancer.

	Patients	Death	%	Crude HR (95% CI)	p	Adjusted HR (95% CI) [a]	p
Smoking							
Never	12,544	3495	27.86	Ref.		Ref.	
Quit/Current	6272	1889	30.12	1.11 (1.05–1.19)	0.0009	1.10 (1.03–1.18)	0.0056
Smoking count							
0	12,544	3495	27.86	Ref.		Ref.	
1–10/day	1757	518	2948	1.03 (0.93–1.15)	0.5581	1.03 (0.92–1.15)	0.6435
11–20/day	3297	1008	30.57	1.17 (1.08–1.27)	0.0001	1.16 (1.07–1.26)	0.0006
>20/day	1218	363	29.80	1.08 (0.95–1.23)	0.2270	1.07 (0.94–1.22)	0.3144
Trend test						p = 0.3686	
Smoking years							
0	12,544	3495	27.86	Ref.		Ref.	
1–10	1248	338	27.08	1.01 (0.89–1.15)	0.8435	1.01 (0.88–1.15)	0.9426
11–30	2528	692	27.37	1.12 (1.02–1.23)	0.0184	1.11 (1.01–1.23)	0.0356
>30	2496	859	34.42	1.15 (1.06–1.26)	0.0014	1.14 (1.04–1.25)	0.0044
Trend test						p = 0.0474	

[a] Adjusted for age (continuous), sex, drinking habit, residence in remote areas, cancer subsite, cancer clinical stage, cancer grade, and CCI group.

3.3. Cigarette Smoking and Mortality Risk Stratified by Sex

The data presented in Table 3 revealed the risk of mortality associated with smoking in patients with CRC stratified by sex. The proportions of male and female smokers were the same (33.3%), but the male smoking population was 9.47 times of the female. Smoking men had a 1.09-fold higher mortality risk (95% CI = 1.02–1.18; p = 0.0156) than nonsmoking men did. A further analysis revealed a significantly higher risk of mortality in men who smoked 11–20 cigarettes per day (HR = 1.16; 95% CI = 1.06–1.26; p = 0.0011) and who smoked for more than 10 years (HR = 1.11; 95% CI = 1.01–1.24; p = 0.0390 for men smoking for 11–30 years; HR = 1.14; 95% CI = 1.04–1.25; p = 0.0076 for those smoking for >30 years) than in those who were nonsmokers. For women, a 1.59-fold higher mortality risk was observed only in those who smoked for 1–10 years (95% CI = 1.03–2.45; p = 0.0367) compared with nonsmoking women. However, the increase in risk was not significant in the other levels of smoking intensity.

Table 3. Cigarette smoking associated with mortality risk of colorectal cancer stratified by sex.

	Men					Women				
	Patients	Death	%	Adjusted HR (95% CI) [a]	p	Patients	Death	%	Adjusted HR (95% CI) [a]	p
Smoking Never	11,346	3213	28.32	Ref.		1198	282	23.54	Ref.	
Quit/Current	5673	1753	30.90	1.09 (1.02–1.18)	0.0156	599	136	22.70	1.26 (0.96–1.66)	0.1032
Smoking count										
0	11,346	3213	28.32	Ref.		1198	282	23.54	Ref.	
1–10/day	1484	455	30.66	1.00 (0.89–1.12)	0.9766	273	63	23.08	1.35 (0.93–1.96)	0.1093
11–20/day	3027	951	31.42	1.16 (1.06–1.26)	0.0011	270	57	21.11	1.17 (0.79–1.74)	0.4235
>20/day	1162	347	29.86	1.06 (0.93–1.22)	0.3752	56	16	28.57	1.20 (0.61–2.36)	0.5938
Trend test				p = 0.4186					p = 0.6222	
Smoking year										
0	11,346	3213	28.32	Ref.		1198	282	23.54	Ref.	
1–10	1057	286	27.06	0.96 (0.83–1.10)	0.5430	191	52	27.23	1.59 (1.03–2.45)	0.0367
11–30	2242	645	28.77	1.11 (1.01–1.24)	0.0390	286	47	16.43	1.04 (0.70–1.55)	0.8407
>30	2374	822	34.63	1.14 (1.04–1.25)	0.0076	122	37	30.33	1.28 (0.79–2.09)	0.3108
Trend test				p = 0.1460					p = 0.8621	

[a] Adjusted for age (continuous), drinking habit, residence in remote areas, cancer subsite, cancer clinical stage, cancer grade, and CCI group.

3.4. Cigarette Smoking and Mortality Risk Stratified by Cancer Subsite

The risk of mortality associated with smoking with respect to the CRC subsite is presented in Table 4. Smoking patients were associated with a significantly higher mortality risk than nonsmoking patients were for colon (HR = 1.12; 95% CI = 1.03–1.22; p = 0.0096) but not rectal cancers (HR = 1.08; 95% CI = 0.95–1.22; p = 0.2339). Furthermore, patients with colon cancer who smoked more than 10 cigarettes (HR = 1.15; 95% CI = 1.04–1.28; p = 0.0072 for patients smoking 11–20 cigarettes; HR = 1.18; 95% CI = 1.01–1.39; p = 0.0376 for those smoking >20 cigarettes) daily and who smoked for more than 10 years (HR = 1.13; 95% CI = 1.00–1.28; p = 0.0447 for patients smoking for 11–30 years; HR = 1.18; 95% CI = 1.05–1.32; p = 0.0046 for those smoking for >30 years) had a significantly higher mortality risk than nonsmoking patients did. A significant trend was also identified for an increased mortality risk due to smoking intensity (p = 0.0463). By contrast, no significant increase in mortality risk was observed in patients with rectal cancer except in those smoking 11–20 cigarettes per day (HR = 1.17; 95% CI = 1.01–1.35; p = 0.0337).

Table 4. Cigarette smoking associated with mortality risk of colorectal cancer stratified by cancer subsite.

	Colon					Rectum				
	Patients	Death	%	Adjusted HR (95% CI) [a]	p	Patients	Death	%	Adjusted HR (95% CI) [a]	p
Smoking										
Never	7999	2229	27.87	Ref.		4545	1266	27.85	Ref.	
Quit/Current	4007	1206	30.10	1.12 (1.03–1.22)	0.0096	2265	683	30.15	1.08 (0.95–1.22)	0.2339
Smoking count										
0	7999	2229	27.87	Ref.		4545	1266	27.85	Ref.	
1–10/day	1134	325	28.66	1.02 (0.89–1.17)	0.7660	623	193	30.98	1.03 (0.86–1.25)	0.7316
11–20/day	2117	647	30.56	1.15 (1.04–1.28)	0.0072	1180	361	30.59	1.17 (1.01–1.35)	0.0337
>20/day	756	234	30.95	1.18 (1.01–1.39)	0.0376	462	129	27.92	0.88 (0.70–1.12)	0.2961
Trend test				p = 0.0463					p = 0.7617	
Smoking year										
0 years	7999	2229	27.87	Ref.		4545	1266	27.85	Ref.	
1–10 years	823	219	26.61	0.98 (0.83–1.15)	0.8084	425	119	28.00	1.06 (0.84–1.33)	0.6220
11–30 years	1636	453	27.69	1.13 (1.00–1.28)	0.0447	892	239	26.79	1.08 (0.90–1.28)	0.4154
>30 years	1548	534	34.50	1.18 (1.05–1.32)	0.0046	948	325	34.28	1.09 (0.93–1.27)	0.3092
Trend test				p = 0.0889					p = 0.0713	

[a] Adjusted for age (continuous), sex, drinking habit, residence in remote areas, cancer clinical stage, cancer grade, and CCI group.

3.5. Cigarette Smoking and Mortality Risk Stratified by Age

The effects of smoking on the mortality risk were assessed with the stratification of the patients' ages (Table 5). For patients younger than 60, an increased CRC mortality risk was not associated with smoking, with the exception of those who smoked for more than 30 years (HR = 1.43; 95% CI = 1.10–1.87; p = 0.0074). By contrast, smoking significantly increased the risk of mortality in patients with CRC who were older than 60 (HR = 1.12; 95% CI = 1.03–1.21; p = 0.0061). Higher risks were observed in such patients who smoked 11–20 cigarettes per day (HR = 1.16; 95% CI = 1.05–1.27; p = 0.0034) and who smoked for more than 10 years (HR = 1.15; 95% CI = 1.02–1.30; p = 0.0190 for patients who smoked for 11–30 years; HR = 1.12; 95% CI = 1.02–1.24; p = 0.0209 for those who smoked for more than 30 years).

Table 5. Cigarette smoking associated with mortality risk of colorectal cancer stratified by age.

	Age ≤ 60					Age > 60				
	Patients	Death	%	Adjusted HR (95% CI) [a]	p	Patients	Death	%	Adjusted HR (95% CI) [a]	p
Smoking										
Never	4117	829	20.14	Ref.		8427	2666	31.64	Ref.	
Quit/Current	2055	445	21.65	1.07 (0.92–1.23)	0.3971	4217	1444	34.24	1.12 (1.03–1.21)	0.0061
Smoking count										
0	4117	829	20.14	Ref.		8427	2666	31.64	Ref.	
1–10/day	590	125	21.19	0.97 (0.77–1.23)	0.8078	1167	393	33.68	1.05 (0.92–1.19)	0.4655
11–20/day	1046	232	22.18	1.19 (0.99–1.42)	0.0616	2251	776	34.47	1.16 (1.05–1.27)	0.0034

Table 5. Cont.

	Age ≤ 60					Age > 60				
	Patients	Death	%	Adjusted HR (95% CI) [a]	p	Patients	Death	%	Adjusted HR (95% CI) [a]	p
>20/day	419	88	21.00	0.93 (0.71–1.21)	0.5737	799	275	34.42	1.12 (0.97–1.31)	0.1274
Trend test				p = 0.9888					p = 0.1497	
Smoking year										
0	4117	829	20.14	Ref.		8427	2666	31.64	Ref.	
1–10	525	118	22.48	0.92 (0.72–1.17)	0.4871	723	220	30.43	1.04 (0.89–1.22)	0.6071
11–30	1200	242	20.17	1.03 (0.86–1.24)	0.7198	1328	450	33.89	1.15 (1.02–1.30)	0.0190
>30	330	85	25.76	1.43 (1.10–1.87)	0.0074	2166	774	35.73	1.12 (1.02–1.24)	0.0209
Trend test				p = 0.2077					p = 0.1265	

[a] Adjusted for age (continuous), sex, drinking habit, residence in remote areas, cancer subsite, cancer clinical stage, cancer grade, and CCI group.

4. Discussion

Through the combined analysis of data from nationwide health insurance and cancer registries, we demonstrated that cigarette smoking was associated with a significantly increased risk of mortality in patients with CRC. The increased risk was more prominent in patients with higher levels of smoking intensity and duration. This pattern was especially present in men, patients with colon cancer, and patients older than 60. A dose–response effect on the risk of mortality was also observed with smoking duration in the whole population and with smoking amount in patients with colon cancer. Although the increase in the mortality risk was moderate in most of the analyzed categories, its significance merits further consideration to improve the prognosis of CRC.

Despite widespread skepticism towards an association between cigarette smoking and CRC, accumulating evidence has suggested an increased risk of incidence incurred with smoking [5]. In the Iowa Women's Health Study (IWHS), ever smokers had a moderately increased CRC risk (RR of approximately 1.20) compared with never smokers [11,27]. In the Cancer Prevention Study II Nutrition Cohort, the incidence of CRC was approximately 30% higher in current smokers than in never smokers [18]. Two meta-analyses demonstrated that the pooled RR increased from 15% to 20% in ever smokers compared with never smokers [1,16].

Furthermore, cigarette smoking was associated with an increased risk of mortality in patients with CRC. In the IWHS, ever smokers had an increased risk of overall mortality (RR = 1.31) compared with never smokers, which was similar to observations of CRC incidence [11]. In a previous meta-analysis, current smokers exhibited a significantly higher risk of CRC mortality (RR = 1.58) compared with nonsmokers [16]. In addition to all-cause mortality, disease-specific mortality was affected by current smoking [23,24]. Further evidence of this was presented in a meta-analysis that demonstrated that smokers had a 26% higher risk of all-cause mortality than never smokers did. Notably, 30-day mortality was reported to be higher by between 49% and 100% [4]. Compared with these previous studies, the mortality risk increased only moderately, though significantly, in smokers in our study. Factors such as components in cigarettes or differences in the study population might be implicated.

Our results indicated an increased risk of mortality in patients who smoked more than 10 cigarettes per day and who smoked for more than 10 years. This amount and the duration were much lower than previously reported. In the Chicago Heart Association cohort, a significant association between smoking and an increased CRC mortality was observed only in patients who smoked more than 20 cigarettes per day [19]. Smoking more than 15 cigarettes per day and having a 20-pack-year history were reported by Walter et al. to affect CRC survival [4]. In addition to differences in the characteristics of cigarettes and study populations, the lower threshold of smoking intensity for an increasing CRC mortality risk in our study may be attributable to the numerous events that may increase the detectability of differences in risks.

The mechanisms underlying the association between smoking and CRC mortality are multifold and incompletely understood. Cigarette smoke contains more than 60 carcinogens [7,17,29]. Of them, nicotine and 4-(methylnitrosamino)-1-(3-pyridyl)-1-butanone may enhance metastasis, which is the leading cause of death in patients with CRC, by enhancing cell migration and epithelial–mesenchymal transformation [6,30,31]. Nicotine may also interfere with the antiproliferative and proapoptotic effects of chemotherapeutic agents [4,32,33]. Tobacco smoking may cause a mutation of the GSTM1 gene, resulting in the impaired detoxification of tobacco carcinogens and enhancement of carcinogens' tumorigenic actions. Smoking may also induce aberrant promoter DNA methylation and silence regulatory genes in tumor progression. Consequent genetic alterations, such as a high microsatellite instability (MSI), the CpG island methylator phenotype, and the BRAF V600E mutation, may impair patient survival [13].

In previous studies, risk factors associated with an increased CRC mortality in smokers included an active smoking status, increased smoking amount or duration, and younger age at initiation [4,9,13,18]. The effects of smoking were also more significant in patients younger than 50 [19,24]. Notably, in our study, smoking patients younger than 60 had a lower risk of mortality. An exception to this was the increased risk in those who smoked for more than 30 years, indicating effects of prolonged smoking duration and younger age at initiation. By contrast, a generally significant association was noted between smoking and an increased risk of mortality in patients older than 60. This contradicted the observations by Colangelo et al. that the association between CRC and smoking mortality was significant only in those younger than 50 [19]. Whether this variance can be explained by other unanalyzed factors, such as genetic alterations, requires further elucidation.

For the effect of sex, Colangelo et al. reported that the risk for CRC mortality was higher for women than for men at the same level of smoking exposure, a phenomenon similar to that observed in patients with lung cancer [19]. However, other studies have reported discordant results. The association between smoking and the risk of CRC mortality was higher in men in a study conducted in Canada [13]; the association was even greater in patients older than 60. Walter et al. and Phipps et al. also reported a greater risk of recurrence or mortality in male smokers [4,24]. In our study, the increased risk in male smokers remained significant and relatively constant at most levels of smoking amount and duration. By contrast, the increases in risk in female smokers were mostly nonsignificant. Although our results may suggest a higher CRC mortality risk in male smokers, the disproportionately low number of female smokers when compared with that of male smokers may attenuate the association in females [4,9,11,18,19,21].

Tumor-related factors associated with an increased risks of recurrence or mortality in smokers include a T3 tumor, one to three affected lymph nodes, nonmetastatic diseases, a mutated KRAS status, and a wild-type BRAF status [4,24]. The effect of MSI remains under debate; some studies have suggested that the associations of smoking with all-cause CRC mortality were higher among patients with microsatellite-stable or MSI-low tumors, whereas others have reported a similar association with MSI-high tumors [4,13,24]. Data regarding genetic analyses of CRC specimens were not available in our database, which precludes the further exploration of the mechanisms underlying the association between cigarette smoking and an increased risk of CRC mortality.

Clinically, cigarette smoking is associated with later stages of CRC at diagnosis, which leads to a poorer prognosis and survival [34]. However, the increased risk persisted in our study despite matching for cancer stage. In addition to a proneoplastic effect, tobacco smoking constitutes a primary risk factor for cardiovascular and pulmonary diseases [32]. Therefore, smoking patients with CRC may incur additional risk or mortality from these causes. A prolonged induction period of more than 35 years is required for smoking to increase the risk of incident CRC [10,11,14,20]. The shorter duration of smoking associated with an increased CRC mortality risk in our study may support the involvement of smoking-induced comorbidities.

Studies have indicated that colon and rectal cancer may have partly different etiologic pathways and should be considered to be two separate entities that differ in susceptibility to carcinogens [11,17]. However, no consensus has been reached regarding whether the risk of incident colon or rectal cancer is more strongly associated with smoking [1,10–12,16–18,20,21,27,35–39]. Similarly, the association between smoking and CRC subsite mortality has been the topic of debate; several studies have reported that smoking was more significantly associated with a worse survival in patients with colon cancer than in those with rectal cancer [4,13,24]. However, others have reported a similar association between smoking and colon and rectal cancer mortality [9]. In our study, smoking was associated with an increased risk of mortality in patients with colon but not rectal cancers, which implies a higher susceptibility in patients with colon cancer. A significant dose–response relationship also supports the stronger association between smoking and colon cancer mortality.

The most pronounced advantage of our study was the sample size of the nationwide population-based cohort study. The number of events regarding the association between smoking and CRC mortality in our study was greater than those in previous studies [4,9,11,13,19]. We chose ever smoking as the main exposure risk because the effects of smoking may persist after changes in smoking behavior [4,39]. Studies have also reported a similar CRC risk for former and current smokers [15,21]. To obviate the influence of potential confounders, we performed propensity score matching to generate the study cohort. We further adjusted for factors, such as the alcohol consumption and body mass index, because they have been closely associated with both smoking and cancer risk [5,9,10]. The results from this and other studies demonstrate that the effects of smoking in CRC were much smaller than those in cancers of the respiratory and upper gastrointestinal tracts [16]. Nevertheless, quitting smoking for at least 20 years may still significantly reduce the risk of CRC incidence and adverse outcomes, suggesting smoking as a potentially modifiable risk factor of CRC prognosis [4,9,13,18].

It might seem peculiar that patients in the highest smoking amount category did not always have an increased risk of mortality in this study, including various subgroup analyses, as did patients in the highest smoking duration category. This might be attributable to the lower thresholds of smoking duration and amount required to increase the risk of CRC mortality in our study population. Furthermore, we speculate that the differential relationship between smoking intensity or smoking duration and CRC survival may also contribute to this phenomenon, that is, a threshold relationship for smoking intensity and a dose–response relationship for smoking duration. The relatively small number of patients in the highest smoking amount category in the whole cohort and in subgroups might also be accountable. Lastly, it might be postulated that the impact of the smoking duration on the risk of CRC mortality outweighs that of smoking intensity in our study population.

The limitation of this study stemmed largely from the use of administrative databases. The self-reported and retrospective collection of information on smoking and other variables was prone to recall and reporting biases. Data regarding family history of CRC, dietary information, physical activity, CRC screening, and use of cyclooxygenase inhibitors were not comprehensively recorded. Most importantly, other measures of smoking behavior, such as age at initiation, cumulative cigarette pack years, and passive smoking, were not collected. These factors may compromise the accuracy of the analysis. Furthermore, although we performed propensity score matching and adjusted for multiple covariates associated with smoking and CRC prognosis, the possibility of residual confounding cannot be excluded. The misclassification of anatomical subsites of CRC may have occurred, especially for tumors located in the junction of the sigmoid colon and the rectum. Finally, data regarding the molecular derangements of cancer were not available. These factors preclude a further detailed analysis of the differential effects of smoking on subsite CRC mortality.

5. Conclusions

Our study demonstrated that cigarette smoking was associated with a significantly, though moderately, increased risk of mortality in Asian patients with CRC. The smoking status can plausibly be considered in the risk stratification of CRC, and smoking cessation can be incorporated into comprehensive treatment planning for patients with CRC.

Author Contributions: Conceptualization, Y.-M.H., P.-L.W., C.-H.H. and C.-C.Y.; Methodology, C.-H.H. and C.-C.Y.; Validation, Y.-M.H., P.-L.W. and C.-C.Y.; Formal Analysis, C.-H.H.; Writing—Original Draft Preparation, Y.-M.H., P.-L.W., C.-H.H. and C.-C.Y.; Writing—Review and Editing, Y.-M.H., P.-L.W., C.-H.H. and C.-C.Y.; Supervision, P.-L.W.; Project Administration, P.-L.W. and C.-C.Y.; Funding Acquisition, P.-L.W., C.-H.H. and C.-C.Y. All authors have read and agreed to the published version of the manuscript.

Funding: This research was funded by the Health and Welfare Surcharge of Tobacco Products, grant numbers MOHW107-TDU-B-212-114020, MOHW108-TDU-B-212-124020, MOHW109-TDU-B-212-134020, and MOHW110-TDU-B-212-144020.

Institutional Review Board Statement: This study was conducted in accordance with the guidelines of the Declaration of Helsinki and was approved by the Research Ethics Committee of Chi Mei Hospital (IRB no. 10702-E04).

Informed Consent Statement: Requirement for patient informed consent was waived by the Research Ethics Committee of Chi Mei Hospital.

Data Availability Statement: The data sources were the Taiwan Nation Health Insurance Database and Taiwan Cancer Registry. The data are available with permission from the Taiwan Health and Welfare Data Science Center (https://dep.mohw.gov.tw/DOS/np-2497-113.html, accessed on 16 November 2021). Restrictions apply to the availability of these data, which were used under license for this study.

Acknowledgments: We are grateful to the Health Data Science Center of National Cheng Kung University Hospital for providing administrative and technical support. The authors also thank Yu-Cih Wu and Yi-Chen Chen for their assistance in advancing this project.

Conflicts of Interest: The authors declare no conflict of interest.

References

1. Botteri, E.; Borroni, E.; Sloan, E.K.; Bagnardi, V.; Bosetti, C.; Peveri, G.; Santucci, C.; Specchia, C.; van den Brandt, P.; Gallus, S.; et al. Smoking and Colorectal Cancer Risk, Overall and by Molecular Subtypes: A Meta-Analysis. *Am. J. Gastroenterol.* **2020**, *115*, 1940–1949. [CrossRef] [PubMed]
2. Siegel, R.L.; Miller, K.D.; Jemal, A. Cancer statistics, 2020. *CA Cancer J. Clin.* **2020**, *70*, 7–30. [CrossRef]
3. Sung, H.; Ferlay, J.; Siegel, R.L.; Laversanne, M.; Soerjomataram, I.; Jemal, A.; Bray, F. Global Cancer Statistics 2020: GLOBOCAN Estimates of Incidence and Mortality Worldwide for 36 Cancers in 185 Countries. *CA Cancer J. Clin.* **2021**, *71*, 209–249. [CrossRef] [PubMed]
4. Walter, V.; Jansen, L.; Hoffmeister, M.; Ulrich, A.; Chang-Claude, J.; Brenner, H. Smoking and survival of colorectal cancer patients: Population-based study from Germany. *Int. J. Cancer* **2015**, *137*, 1433–1445. [CrossRef] [PubMed]
5. Wakai, K.; Hayakawa, N.; Kojima, M.; Tamakoshi, K.; Watanabe, Y.; Suzuki, K.; Hashimoto, S.; Tokudome, S.; Toyoshima, H.; Ito, Y.; et al. Smoking and colorectal cancer in a non-Western population: A prospective cohort study in Japan. *J. Epidemiol.* **2003**, *13*, 323–332.e1-5. [CrossRef]
6. Wei, P.L.; Kuo, L.J.; Huang, M.T.; Ting, W.C.; Ho, Y.S.; Wang, W.; An, J.; Chang, Y.J. Nicotine enhances colon cancer cell migration by induction of fibronectin. *Ann. Surg. Oncol.* **2011**, *18*, 1782–1790. [CrossRef] [PubMed]
7. Wong, H.P.; Yu, L.; Lam, E.K.; Tai, E.K.; Wu, W.K.; Cho, C.H. Nicotine promotes cell proliferation via alpha7-nicotinic acetylcholine receptor and catecholamine-synthesizing enzymes-mediated pathway in human colon adenocarcinoma HT-29 cells. *Toxicol. Appl. Pharmacol.* **2007**, *221*, 261–267. [CrossRef]
8. NIH State-of-the-Science Conference Statement on Tobacco Use: Prevention, Cessation, and Control. *NIH Consens. State Sci. Statements* **2006**, *23*, 1–26.
9. Chao, A.; Thun, M.J.; Jacobs, E.J.; Henley, S.J.; Rodriguez, C.; Calle, E.E. Cigarette smoking and colorectal cancer mortality in the cancer prevention study II. *J. Natl. Cancer Inst.* **2000**, *92*, 1888–1896. [CrossRef]
10. Giovannucci, E.; Colditz, G.A.; Stampfer, M.J.; Hunter, D.; Rosner, B.A.; Willett, W.C.; Speizer, F.E. A prospective study of cigarette smoking and risk of colorectal adenoma and colorectal cancer in U.S. women. *J. Natl. Cancer Inst.* **1994**, *86*, 192–199. [CrossRef]

11. Limburg, P.J.; Vierkant, R.A.; Cerhan, J.R.; Yang, P.; Lazovich, D.; Potter, J.D.; Sellers, T.A. Cigarette smoking and colorectal cancer: Long-term, subsite-specific risks in a cohort study of postmenopausal women. *Clin. Gastroenterol. Hepatol.* **2003**, *1*, 202–210. [CrossRef]
12. Paskett, E.D.; Reeves, K.W.; Rohan, T.E.; Allison, M.A.; Williams, C.D.; Messina, C.R.; Whitlock, E.; Sato, A.; Hunt, J.R. Association between cigarette smoking and colorectal cancer in the Women's Health Initiative. *J. Natl. Cancer Inst.* **2007**, *99*, 1729–1735. [CrossRef] [PubMed]
13. Zhu, Y.; Yang, S.R.; Wang, P.P.; Savas, S.; Wish, T.; Zhao, J.; Green, R.; Woods, M.; Sun, Z.; Roebothan, B.; et al. Influence of pre-diagnostic cigarette smoking on colorectal cancer survival: Overall and by tumour molecular phenotype. *Br. J. Cancer* **2014**, *110*, 1359–1366. [CrossRef] [PubMed]
14. Giovannucci, E. An updated review of the epidemiological evidence that cigarette smoking increases risk of colorectal cancer. *Cancer Epidemiol. Biomark. Prev.* **2001**, *10*, 725–731.
15. Liang, P.S.; Chen, T.Y.; Giovannucci, E. Cigarette smoking and colorectal cancer incidence and mortality: Systematic review and meta-analysis. *Int. J. Cancer* **2009**, *124*, 2406–2415. [CrossRef]
16. Tsoi, K.K.; Pau, C.Y.; Wu, W.K.; Chan, F.K.; Griffiths, S.; Sung, J.J. Cigarette smoking and the risk of colorectal cancer: A meta-analysis of prospective cohort studies. *Clin. Gastroenterol. Hepatol.* **2009**, *7*, 682–688. [CrossRef]
17. Cheng, J.; Chen, Y.; Wang, X.; Wang, J.; Yan, Z.; Gong, G.; Li, G.; Li, C. Meta-analysis of prospective cohort studies of cigarette smoking and the incidence of colon and rectal cancers. *Eur. J. Cancer Prev.* **2015**, *24*, 6–15. [CrossRef]
18. Hannan, L.M.; Jacobs, E.J.; Thun, M.J. The association between cigarette smoking and risk of colorectal cancer in a large prospective cohort from the United States. *Cancer Epidemiol. Biomark. Prev.* **2009**, *18*, 3362–3367. [CrossRef]
19. Colangelo, L.A.; Gapstur, S.M.; Gann, P.H.; Dyer, A.R. Cigarette smoking and colorectal carcinoma mortality in a cohort with long-term follow-up. *Cancer* **2004**, *100*, 288–293. [CrossRef]
20. Parajuli, R.; Bjerkaas, E.; Tverdal, A.; Le Marchand, L.; Weiderpass, E.; Gram, I.T. Smoking increases rectal cancer risk to the same extent in women as in men: Results from a Norwegian cohort study. *BMC Cancer* **2014**, *14*, 321. [CrossRef]
21. Parajuli, R.; Bjerkaas, E.; Tverdal, A.; Selmer, R.; Le Marchand, L.; Weiderpass, E.; Gram, I.T. The increased risk of colon cancer due to cigarette smoking may be greater in women than men. *Cancer Epidemiol. Biomark. Prev.* **2013**, *22*, 862–871. [CrossRef]
22. Rex, D.K.; Johnson, D.A.; Anderson, J.C.; Schoenfeld, P.S.; Burke, C.A.; Inadomi, J.M. American College of Gastroenterology guidelines for colorectal cancer screening 2009 [corrected]. *Am. J. Gastroenterol.* **2009**, *104*, 739–750. [CrossRef] [PubMed]
23. Munro, A.J.; Bentley, A.H.; Ackland, C.; Boyle, P.J. Smoking compromises cause-specific survival in patients with operable colorectal cancer. *Clin. Oncol.* **2006**, *18*, 436–440. [CrossRef]
24. Phipps, A.I.; Baron, J.; Newcomb, P.A. Prediagnostic smoking history, alcohol consumption, and colorectal cancer survival: The Seattle Colon Cancer Family Registry. *Cancer* **2011**, *117*, 4948–4957. [CrossRef]
25. Park, S.M.; Lim, M.K.; Shin, S.A.; Yun, Y.H. Impact of prediagnosis smoking, alcohol, obesity, and insulin resistance on survival in male cancer patients: National Health Insurance Corporation Study. *J. Clin. Oncol.* **2006**, *24*, 5017–5024. [CrossRef]
26. Yu, G.P.; Ostroff, J.S.; Zhang, Z.F.; Tang, J.; Schantz, S.P. Smoking history and cancer patient survival: A hospital cancer registry study. *Cancer Detect. Prev.* **1997**, *21*, 497–509. [PubMed]
27. Limsui, D.; Vierkant, R.A.; Tillmans, L.S.; Wang, A.H.; Weisenberger, D.J.; Laird, P.W.; Lynch, C.F.; Anderson, K.E.; French, A.J.; Haile, R.W.; et al. Cigarette smoking and colorectal cancer risk by molecularly defined subtypes. *J. Natl. Cancer Inst.* **2010**, *102*, 1012–1022. [CrossRef]
28. Walter, V.; Jansen, L.; Hoffmeister, M.; Brenner, H. Smoking and survival of colorectal cancer patients: Systematic review and meta-analysis. *Ann. Oncol.* **2014**, *25*, 1517–1525. [CrossRef] [PubMed]
29. Hoffmann, D.; Hoffmann, I. The changing cigarette, 1950–1995. *J. Toxicol. Environ. Health* **1997**, *50*, 307–364. [CrossRef]
30. Hajiasgharzadeh, K.; Somi, M.H.; Sadigh-Eteghad, S.; Mokhtarzadeh, A.; Shanehbandi, D.; Mansoori, B.; Mohammadi, A.; Doustvandi, M.A.; Baradaran, B. The dual role of alpha7 nicotinic acetylcholine receptor in inflammation-associated gastrointestinal cancers. *Heliyon* **2020**, *6*, e03611. [CrossRef]
31. Wei, P.L.; Chang, Y.J.; Ho, Y.S.; Lee, C.H.; Yang, Y.Y.; An, J.; Lin, S.Y. Tobacco-specific carcinogen enhances colon cancer cell migration through alpha7-nicotinic acetylcholine receptor. *Ann. Surg.* **2009**, *249*, 978–985. [CrossRef] [PubMed]
32. Cucina, A.; Dinicola, S.; Coluccia, P.; Proietti, S.; D'Anselmi, F.; Pasqualato, A.; Bizzarri, M. Nicotine stimulates proliferation and inhibits apoptosis in colon cancer cell lines through activation of survival pathways. *J. Surg. Res.* **2012**, *178*, 233–241. [CrossRef] [PubMed]
33. Dinicola, S.; Morini, V.; Coluccia, P.; Proietti, S.; D'Anselmi, F.; Pasqualato, A.; Masiello, M.G.; Palombo, A.; De Toma, G.; Bizzarri, M.; et al. Nicotine increases survival in human colon cancer cells treated with chemotherapeutic drugs. *Toxicol. In Vitro* **2013**, *27*, 2256–2263. [CrossRef]
34. Longnecker, M.P.; Clapp, R.W.; Sheahan, K. Associations between smoking status and stage of colorectal cancer at diagnosis in Massachusetts between 1982 and 1987. *Cancer* **1989**, *64*, 1372–1374. [CrossRef]
35. Ho, J.W.; Lam, T.H.; Tse, C.W.; Chiu, L.K.; Lam, H.S.; Leung, P.F.; Ng, K.C.; Ho, S.Y.; Woo, J.; Leung, S.S.; et al. Smoking, drinking and colorectal cancer in Hong Kong Chinese: A case-control study. *Int. J. Cancer* **2004**, *109*, 587–597. [CrossRef]
36. Shimizu, N.; Nagata, C.; Shimizu, H.; Kametani, M.; Takeyama, N.; Ohnuma, T.; Matsushita, S. Height, weight, and alcohol consumption in relation to the risk of colorectal cancer in Japan: A prospective study. *Br. J. Cancer* **2003**, *88*, 1038–1043. [CrossRef]

37. Slattery, M.L.; Curtin, K.; Anderson, K.; Ma, K.N.; Ballard, L.; Edwards, S.; Schaffer, D.; Potter, J.; Leppert, M.; Samowitz, W.S. Associations between cigarette smoking, lifestyle factors, and microsatellite instability in colon tumors. *J. Natl. Cancer Inst.* **2000**, *92*, 1831–1836. [CrossRef] [PubMed]
38. Dénes, M.I.; Borz, C.; Török, Á.; Kántor, T.; Nădășan, V.; Csibi, M.; Ábrám, Z. The Role of Smoking in the Development of Colorectal Cancer. *Acta Marisiensis-Ser. Med.* **2016**, *62*, 400–402. [CrossRef]
39. Tsong, W.H.; Koh, W.P.; Yuan, J.M.; Wang, R.; Sun, C.L.; Yu, M.C. Cigarettes and alcohol in relation to colorectal cancer: The Singapore Chinese Health Study. *Br. J. Cancer* **2007**, *96*, 821–827. [CrossRef]

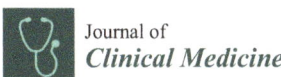

Article

Clinical Differences in c-Myc Expression in Early-Stage Gastric Neoplasia: A Retrospective Study Based on the WHO Classification

Noriyuki Arakawa [1,*], Atsushi Irisawa [2], Kazuyuki Ishida [3], Takuya Tsunoda [1], Yoshiko Yamaguchi [4], Goro Shibukawa [5], Makoto Eizuka [6], Shunzo Tokioka [1] and Hiroto Wakabayashi [1]

[1] Department of Gastroenterology, Takeda General Hospital, Aizuwakamatsu 965-8585, Japan; tsunotaku@takeda.or.jp (T.T.); shunzo.tokioka.1103@gmail.com (S.T.); wakaba@takeda.or.jp (H.W.)
[2] Department of Gastroenterology, Dokkyo Medical University School of Medicine, Mibu 321-0293, Japan; irisawa@dokkyomed.ac.jp
[3] Department of Pathology, Dokkyo Medical University School of Medicine, Mibu 321-0293, Japan; ishida-k@dokkyomed.ac.jp
[4] Department of Pathology, Takeda General Hospital, Aizuwakamatsu 965-8585, Japan; yyamaguchi@takeda.or.jp
[5] Department of Gastroenterology, Aizu Medical Center, Fukushima Medical University, Aizuwakamatsu 969-3492, Japan; goro4649@aol.com
[6] Department of Molecular Diagnostic Pathology, Iwate Medical University School of Medicine, Iwate 028-3694, Japan; m10_makoeizuka@yahoo.co.jp
* Correspondence: imu_nori0111@yahoo.co.jp; Tel.: +81-242-27-5511

Abstract: c-Myc is an oncogene that is dysregulated in various cancers. Early gastric neoplasia with c-Myc expression has been reported as a more malignant lesion. This study clarifies the differences in c-Myc expression in early gastric neoplasia based on the WHO classification. Samples from 100 patients with differentiated-type early gastric neoplasia, who underwent endoscopic submucosal dissection between March 2020 and January 2021, were stained for c-Myc. One hundred lesions were classified as low-grade dysplasia, high-grade dysplasia, or intramucosal adenocarcinoma. The staining intensity and extent were scored. A hierarchical cluster analysis for a clinicopathological analysis among the groups, the chi-square test, Bonferroni correction, and residual analysis were performed. Subgroup one and two consisted of 39 patients; while subgroup three consisted of 22. Significant differences among various characteristics were observed between these subgroups. The frequency of low-grade dysplasia was significantly higher, while that of high-grade dysplasia was significantly lower in subgroup three. The frequency of intramucosal adenocarcinoma was significantly higher in subgroup one. The c-Myc positivity rate was significantly higher in subgroup one compared with that in subgroup three. c-Myc expression distinctly differed in early gastric neoplasia. c-Myc-negative low-grade dysplasia may be separately categorized from c-Myc-positive low-grade dysplasia, high-grade dysplasia, and intramucosal adenocarcinoma.

Keywords: gastric cancer; c-Myc; genetic linkage analysis

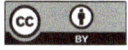

1. Introduction

The use of a genetic analysis to clarify the molecular pathogenesis of gastric cancer has greatly increased in recent years [1]. In Europe and the United States, gastric cancer is diagnosed based on the WHO classification. The intramucosal invasive neoplasia is treated by a mucosectomy or gastrectomy due to the metastatic potential of lesions invading the lamina propria [2]. In Japan, not only an intramucosal adenocarcinoma (IMA), but also low-grade dysplasia (LGD) and high-grade dysplasia (HGD) are targeted for resection. By analyzing the copy number alterations (CNAs) of early-stage gastric cancer, the authors identify several genes that may be related to the early stages of cancer. Among them, a gain in c-Myc (8q24.21) is a genetic abnormality that occurs in the early stage of the disease and may be a driver gene [3]. The CNA analysis of 84 cases of gastric intramucosal epithelial tumors showed that the frequency of 8q gain was increased in HGD and IMA rather than in LGD [4]. It is suggested that the amplification level of c-Myc differs depending on the nuclear and structural atypia. In addition, the gain of a gene has been reported to correlate with an increased protein expression [5].

c-Myc, an oncogene that is dysregulated in various cancers, is involved in carcinogenesis and cancer progression. This gene has also been associated with a variety of biological phenomena, including the promotion of disordered cell growth, neoangiogenesis, metastasis, anaerobic metabolism, and genomic instability [6].

Considering the results of the genetic analysis reported previously, lesions with c-Myc expression in early gastric neoplasia are likely malignant. However, there have been no reports discussing c-Myc expression with a focus on the WHO classification. This study was conducted to clarify the differences in c-Myc expression in early gastric neoplasia based on the WHO classification.

2. Materials and Methods

2.1. Study Design

This was a retrospective study conducted in a single center and approved by the Clinical Research Ethics Committee of Takeda General Hospital and registered with the University Hospital Medical Information Network (registration number UMIN000044040). Written informed consent was obtained from each patient included in the study, which was performed in accordance with the Declaration of Helsinki. The primary endpoint of the study was hierarchical cluster analysis based on the scores obtained by c-Myc staining to clarify the characteristics of each group. The secondary endpoints of the study were the c-Myc expression rates in early gastric neoplasia based on the WHO classification.

2.1.1. Patients

We evaluated 107 patients who underwent endoscopic submucosal dissection at the Department of Gastroenterology, Takeda General Hospital, between March 2020 and January 2021, and were diagnosed with differentiated-type early gastric neoplasia based on histopathological examination. A total of 100 cases was included, excluding mixed tissue types (cases in which a component of the secondary tissue type accounted for more than 10% of the total, or cases in which the component of the secondary tissue type was small but included poorly differentiated cancer).

2.1.2. Immunohistochemistry

Lesions removed by endoscopic submucosal dissection were fixed in 10% buffered formalin, and the specimens were prepared by total segmentation. The pathological diagnosis was determined following hematoxylin and eosin staining according to the gastric cancer treatment protocol, and the WHO classification was determined [2,7]. One hundred lesions were classified as LGD (Figure 1), HGD (Figure 2), or IMA (Figure 3) using the WHO classification criteria. The WHO classification for intramucosal lesions was used for cases of submucosal invasive cancer. Immunostaining was performed on representative sections following speculum examination. Immunostaining was performed using an automated immunostainer (Histostainer, Nichirei, Tokyo, Japan) and the anti-c-Myc antibody (clone EP121, Nichirei). Staining was evaluated by scoring the intensity and extent of staining (as described below) [8,9]. c-Myc expression was evaluated for nuclear rather than cytoplasmic staining. The staining intensity was classified as negative (0 points), weak (1 point), moderate (2 points), or strong (3 points). The staining field was defined as follows: less than 10% (0 points), 11–25% (1 point), 26–50% (2 points), and >50% (3 points). The obtained values were multiplied and scores of >4 points were considered as positive, whereas scores of <4 points were considered as negative. The stained area was measured using the ImageJ software (v.1.52a, National Institutes of Health, Bethesda, MD, USA) [10]. An example of the stain interpretation is shown in Figure 4.

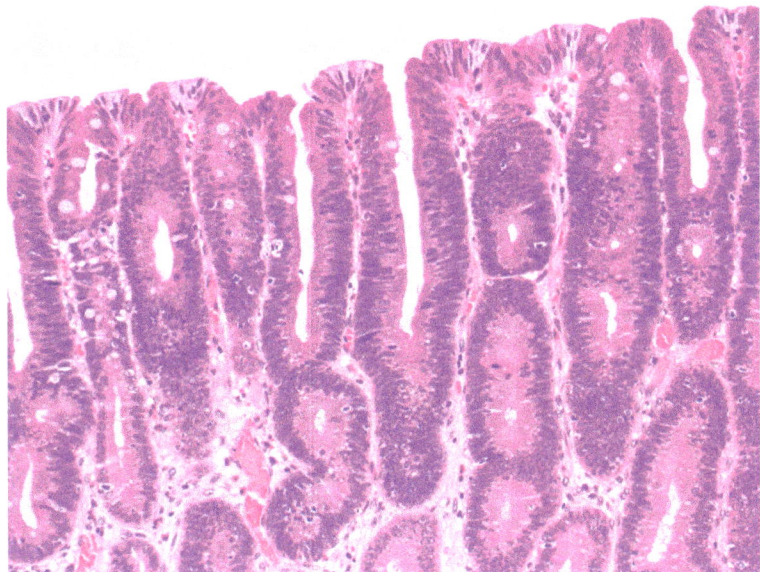

Figure 1. Low-grade dysplasia. Glands are slightly crowed with a regular shape and size. The nuclei are cigar shaped and basally oriented.

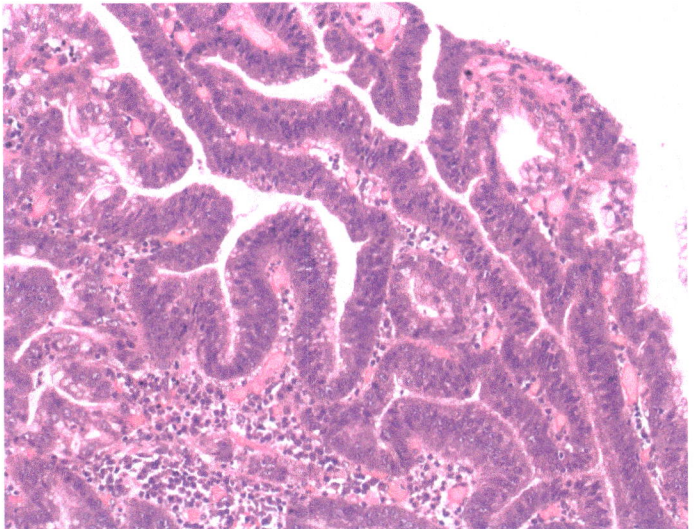

Figure 2. High-grade dysplasia. Glands have a variable size and shape. The nuclei are irregular in shape and size.

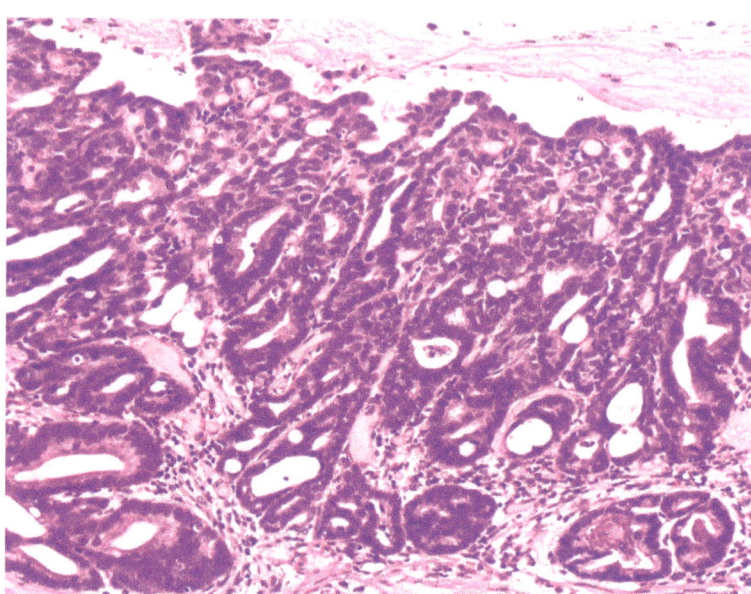

Figure 3. Intramucosal adenocarcinoma. Glands have a complex architecture with irregular branching and glandular anastomosis. Invasion into the lamina propria with no evident desmoplastic reaction.

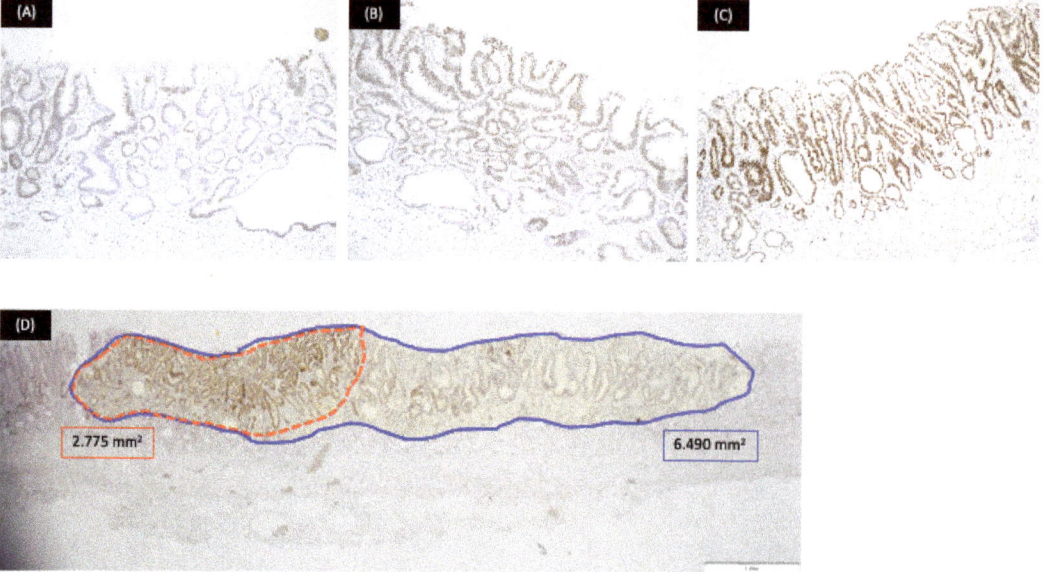

Figure 4. Example of stain interpretation. (**A**): Staining intensity: 1 point (c-Myc; ×40); (**B**): staining intensity: 2 points (c-Myc; ×40); (**C**): staining intensity: 3 points (c-Myc; ×40); (**D**): stained area was measured using the ImageJ software. Red and blue frames show c-Myc positive and gastric neoplasia areas, respectively.

2.1.3. Statistical Analysis

Hierarchical cluster analysis was performed using the obtained data [11]. The chi-square test, Bonferroni correction, and residual analysis were used for the statistical analyses

3. Results

3.1. Clinical Pathological Evaluation

The clinicopathological results of the 100 cases of early gastric neoplasia evaluated based on the WHO classification are shown in Table 1. In terms of the invasion depth, the frequency of T1a was higher in LGD (100%) and that of T1b was higher in IMA (25%) ($p < 0.01$) among the groups. In terms of the gross morphology, the elevated type was more frequent in LGD (70.8%), the mixed type was more frequent in HGD (11.1%), and the depressed type was more frequent in IMA (87.5%) ($p < 0.01$). The c-Myc positivity rate was higher in HGD (94.4%) and IMA (100%) compared with that in LGD (41.7%) ($p < 0.01$).

Table 1. Clinicopathological findings of early gastric neoplasia patients.

	LGD	HGD	IMA	p Value
Total	48	36	16	
Age (range)	78 (57–87)	79.5 (62–94)	78.5 (64–92)	N.S
Sex (Man/Woman)	30/18	22/14	12/4	N.S
Locus				
Upper	13	10	4	N.S
Middle	22	8	6	N.S
Lower	13	18	6	N.S
Depth (%)				
T1a	48 (100)	32 (88.9)	12 (75)	<0.01, N.S, <0.01
T1b	0 (0)	4 (11.1)	4 (25)	<0.01, N.S, <0.01
Macroscopy (%)				
elevated	34 (70.8)	18 (50)	2 (12.5)	<0.01, N.S, <0.01
depressed	14 (29.2)	14 (38.9)	14 (87.5)	<0.05, N.S, <0.01
Mixed	0 (0)	4 (11.1)	0 (0)	<0.05, <0.01, N.S
c-Myc expression (%)				
positive	20 (41.7)	34 (94.4)	16 (100)	<0.01, <0.01, <0.01
negative	28 (58.3)	2 (5.6)	0 (0)	<0.01, <0.01, <0.01

Low-grade dysplasia; LGD, high-grade dysplasia; HGD, intramucosal adenocarcinoma; IMA, not significant; N.S.

3.2. Hierarchical Cluster Analysis

A hierarchical cluster analysis was performed based on the staining intensity, staining range, and score (Figure 5). Subgroups one, two, and three consisted of 39, 39, and 22 patients, respectively. Clinicopathological analyses were performed among the subgroups (Table 2).

Table 2. Clinicopathological findings based on Hierarchical cluster analysis.

	Subgroup1	Subgroup2	Subgroup3	p Value
Total	39	39	22	
Age (range)	78 (63–93)	78 (57–94)	78 (68–88)	N.S
Sex (Man/Woman)	29/10	23/16	12/10	N.S
Locus (%)				
Upper	16 (41)	10 (25.6)	2 (9.1)	<0.05, N.S, <0.05
Middle	8 (20.5)	16 (41.0)	12 (54.5)	<0.01, N.S, <0.01
Lower	15 (38.5)	13 (33.3)	8 (36.4)	N.S, N.S, N.S
Depth (%)				
T1a	33 (84.6)	37 (94.9)	22 (100)	<0.05, N.S, N.S
T1b	6 (15.4)	2 (5.1)	0 (0)	<0.05, N.S, N.S

Table 2. Cont.

	Subgroup1	Subgroup2	Subgroup3	p Value
Macroscopy (%)				
elevated	14 (35.9)	22 (56.4)	18 (81.8)	<0.01, N.S, <0.01
depressed	22 (56.4)	16 (41.0)	4 (18.2)	<0.05, N.S, <0.05
Mixed	3 (7.7)	1 (2.6)	0 (0)	N.S, N.S, N.S
WHO (%)				
IMA	14 (35.9)	2 (5.1)	0 (0)	<0.01, <0.05, <0.05
HGD	17 (43.6)	17 (43.6)	2 (9.1)	N.S, N.S, <0.01
LGD	8 (20.5)	20 (51.3)	20 (90.9)	<0.01, N.S, <0.01
c-Myc expression (%)				
positive	39 (100)	31 (79.5)	0 (0)	<0.01, N.S, <0.01
negative	0 (0)	8 (20.5)	22 (100)	<0.01, N.S, <0.01

Low-grade dysplasia; LGD, high-grade dysplasia; HGD, intramucosal adenocarcinoma; IMA, not significant; N.S.

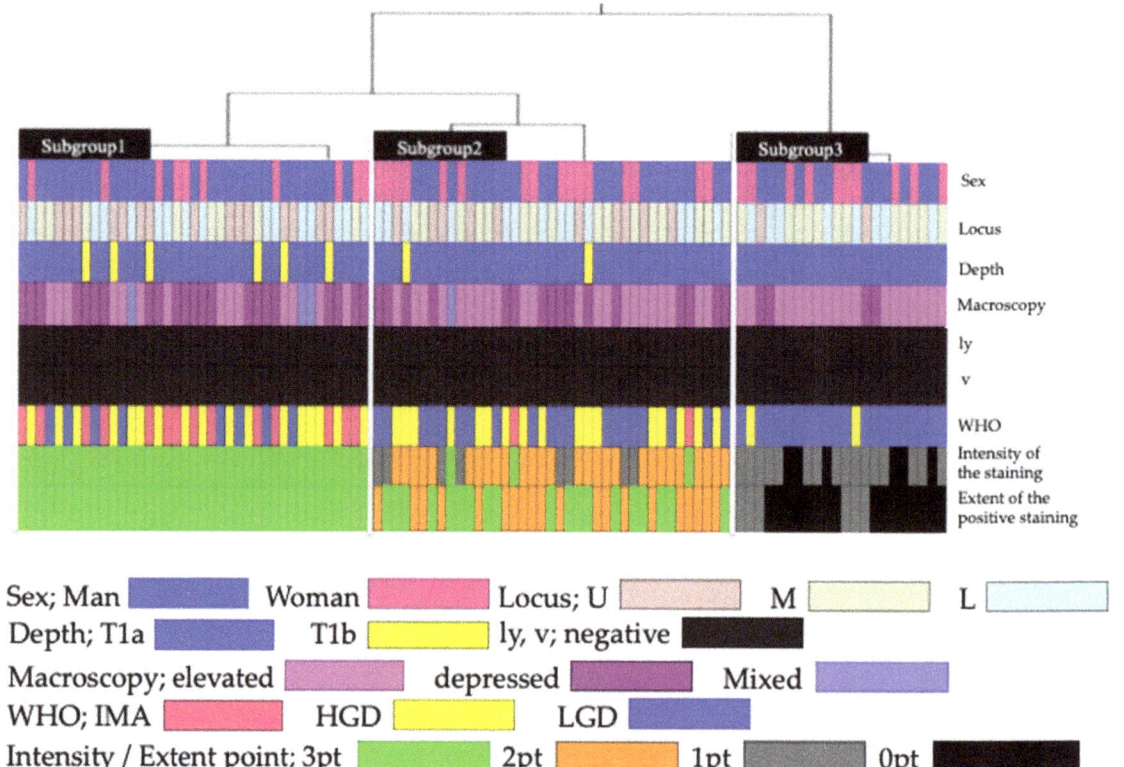

Figure 5. Hierarchical cluster analysis based on c-Myc expression. U: upper; M: middle; L: lower; ly: lymphatic invasion; v: venous invasion; LGD: low-grade dysplasia; HGD: high-grade dysplasia; IMA: intramucosal adenocarcinoma.

An origin in the upper part of the body was significantly more frequent in subgroup one (41%) ($p < 0.05$), and the origin was proximal to the midline of the body significantly more frequently in subgroup three (54.5%) ($p < 0.01$). In terms of the invasion depth, the frequency of T1b was significantly higher in subgroup one (15.4%) ($p < 0.05$). In terms of the gross morphology, the elevated type was significantly more frequent in subgroup three (81.8%) ($p < 0.01$), and the depressed type was significantly more frequent in subgroup one (56.4%) ($p < 0.05$).

The frequency of LGD was significantly higher in subgroup three (90.9%) than in subgroup one (20.5%) and subgroup two (51.3%) ($p < 0.01$). The frequency of IMA was significantly higher in subgroup one (35.9%) than in subgroup two (5.1%) and subgroup three (0%) ($p < 0.01$). The frequency of HGD was significantly lower in subgroup three (9.1%) than in subgroup one (43.6%) and subgroup two (43.6%).

The c-Myc positivity rate was significantly higher in subgroup one (100%) than in subgroup three (0%) ($p < 0.01$), while that in subgroup two (79.5%) did not differ significantly from that in the other groups.

4. Discussion

The molecular pathogenic mechanisms of cancer can be broadly classified into genomic and epigenomic abnormalities [12]. Genomic abnormalities include the loss of heterozygosity, mutations, and CNA. In recent years, many genes that may be key drivers of gastric cancer have been reported. In 2018, Nanki et al. [13] reported that most gastric cancers depend on the growth factor Wnt. Abnormal Wnt signaling induces the nuclear heteroaccumulation of β-catenin, which in turn induces abnormal cell proliferation via the overexpression of oncogenes, such as cyclin D1 and c-Myc. As a result of the CNA analysis of early gastric cancer, a gain of c-Myc was frequently observed, which may be closely related to abnormalities in Wnt signaling [3,4]. The current study was conducted to clarify the biological importance of c-Myc expression in early gastric neoplasia based on the WHO classification.

The cluster analysis was performed based on the c-Myc staining results. Each cluster showed independent clinicopathological features, which could be classified into three patterns in terms of c-Myc expression: subgroup one, characterized by a high c-Myc expression, high frequency of IMA, and depressed gross morphology; subgroup three, characterized by a low c-Myc expression, and most cases involving LGD and an elevated gross morphology; subgroup two, exhibiting intermediate characteristics between subgroups one and three, with no significant differences. Notably, the positive rate of c-Myc expression was 100% for IMA, 94.4% for HGD, and 41.7% for LGD. In early gastric neoplasia, c-Myc expression was correlated with nuclear and structural atypia. The incidence of immunostaining in early gastric cancer was reported as 18.1–100% [14–20]. However, these studies included both differentiated and poorly differentiated adenocarcinomas and were not evaluated using the WHO classification.

Nakayama et al. [21] reported highly interesting data on c-Myc expression. They used laser microdissection to extract DNA from intramucosal carcinoma, submucosal invasive carcinoma, and advanced carcinoma, and performed a CNA analysis by array comparative genomic hybridization. Myc loss and TP53 gain are defined as dormant patterns, whereas Myc gain and/or TP53 loss are defined as aggressive patterns. The results of the genealogical analysis suggested that differentiated adenocarcinomas with dormant patterns rarely develop into advanced cancer. In addition, some intramucosal carcinomas showed an aggressive pattern. This disease state may have undergone an epigenetic change (methylation) that was, subsequently, corrected. The c-Myc expression rate of LGD in this study was 41.7%. LGD with c-Myc expression is referred to as aggressive LGD, and LGD without c-Myc expression is referred to as dormant LGD. Aggressive LGD may readily progress to HGD and IMA.

In gastric cancer, c-Myc expression is an indicator of malignancy and poor prognosis [14], but is not necessarily high in patients with advanced gastric cancer. The level of the c-Myc messenger RNA expression has been reported as higher in early gastric cancer than in advanced gastric cancer [22]. c-Myc has been shown to further increase the expression level of genes with some level of expression and to alter the characteristics of cancer cells [23,24]. Therefore, the expression of c-Myc is thought to be a genetic abnormality in the early stages of carcinogenesis.

Presently, there are no reports, including basic research studies, on the potential of c-Myc as a therapeutic target in advanced gastric cancer. This is because c-Myc is a nuclear molecule and has no target-binding site for small molecules, making it unsuitable for drug design [25]. In contrast, BET inhibitors (JQ1, ARV-825), which indirectly inhibit c-Myc, have been reported in hematopoietic tumors [26,27]. Further studies are required to determine whether BET inhibitors can be used to treat solid tumors, including gastric cancer.

5. Conclusions

We observed a clear clinicopathological difference in c-Myc expression in early gastric neoplasia based on the WHO classification. These results suggested that the dormant LGD tumor group belongs to a different category than aggressive LGD, HGD, and IMA. The expression of c-Myc is thought to be a key element in the early stages of carcinogenesis. When biopsies are taken by upper endoscopy and proliferative LGD is diagnosed, c-Myc staining can be used as a supplementary tool to determine whether the tumor is aggressive. However, gastric cancer is considered to have a strong heterogeneity and should be carefully evaluated.

Author Contributions: N.A. and A.I. collected the data and wrote the paper. A.I., K.I., Y.Y., G.S., M.E., S.T. and H.W. provided clinical advice, Resources, T.T. and G.S. All authors have read and agreed to the published version of the manuscript.

Funding: This research received no external funding.

Institutional Review Board Statement: The study was conducted according to the guidelines of the Declaration of Helsinki and approved by the Clinical Research Ethics Committee of Takeda General Hospital and registered with the University Hospital Medical Information Network (registration number UMIN000044040).

Informed Consent Statement: Informed consent was obtained from all subjects involved in the study.

Data Availability Statement: The data that support the findings of this study are available from the corresponding author, N.A., upon reasonable request.

Acknowledgments: We thank members of the Department of Pathology, Takeda General Hospital, for their support.

Conflicts of Interest: The authors declare no conflict of interest.

References

1. Cancer Genome Atlas Research Network. Comprehensive Molecular Characterization of Gastric Adenocarcinoma. *Nature* **2014**, *513*, 202–209. [CrossRef]
2. The WHO Classification Tumours Editorial Board. *WHO Classification of Tumours: Digestive System Tumours*, 5th ed.; IARC Press: Lyon, France, 2019.
3. Arakawa, N.; Sugai, T.; Habano, W.; Eizuka, M.; Sugimoto, R.; Akasaka, R.; Toya, Y.; Yamamoto, E.; Koeda, K.; Sasaki, A.; et al. Genome-wide analysis of DNA copy number alterations in early and advanced gastric cancers. *Mol. Carcinog.* **2017**, *56*, 527–537. [CrossRef]
4. Sugai, T.; Eizuka, M.; Arakawa, N.; Osakabe, M.; Habano, W.; Fujita, Y.; Yamamoto, E.; Yamano, H.; Endoh, M.; Matsumoto, T.; et al. Molecular profiling and comprehensive genome-wide analysis of somatic copy number alterations in gastric intramucosal neoplasias based on microsatellite status. *Gastric Cancer* **2018**, *21*, 765–775. [CrossRef]
5. Dang, C.V. MYC on the Path to Cancer. *Cell* **2012**, *149*, 22–35. [CrossRef]
6. Eilers, M.; Eisenman, R.N. Myc's Broad Reach. *Genes Dev.* **2008**, *22*, 2755–2766. [CrossRef]
7. Japanese Gastric Cancer Association. *Japanese Classification of Gastric Carcinoma*, 15th ed.; Kanehara Shuppan: Tokyo, Japan, 2017. (In Japanese)
8. Chiurillo, M.A. Role of the Wnt/β-catenin pathway in gastric cancer: An in-depth literature review. *World J. Exp. Med.* **2015**, *5*, 84–102. [CrossRef]
9. Oliveira, L.A.; Oshima, C.T.F.; Soffner, P.A.; Silva, M.S.; Lins, R.R.; Malinverni, A.C.M.; Waisberg, J. The Canonical Wnt Pathway in Gastric Carcinoma. *Arq. Bras. Cir. Dig.* **2019**, *32*, e1414. [CrossRef]
10. Schneider, C.A.; Rasband, W.S.; Eliceiri, K.W. NIH Image to ImageJ: 25 Years of image analysis. *Nat. Methods* **2012**, *9*, 671–675. [CrossRef]
11. Kanda, Y. Investigation of the Freely Available Easy-to-Use Software 'EZR' for Medical Statistics. *Bone Marrow Transplant.* **2013**, *48*, 452–458. [CrossRef]
12. Lengauer, C.; Kinzler, K.W.; Vogelstein, B. Genetic instability in colorectal cancers. *Nature* **1997**, *386*, 623–627. [CrossRef]

13. Nanki, K.; Toshimitsu, K.; Takano, A.; Fujii, M.; Shimokawa, M.; Ohta, Y.; Matano, M.; Seino, T.; Nishikori, S.; Ishikawa, K.; et al. Divergent Routes toward Wnt and R-spondin Niche Independency during Human Gastric Carcinogenesis. *Cell* **2018**, *174*, 856–869.e17. [CrossRef]
14. Han, S.; Kim, H.Y.; Park, K.; Cho, H.J.; Lee, M.S.; Kim, H.J.; Kim, Y.D. c-Myc expression is related with cell proliferation and associated with poor clinical outcome in human gastric cancer. *J. Korean Med. Sci.* **1999**, *14*, 526–530. [CrossRef]
15. Sanz-Ortega, J.; Steinberg, S.M.; Moro, E.; Saez, M.; Lopez, J.A.; Sierra, E.; Sanz-Esponera, J.; Merino, M.J. Comparative study of tumor angiogenesis and immunohistochemistry for p53, c-ErbB2, c-myc and EGFr as prognostic factors in gastric cancer. *Histol. Histopathol.* **2000**, *15*, 455–462.
16. Xu, A.-G.; Li, S.-G.; Liu, J.-H.; Gan, A.-H. Function of apoptosis and expression of the proteins Bcl-2, p53 and C-myc in the development of gastric cancer. *World J. Gastroenterol.* **2001**, *7*, 403–406. [CrossRef] [PubMed]
17. Ishii, H.H.; Gobé, G.C.; Pan, W.; Yoneyama, J.; Ebihara, Y. Apoptosis and cell proliferation in the development of gastric carcinomas: Associations with c-myc and p53 protein expression. *J. Gastroenterol. Hepatol.* **2002**, *17*, 966–972. [CrossRef]
18. Raiol, L.C.C.; Silva, E.C.F.; da Fonseca, D.M.; Leal, M.F.; Guimarães, A.C.; Calcagno, D.Q.; Khayat, A.S.; Assumpção, P.P.; de Arruda Cardoso Smith, M.; Burbano, R.R. Interrelationship between MYC gene numerical aberrations and protein expression in individuals from northern Brazil with early gastric adenocarcinoma. *Cancer Genet. Cytogenet.* **2008**, *181*, 31–35. [CrossRef]
19. Calcagno, D.Q.; Freitas, V.M.; Leal, M.F.; De Souza, C.R.T.; Demachki, S.; Montenegro, R.C.; Assumpção, P.P.; Khayat, A.S.; de Smith, M.D.A.C.; dos Santos, A.K.C.R.; et al. MYC, FBXW7 and TP53 copy number variation and expression in Gastric Cancer. *BMC Gastroenterol.* **2013**, *13*, 141. [CrossRef]
20. Khaleghian, M.; Jahanzad, I.; Shakoori, A.; Razavi, A.E.; Azimi, C. Association between Amplification and Expression of C-MYC Gene and Clinicopathological Characteristics of Stomach Cancer. *Iran. Red Crescent Med. J.* **2016**, *18*, e21221. [CrossRef]
21. Nakayama, T.; Ling, Z.Q.; Mukaisho, K.; Hattori, T.; Sugihara, H. Lineage Analysis of Early and Advanced Tubular Adenocarcinomas of the Stomach: Continuous or Discontinuous? *BMC Cancer* **2010**, *10*, 311. [CrossRef]
22. Onoda, N.; Maeda, K.; Chung, Y.S.; Yano, Y.; Matsui-Yuasa, I.; Otani, S.; Sowa, M. Overexpression of c-myc messenger RNA in primary and metastatic lesions of carcinoma of the stomach. *J. Am. Coll. Surg.* **1996**, *182*, 55–59.
23. Lin, C.Y.; Lovén, J.; Rahl, P.B.; Paranal, R.M.; Burge, C.B.; Bradner, J.E.; Lee, T.I.; Young, R.A. Transcriptional Amplification in Tumor Cells with Elevated c-Myc. *Cell* **2012**, *151*, 56–67. [CrossRef]
24. Nie, Z.; Hu, G.; Wei, G.; Cui, K.; Yamane, A.; Resch, W.; Wang, R.; Green, D.R.; Tessarollo, L.; Casellas, R.; et al. c-Myc Is a Universal Amplifier of Expressed Genes in Lymphocytes and Embryonic Stem Cells. *Cell* **2012**, *151*, 68–79. [CrossRef] [PubMed]
25. Whitfield, J.; Beaulieu, M.-E.; Soucek, L. Strategies to Inhibit Myc and Their Clinical Applicability. *Front. Cell Dev. Biol.* **2017**, *5*, 10. [CrossRef] [PubMed]
26. Delmore, J.E.; Issa, G.C.; Lemieux, M.E.; Rahl, P.B.; Shi, J.; Jacobs, H.M.; Kastritis, E.; Gilpatrick, T.; Paranal, R.M.; Qi, J.; et al. BET Bromodomain Inhibition as a Therapeutic Strategy to Target c-Myc. *Cell* **2011**, *146*, 904–917. [CrossRef]
27. Lu, J.; Qian, Y.; Altieri, M.; Dong, H.; Wang, J.; Raina, K.; Hines, J.; Winkler, J.D.; Crew, A.P.; Coleman, K.; et al. Hijacking the E3 Ubiquitin Ligase Cereblon to Efficiently Target BRD4. *Chem. Biol.* **2015**, *22*, 755–763. [CrossRef]

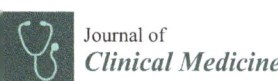

Article

Association of Regular Endoscopic Screening with Interval Gastric Cancer Incidence in the National Cancer Screening Program

Choong-Kyun Noh [1,†], Eunyoung Lee [2,3,4,†], Gil Ho Lee [1], Sun Gyo Lim [1], Bumhee Park [2,3,4], Sung Jae Shin [1], Jae Youn Cheong [1] and Kee Myung Lee [1,*]

[1] Department of Gastroenterology, Ajou University School of Medicine, Suwon 16499, Korea; cknoh23@gmail.com (C.-K.N.); micorie@hanmail.net (G.H.L.); mdlsk75@gmail.com (S.G.L.); shsj9128@ajou.ac.kr (S.J.S.); jaeyoun620@gmail.com (J.Y.C.)
[2] Department of Biomedical Informatics, Ajou University School of Medicine, Suwon 16499, Korea; eylee@aumc.ac.kr (E.L.); bhpark@ajou.ac.kr (B.P.)
[3] Office of Biostatistics, Ajou Research Institute for Innovative Medicine, Ajou University Medical Center, Suwon 16499, Korea
[4] Department of Medical Sciences, Biomedical Informatics, Graduate School of Ajou University, Suwon 16499, Korea
* Correspondence: lkm5104@ajou.ac.kr; Tel.: +82-31-219-5119; Fax: +82-31-219-5999
† These authors contributed equally to this work.

Abstract: Although regular endoscopic screening may help in early detection of gastric cancer, interval cancer remains a problem in the screening program. This study evaluated the association between regular endoscopic screening and interval cancer detection in the Korean National Cancer Screening Program (KNCSP). We defined three groups (regularly, irregularly, and not screened) according to the screening interval, and the trends in the interval cancer rate (ICR) between the groups were tested using the Cochran–Armitage test. The influence of regular endoscopic screening on the risk of interval cancer was evaluated using multivariable logistic regression. Among the 11,642,410 participants who underwent endoscopy, the overall ICR was 0.36 per 1000 negative screenings. The ICR of the not screened group (0.41) was the highest among the three groups and the risk of interval cancer in this group was 1.68 times higher ($p < 0.001$) than that in the regularly screened group. Women in their 40s who had regular screening with no history of intestinal metaplasia and gastric polyps would have the lowest probability of having interval cancer (0.005%). Regular participation in endoscopic screening programs for reducing the risk of interval cancer may help to improve the quality of screening programs.

Keywords: gastric cancer; interval cancer; screening; endoscopy; national cancer screening program

1. Introduction

Gastric cancer is considered as an important contributor to the global cancer burden, accounting for the fifth highest incidence among cancers and the third highest cause of cancer-related mortality [1]. In 2018, there were over 1,000,000 new patients diagnosed with gastric cancer and 783,000 deaths [1]. Particularly, the incidence of gastric cancer is high in Eastern Asia, including South Korea and Japan [1].

Generally, early gastric cancer involves small-sized lesions with no apparent symptoms. Once the disease progresses because of the late detection of the lesion, the mortality of cancer patients increases. Hence, it is crucial to detect gastric cancer in the early stage, followed by appropriate treatments, for which some Asian countries have operated screening programs for gastric cancer. Some studies have reported that a screening program reduced gastric cancer-related mortality [2–4]. However, the efficiency of the screening program is still controversial [5,6].

Screening programs need to detect cancer early and control screening quality. A significant factor to determine the quality of screening programs is to achieve a reduction in interval cancer [7]. Interval cancer refers to cancer that was negative in the screening test and was detected before the next screening surveillance examination [7]. While upper endoscopy is highly useful for the early detection of gastric cancer [8–10], interval cancer is an issue that needs to be solved in the screening program.

Unlike colonoscopy, which has predictors for interval cancer risk [7], there is no effective way for an upper endoscopy to reduce the incidence of interval cancer because it lacks clear quality indicators. Screening programs are composed of a survey on baseline information and examinations for detecting cancer. The survey questionnaire includes the examination history. We hypothesized that regular participation in a screening program, rather than irregular participation would reduce the incidence of interval cancer by providing endoscopists with accurate information, thus increasing the accuracy of the examination. Accordingly, this study aimed to evaluate risk factors of interval cancer in screening participants and to assess reductions in the number of interval gastric cancer cases with a two-year interval of regular endoscopic screening using the large cohort database from the Korean National Cancer Screening Program (KNCSP). Additionally, we report the incidence probability of interval cancer by the identified risk factors.

2. Methods

2.1. Study Population

This is a retrospective, large population-based cohort study using the KNCSP database. The total cohort was selected from the two most recent KNCSP cycles that we obtained: one cycle of 2013–2014 and the other cycle of 2015–2016. The data of the first cycle was used as the reference cohort for confirming the consecutive screening of participants. Based on this data and the answers to the questionnaire of history of endoscopy from the data of the second cycle, the cohort of the second cycle was divided into three groups: the regularly screened group (group 1) was defined as those who reported their last endoscopy within the past two years; the irregularly screened group (group 2) was defined as those who reported their last endoscopy within the past 2–10 years; and the not screened group (group 3) was defined as those who reported no endoscopy in the past ten years or no experience in their lifetime. Individuals who newly participated in the 2015–2016 cycle were also divided into three groups according to their endoscopy history with/without KNCSP invitation. Exclusion criteria for participants were as follows: (1) previously diagnosed gastric cancer; (2) upper gastrointestinal (UGI) series only; (3) disqualified from the KNCSP; (4) did not return for subsequent screening; (5) participants who received a gastric cancer diagnosis in the 2013–2014 cycle; and (6) participants who received negative results but were diagnosed with ulcer were confirmed subsequent gastric cancer diagnosis within eight weeks. The study protocol was approved by the Ajou University hospital's institutional review board (approval No. AJIRB-MED-MDB-19-109), which waived the requirement for individual informed consent owing to the use of a de-identified dataset.

2.2. The KNCSP and Data Collection

The specific KNCSP protocol is described in the Supplement method [11,12]. Participant data were extracted from the KNCSP database in 2015–2016. The KNCSP data included demographic characteristics, a brief history of endoscopy, and medical history using questionnaires; endoscopy, biopsy, and comprehensive cancer screening results; and screening sites and providers. We defined screening results as positive if endoscopic results were recorded as possible gastric cancer, early gastric cancer, or advanced gastric cancer, or if biopsy results were recorded as low-grade dysplasia, high-grade dysplasia, suspicious gastric cancer, or gastric cancer. We tracked and checked interval gastric cancer cases up to 31 December 2017 by linking individual medical records from the National Health Insurance Sharing Service-National Health Information Database (NHIS-NHID). We defined interval gastric cancer when participants received a diagnosis code for gastric cancer (International Classification of Diseases, 10th revision, C16.xx) within one year of endoscopy screening (negative screening results) [13,14]. Missed cancer is an important component of interval cancer that determines screening quality. Therefore, the observation period to detect interval cancer was defined as "within one year" of negative screening results. Interval cancer was found by additional examinations performed at different centers from the screening program for various reasons, including symptom development.

2.3. Statistical Analyses

Participants' demographics, medical history, and screening characteristics between the three groups were summarized and compared using the chi-squared test. The interval cancer rate (ICR) per 1000 negative screenings was computed as the number of interval cancer divided by the number of negative screenings and was presented with 95% confidence intervals (CIs). The trend in the ICR was tested with a one-sided Cochran–Armitage test. The multivariable logistic regression analysis was conducted for identifying risk factors associated with interval cancer. Additionally, a stepwise selection method was used for selecting the best subset of risk factors for predicting interval cancers among the risk factor candidates, including screening regularity (three groups), sex, age groups, and history of gastric diseases. The odds ratios (ORs) were provided with the corresponding 95% CIs. Based on the estimated parameter of multivariable logistic regression analysis, the probability of interval cancer was also predicted. All the reported p-values were two-sided, and p-values of <0.05 were considered statistically significant. Analyses were performed using SAS version 9.4 (SAS Institute Inc., Cary, NC, USA).

3. Results

3.1. Study Population and Baseline Characteristics

The total cohort comprised of 21,535,222 participants who underwent endoscopy in the screening program between 2013 and 2016 (mean [standard deviation] age, 55.61 [10.61] years; 11,761,709 [54.62%] women). Among them, 9,892,812 individuals (45.94%) participated in the first cycle of 2013–2014 and 11,642,410 (54.06%) in the second cycle of 2015–2016 (Figure 1). Participants were divided into three groups based on screening intervals and regularity. The regular screened group (n = 8,085,011, 69.44%) was the most prevalent, followed by the irregular screened group (n = 1,969,863, 16.92%) and the not screened group (n = 1,587,536, 13.64%). All three groups had differences in all the characteristics ($p < 0.001$ for all). There were more men and younger (40–49 years) participants in the not screened group than in other screened groups. Most notably, history of gastric diseases, including atrophic gastritis, intestinal metaplasia, ulcer, and gastric polyp, were more common in the regularly screened group than in other groups (Table 1). The overall gastric cancer detection rates of the 2013–2014 cycle and 2015–2016 cycle were 0.29 (per 100, 95% CI, 0.17–0.29) and 0.27 (per 100, 95% CI, 0.26–0.27), respectively (Supplementary Table S1).

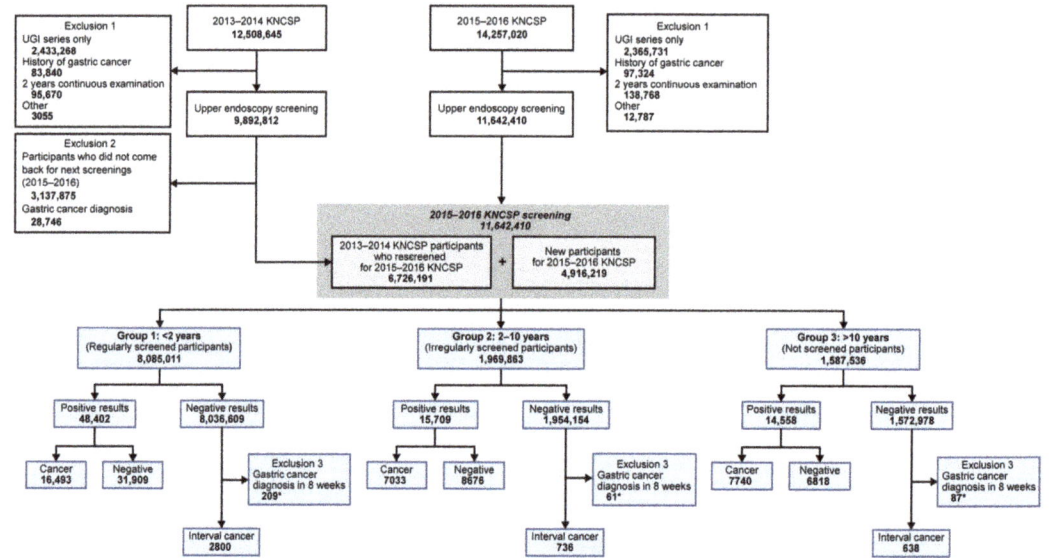

Figure 1. Flow diagram for selection of enrolled participants in this study. Among the participants from the first cycle (9,892,812, 2013–2014), 6,726,191 (67.99%) were re-screened in the next cycle of 2015–2016, and 3,137,875 (31.72%) did not return for screening. In the second cycle, 4,916,219 were newcomers who did not participate in the previous cycle. KNCSP, Korean National Cancer Screening Program. * Participants who received negative results but were diagnosed with ulcer were confirmed subsequent gastric cancer diagnosis within eight weeks.

Table 1. Sociodemographics of the screening participants and characteristics of screenings based on participation interval for screening endoscopy.

Characteristics	Group 1 (<2 Years) n = 8,085,011	Group 2 (2–10 Years) n = 1,969,863	Group 3 (>10 Years) n = 1,587,536	p Value [a]
Sex, No. (%)				<0.001
Male	3,629,799 (44.90)	888,042 (45.08)	816,937 (51.46)	
Female	4,455,212 (55.10)	1,081,821 (54.92)	770,599 (48.54)	
Age (year), No. (%)				<0.001
40–49	2,190,059 (27.09)	696,934 (35.38)	800,614 (50.43)	
50–59	2,635,522 (32.60)	640,236 (32.50)	442,263 (27.86)	
60–69	2,113,188 (26.14)	389,015 (19.75)	220,777 (13.91)	
70–79	1,002,090 (12.39)	198,231 (10.06)	98,010 (6.17)	
≥80	144,152 (1.78)	45,447 (2.31)	25,872 (1.63)	
Hospital type, No. (%)				<0.001
General hospital (≥100 beds)	2,444,925 (30.24)	529,594 (26.88)	495,716 (31.23)	
Hospital (30–99 beds)	1,459,087 (18.05)	392,878 (19.94)	333,562 (21.01)	
Clinics (<30 beds)	4,180,999 (51.71)	1,047,391 (53.17)	758,258 (47.76)	
Screening location, No. (%)				<0.001
Capital area [b]	3,955,485 (48.92)	936,039 (47.52)	828,406 (52.18)	
Non-capital area	4,129,526 (51.08)	1,033,824 (52.48)	759,130 (47.82)	

Table 1. Cont.

Characteristics	Group 1 (<2 Years) n = 8,085,011	Group 2 (2–10 Years) n = 1,969,863	Group 3 (>10 Years) n = 1,587,536	p Value [a]
History of gastric disease [c], No. (%)				
Atrophic gastritis	1,169,183 (14.46)	194,925 (9.90)	53,616 (3.38)	<0.001
Intestinal metaplasia [d]	77,059 (0.95)	5392 (0.27)	1686 (0.11)	<0.001
Ulcer	795,076 (9.83)	150,153 (7.62)	62,044 (3.91)	<0.001
Gastric polyp	227,829 (2.82)	33,069 (1.68)	7166 (0.45)	<0.001
Other	824,317 (10.20)	182,383 (9.26)	39,521 (2.49)	<0.001

[a] p Values were calculated by chi-squared test; [b] The capital area includes Seoul, Incheon, and Gyeonggi province; [c] The source of these variables was participants' self-reported questionnaires for the National Cancer Screening Program; [d] Intestinal metaplasia was accompanied by atrophic gastritis.

3.2. ICR and Their Risk Factors in the National Cancer Screening Program

In the cycle of 2015–2016, 4174 participants were diagnosed with gastric cancer within one year of negative screening. Overall, the ICR in this cycle was 0.36 per 1000 negative screenings (95% CI, 0.35–0.37). The ICR for the not screened group (0.41, 95% CI, 0.37–0.44) was the highest among the three groups, which was 1.17 times higher than those for the regularly screened group (0.35, 95% CI, 0.34–0.36). Based on the results of the Cochran–Armitage test for trend, there was an increasing trend in ICR between the three groups ($p < 0.001$) (Table 2).

Table 2. Overall interval cancer rates with 95% confidence intervals arranged group-wise.

Variable	Number	Negative Screening	Interval Cancer	ICR Per 1000 Negative Screenings (95% CI)	p Value [a]
Overall	11,642,410	11,563,741	4174	0.36 (0.35 to 0.37)	N/A
Group 1 (regular rescreened group, <2 years)	8,085,011	8,036,609	2800	0.35 (0.34 to 0.36)	
Group 2 (irregular screened group, 2–10 years)	1,969,863	1,954,154	736	0.38 (0.35 to 0.40)	<0.001
Group 3 (not screened group, >10 years)	1,587,536	1,572,978	638	0.41 (0.37 to 0.44)	

Abbreviations: ICR, interval cancer rates, CI, confidence intervals; [a] p Values were calculated using the Cochran–Armitage test for trend.

The multivariable logistic regression analysis was conducted to identify risk factors associated with interval cancer. The risk factors of screening regularly, sex, age groups, and the presence of intestinal metaplasia and gastric polyps were selected from the stepwise selection method, and they were all significant ($p < 0.001$ for all). The risk of having interval cancer in the not screened group was 1.68 times higher (95% CI, 1.54–1.84) than that in the regularly screened group. As the participants aged, the OR of interval cancer gradually increased from 2.63 (50–59 years; 95% CI, 2.31–2.99) to 14.09 (≥80 years; 95% CI, 11.93–16.65). Men (OR: 2.58; 95% CI, 2.40–2.77), the history of intestinal metaplasia (OR: 1.99; 95% CI, 1.48–2.69), and gastric polyp (OR: 2.44; 95% CI, 2.09–2.86) were significantly associated with interval cancer (Table 3).

Table 3. Multivariable logistic regression analysis of risk factors associated with interval cancer detection in the Korean National Cancer Screening Program for gastric cancer.

Variable	OR (95% CI)	p Value [a]
Group		<0.001
Group 1 (regular screened group, <2 years)	1	
Group 2 (irregular screened group, 2–10 years)	1.27 (1.16 to 1.38)	
Group 3 (not-screened group, >10 years)	1.68 (1.54 to 1.84)	
Sex		<0.001
Female	1	
Male	2.58 (2.40 to 2.77)	
Age group, years		<0.001
40–40	1	
50–59	2.63 (2.31 to 2.99)	
60–69	5.44 (4.81 to 6.15)	
70–79	9.93 (8.75 to 11.26)	
≥80	14.09 (11.93 to 16.65)	
History of intestinal metaplasia [b,c]		<0.001
Absent	1	
Presence	1.99 (1.48 to 2.69)	
History of Gastric polyp [b]		<0.001
Absent	1	
Presence	2.44 (2.09 to 2.86)	

Abbreviations: CI, confidence interval; OR, odds ratio; [a] p Values were calculated using the Wald chi-square test. The multivariable logistic model was selected using the stepwise selection method with group, sex, age group, gastric ulcer, atrophic gastritis, intestinal metaplasia, and gastric polyps. [b] The source of these variables was participants' self-reported questionnaires for the National Cancer Screening Program; [c] Intestinal metaplasia was accompanied by atrophic gastritis.

3.3. The Probability Model for Having Interval Gastric Cancer after Endoscopic Screening

We developed a probability model of interval gastric cancer after endoscopic screening based on the analyzed data. Based on the multivariable logistic regression results, the probability of having interval cancer was computed as:

$$\Pr(interval\ cancer) = \frac{\exp(A)}{1 + \exp(A)}$$

where

$$A = -9.991 + 0.236 x_{group2} + 0.520 x_{group3} + 0.947 x_{male}$$
$$+ 0.966 x_{age50s} + 1.693 x_{age60s} + 2.295 x_{age70s}$$
$$+ 2.646 x_{age80s} + 0.689 x_{intestinal\ metaplasia} + 0.894 x_{polyp}$$

$x_{group2} = 1$ for the irregularly screened group, otherwise 0
$x_{group3} = 1$ for the not screened group, otherwise 0
$x_{male} = 1$ for male, otherwise 0
$x_{age50s} = 1$ for 50–59 years age group, otherwise 0
$x_{age60s} = 1$ for 60–69 years age group, otherwise 0
$x_{age70s} = 1$ for 70–79 years age group, otherwise 0
$x_{age80s} = 1$ for ≥80 years age group, otherwise 0
$x_{intestinal\ metaplasia} = 1$ for the presence of intestinal metaplasia, otherwise 0
$x_{polyp} = 1$ for the presence of gastric polyps, otherwise 0.

Hence, participants who did not undergo endoscopy for cancer screening for >10 years were men in their 80s whom had both intestinal metaplasia and gastric polyps; these participants would have the highest probability of having interval cancer (1.350%). Meanwhile, those who had regular cancer screenings were women in their 40s who did not have intestinal metaplasia and gastric polyps; these participants would have the lowest probability (0.005%). Parameter estimates and its 95% CIs from the multivariable logistic regression are presented in Table 4.

Table 4. Parameter estimates and 95% confidence intervals from multivariable logistic regression analysis estimating the probability of having interval gastric cancer after screening endoscopy.

Parameter	Estimate (95% CI)	p Value
Intercept	−9.99 (−10.12 to −9.87)	<0.001
Group 2 (irregularly screened group, 2–10 years)	0.24 (0.15 to 0.32)	<0.001
Group 3 (not−screened group, >10 years)	0.52 (0.43 to 0.61)	<0.001
Male	0.95 (0.88 to 1.02)	<0.001
Age group (50–59)	0.97 (0.84 to 1.10)	<0.001
Age group (60–69)	1.69 (1.57 to 1.82)	<0.001
Age group (70–79)	2.30 (2.17 to 2.42)	<0.001
Age group (≥80)	2.65 (2.48 to 2.81)	<0.001
History of intestinal metaplasia [a,b]	0.69 (0.39 to 0.99)	<0.001
History of gastric polyp [a]	0.89 (0.74 to 1.05)	<0.001

Abbreviations: CI, confidence interval; OR, odds ratio. [a] The source of these variables was participants' self-reported questionnaires for the National Cancer Screening Program; [b] Intestinal metaplasia was accompanied by atrophic gastritis.

4. Discussion

The interval of an endoscopic screening program directly influences gastric cancer-related survival [15], and individuals with a regular screening interval of <2 years tended to get diagnosed early, thereby being eligible for endoscopic treatment. In contrast, those who had a longer screening interval were more likely to be diagnosed with advanced stages of cancer where endoscopy was not effective [16]. Despite such reports on the relationship between the detection of gastric cancer and screening interval, there has been no study on the relationship between screening programs and interval cancer, which is a quality index of the screening program. With a large national cohort, we found that regular participation in the national cancer screening program was likely to reduce interval cancer. Even with endoscopic screening, the incidence of interval cancer increased when it was performed in a long screening interval (screening interval of <2 years vs. 2–10 years vs. >10 years). Particularly, the OR of those who had no endoscopic screening for 10 years was 1.68 times higher than that of participants who had screening every two years. Additionally, the risk factors for interval cancer were male gender, older age, and the presence of intestinal metaplasia and gastric polyps, based on which a probability model of interval cancer was developed. While the role of endoscopists during endoscopic screening is important, these results obtained using the large cohort database suggested that regular participation in screening should also be considered important.

Gastric cancer is histopathologically evaluated using biopsy of lesions detected with endoscopy, resulting in a definitive diagnosis [17,18]. Endoscopy has high diagnostic accuracy for the detection of gastric cancer [19]. Since it is difficult to suspect gastric cancer owing to the uncertainty of its symptoms in the early stage, endoscopy can play a significant role in the early detection of cancer. Thus, the endoscopic screening program has been operated for gastric cancer. When cancer is detected in an advanced stage, the prognosis of the patient would be poor; hence, the screening program aims to detect and treat cancer in the early stage. Case–control studies have reported that endoscopic screening could reduce gastric cancer-related mortality [3,4,20]. It is expected that endoscopy would be considered more important for the early detection of gastric cancer. In an endoscopic examination that allows direct observation of lesions and biopsy, the occurrence of interval cancer is a significant issue. Interval cancer includes missed lesions and latent lesions, whose number should be reduced by the screening program [21]. Since interval gastric cancer is a new terminology used in countries like South Korea and Japan, where nationwide screening programs for gastric cancer were established, there have been few studies on this subject. Previously, a single-center study characterized interval gastric cancer, found tumor location (lower body), and observed tumor differentiation [22]. However, this study comparatively analyzed interval cancer and the control with a small sample size in a single center; hence, it had a limitation in identifying risk factors.

In our study, the OR of interval cancer increased in participants who irregularly participated in the screening program, who were men, with older age, and with the presence of metaplasia and polyp history. With endoscopy, intestinal metaplasia was found to have irregular surfaces, such as ash-colored nodular change, plaque, patch, a rough mucosal surface, and villous appearance [23,24]. As for missed cancer, with upper endoscopy, unlike colonoscopy, it may be difficult to visually identify early gastric cancer and adenoma owing to irregular surfaces of the gastric mucosa rather than blind spots, which might have led to missing those lesions. Intestinal metaplasia increases with age [25] and is one of the important risk factors for gastric cancer [26]. From such perspectives, our study also showed similar results, wherein male sex, older age, and intestinal metaplasia were associated with interval cancer in participants in the screening program. The presence of gastric polyp history was also an associated factor for interval cancer (OR 2.44). In our study, tumor characteristics of interval cancer could not be identified owing to privacy issues of the KNCSP. It was also impossible to investigate whether polyps progressed to cancer because polyp history, like other factors, was obtained from the questionnaire provided to participants of the KNCSP. A previous study showed that gastric polyps could be a risk factor for cancer [27]; however, our results should be interpreted carefully. Additionally, the relationship between the number of polyps and cancer could not be evaluated. Thus, this relationship should be further investigated if polyp history itself is associated with the occurrence of interval cancer.

Although regular screening can be helpful for the early detection of gastric cancer, it remains unclear why it reduces interval cancer. The KNCSP was composed of a survey and an examination. In a pre-examination survey, previous endoscopic results and history need to be answered in detail, which can be checked by an endoscopist before the examination. Thus, it is speculated that such information of individuals who regularly participated would be more accurate than those who had no regular screening. Such pre-test information would be helpful for the endoscopic exam. Additionally, it is postulated that regular participation in screening would increase the chance of having an examination in the same institution. In such cases, endoscopists could check the previous endoscopic results and they might be able to perform the tests with more accurate information. Moreover, it is possible that individuals who regularly participate in screening are highly interested in their health and might be better in managing their health. However, such reasons cannot explain the association between interval cancer and regular screening. A prospective randomized study would show accurate results; however, it is practically difficult and may be accompanied by ethical issues, which makes it difficult to apply to this study.

There were some limitations to our study. First, the cancer information of individual patients was protected from being disclosed because of privacy issues; hence, it could not be used for analysis. Second, we could not analyze the survival rates associated with cancer stages and their effects in this study due to data unavailability. Third, *Helicobacter pylori* infection plays a significant role in gastric cancer onset [28]. Nevertheless, we were unable to identify the baseline status of *Helicobacter pylori* infection. Fourth, a history of UGI series was not considered. Fifth, our study utilized the KNCSP data of 2013–2016 and investigated up to 2017 to detect the occurrence of interval cancer. Despite limitation in representativeness, it was the most recent accessible data containing a large cohort of 11,642,410 participants who underwent endoscopic screening. Sixth, since several endoscopists participated in the KNCSP, differences in endoscopy quality may exist. Thus, Korea is overcoming this limitation by implementing a quality control program led by the society and government. Seventh, we did not confirm the exact preparation status during screening endoscopy. Finally, potential risk of recall bias exists, as questionnaires were used for data collection.

In summary, using a nationwide cohort, we investigated the baseline characteristics that increased the risk of interval cancer in participants of the screening program. Although guidelines exist to improve the quality of screening programs by increasing the number of endoscopies performed [29,30], interval cancer remains an important issue. To reduce interval cancer, it is important not only to have quality control by endoscopists but also to ensure that regular screening of participants is performed. Based on our results, it is expected that active participation is required to improve the quality of the screening program, and endoscopists should refer to participants' baseline information in clinical practice to reduce the incidence of interval cancer.

Supplementary Materials: The following supporting information can be downloaded at: https://www.mdpi.com/article/10.3390/jcm11010230/s1, Table S1: Overall Screening Performance for Gastric Cancer Between The 2013–2014 and 2015–2016 Korean National Cancer Screening Program Cyclesa.

Author Contributions: C.-K.N. and E.L. contributed equally to this work. Conceptualization: C.-K.N., K.M.L. Acquisition, analysis, or interpretation of data: E.L.; B.P., S.J.S., J.Y.C. Drafting of the manuscript: C.-K.N., E.L. Critical revision of the manuscript for important intellectual content: C.-K.N., E.L., G.H.L., S.G.L., S.J.S., K.M.L. Statistical analysis: E.L., B.P. Administrative, technical, or material support: C.-K.N., E.L., G.H.L. Supervision: S.J.S., J.Y.C., K.M.L. All authors have read and agreed to the published version of the manuscript.

Funding: This research received no external funding.

Institutional Review Board Statement: The study protocol was approved by our institution's review board and ethics committee (approval No. AJIRB-MED- MDB-19-109).

Informed Consent Statement: Institutional review board waived the requirement for individual informed consent owing to the use of a de-identified dataset.

Data Availability Statement: Data cannot be shared publicly because of the sensitive nature of the data collected for this study. Data are available from the Korea National Health Insurance Sharing Service (contact via https://nhiss.nhis.or.kr, contact: +82-33-736-2432 (ext. 2433)) for researchers who meet the criteria for access to confidential data.

Conflicts of Interest: The authors declared no potential conflicts of interest with respect to the research, authorship, and/or publication of this article. The funders had no role in the design of the study; in the collection, analyses, or interpretation of data; in the writing of the manuscript, or in the decision to publish the results.

References

1. Bray, F.; Ferlay, J.; Soerjomataram, I.; Siegel, R.L.; Torre, L.A.; Jemal, A. Global cancer statistics 2018: GLOBOCAN estimates of incidence and mortality worldwide for 36 cancers in 185 countries. *CA Cancer J. Clin.* **2018**, *68*, 394–424. [CrossRef] [PubMed]
2. Leung, W.K.; Wu, M.S.; Kakugawa, Y.; Kim, J.J.; Yeoh, K.G.; Goh, K.L.; Wu, K.C.; Wu, D.C.; Sollano, J.; Kachintorn, U.; et al. Screening for gastric cancer in Asia: Current evidence and practice. *Lancet Oncol.* **2008**, *9*, 279–287. [CrossRef]
3. Jun, J.K.; Choi, K.S.; Lee, H.Y.; Suh, M.; Park, B.; Song, S.H.; Jung, K.W.; Lee, C.W.; Choi, I.J.; Park, E.C.; et al. Effectiveness of the Korean National Cancer Screening Program in reducing gastric cancer mortality. *Gastroenterology* **2017**, *152*, 1319–1328.e7. [CrossRef] [PubMed]
4. Hamashima, C.; Ogoshi, K.; Okamoto, M.; Shabana, M.; Kishimoto, T.; Fukao, A. A community-based, case-control study evaluating mortality reduction from gastric cancer by endoscopic screening in Japan. *PLoS ONE* **2013**, *8*, e79088. [CrossRef]
5. Hamashima, C. Benefits and harms of endoscopic screening for gastric cancer. *World J. Gastroenterol.* **2016**, *22*, 6385–6392. [CrossRef] [PubMed]
6. Kim, G.H.; Liang, P.S.; Bang, S.J.; Hwang, J.H. Screening and surveillance for gastric cancer in the United States: Is it needed? *Gastrointest. Endosc.* **2016**, *84*, 18–28. [CrossRef]
7. Kaminski, M.F.; Regula, J.; Kraszewska, E.; Polkowski, M.; Wojciechowska, U.; Didkowska, J.; Zwierko, M.; Rupinski, M.; Nowacki, M.P.; Butruk, E. Quality indicators for colonoscopy and the risk of interval cancer. *N. Engl. J. Med.* **2010**, *362*, 1795–1803. [CrossRef]
8. Dan, Y.Y.; So, J.B.; Yeoh, K.G. Endoscopic screening for gastric cancer. *Clin. Gastroenterol. Hepatol.* **2006**, *4*, 709–716. [CrossRef] [PubMed]
9. Tashiro, A.; Sano, M.; Kinameri, K.; Fujita, K.; Takeuchi, Y. Comparing mass screening techniques for gastric cancer in Japan. *World J. Gastroenterol.* **2006**, *12*, 4873–4874.

10. Choi, K.S.; Jun, J.K.; Lee, H.Y.; Park, S.; Jung, K.W.; Han, M.A.; Choi, I.J.; Park, E.C. Performance of gastric cancer screening by endoscopy testing through the National Cancer Screening Program of Korea. *Cancer Sci.* **2011**, *102*, 1559–1564. [CrossRef] [PubMed]
11. Shin, H.R.; Won, Y.J.; Jung, K.W.; Kong, H.J.; Yim, S.H.; Lee, J.K.; Noh, H.I.; Lee, J.K.; Pisani, P.; Park, J.G.; et al. Nationwide cancer incidence in Korea, 1999~2001; First result using the national cancer incidence database. *Cancer Res. Treat.* **2005**, *37*, 325–331. [CrossRef] [PubMed]
12. Lee, S.; Jun, J.K.; Suh, M.; Park, B.; Noh, D.K.; Jung, K.W.; Choi, K.S. Gastric cancer screening uptake trends in Korea: Results for the National Cancer Screening Program from 2002 to 2011: A prospective cross-sectional study. *Medicine* **2015**, *94*, e533. [CrossRef] [PubMed]
13. Choi, K.S.; Jun, J.K.; Park, E.C.; Park, S.; Jung, K.W.; Han, M.A.; Choi, I.J.; Lee, H.Y. Performance of different gastric cancer screening methods in Korea: A population-based study. *PLoS ONE* **2012**, *7*, e50041. [CrossRef] [PubMed]
14. Hamashima, C.; Okamoto, M.; Shabana, M.; Osaki, Y.; Kishimoto, T. Sensitivity of endoscopic screening for gastric cancer by the incidence method. *Int. J. Cancer* **2013**, *133*, 653–659. [CrossRef] [PubMed]
15. Mori, Y.; Arita, T.; Shimoda, K.; Yasuda, K.; Yoshida, T.; Kitano, S. Effect of periodic endoscopy for gastric cancer on early detection and improvement of survival. *Gastric Cancer* **2001**, *4*, 132–136. [CrossRef]
16. Nam, S.Y.; Choi, I.J.; Park, K.W.; Kim, C.G.; Lee, J.Y.; Kook, M.C.; Lee, J.S.; Park, S.R.; Lee, J.H.; Ryu, K.W.; et al. Effect of repeated endoscopic screening on the incidence and treatment of gastric cancer in health screenees. *Eur. J. Gastroenterol. Hepatol.* **2009**, *21*, 855–860. [CrossRef]
17. Van Cutsem, E.; Sagaert, X.; Topal, B.; Haustermans, K.; Prenen, H. Gastric cancer. *Lancet* **2016**, *388*, 2654–2664. [CrossRef]
18. Gado, A.; Ebeid, B. Gastric cancer missed at endoscopy. *Alex. J. Med.* **2019**, *49*, 25–27. [CrossRef]
19. Voutilainen, M.E.; Juhola, M.T. Evaluation of the diagnostic accuracy of gastroscopy to detect gastric tumours: Clinicopathological features and prognosis of patients with gastric cancer missed on endoscopy. *Eur. J. Gastroenterol. Hepatol.* **2005**, *17*, 1345–1349. [CrossRef]
20. Matsumoto, S.; Yoshida, Y. Efficacy of endoscopic screening in an isolated island: A case-control study. *Indian J. Gastroenterol.* **2014**, *33*, 46–49. [CrossRef]
21. Kim, B.W. Lessons from interval gastric cancer: Read between the lines. *Gut Liver* **2015**, *9*, 133–134. [CrossRef]
22. Park, M.S.; Yoon, J.Y.; Chung, H.S.; Lee, H.; Park, J.C.; Shin, S.K.; Lee, S.K.; Lee, Y.C. Clinicopathologic characteristics of interval gastric cancer in Korea. *Gut Liver* **2015**, *9*, 166–173. [CrossRef]
23. Lin, B.R.; Shun, C.T.; Wang, T.H.; Lin, J.T. Endoscopic diagnosis of intestinal metaplasia of stomach–accuracy judged by histology. *Hepatogastroenterology* **1999**, *46*, 162–166. [PubMed]
24. Fukuta, N.; Ida, K.; Kato, T.; Uedo, N.; Ando, T.; Watanabe, H.; Shimbo, T.; Study Group for Investigating Endoscopic Diagnosis of Gastric Intestinal Metaplasia. Endoscopic diagnosis of gastric intestinal metaplasia: A prospective multicenter study. *Dig. Endosc.* **2013**, *25*, 526–534. [CrossRef]
25. Joo, Y.E.; Park, H.K.; Myung, D.S.; Baik, G.H.; Shin, J.E.; Seo, G.S.; Kim, G.H.; Kim, H.U.; Kim, H.Y.; Cho, S.I.; et al. Prevalence and risk factors of atrophic gastritis and intestinal metaplasia: A nationwide multicenter prospective study in Korea. *Gut Liver* **2013**, *7*, 303–310. [CrossRef] [PubMed]
26. Leung, W.K.; Sung, J.J. Intestinal metaplasia and gastric carcinogenesis. *Aliment. Pharmacol. Ther.* **2002**, *16*, 1209–1216. [CrossRef]
27. Ginsberg, G.G.; Al-Kawas, F.H.; Fleischer, D.E.; Reilly, H.F.; Benjamin, S.B. Gastric polyps: Relationship of size and histology to cancer risk. *Am. J. Gastroenterol.* **1996**, *91*, 714–717. [PubMed]
28. Uemura, N.; Okamoto, S.; Yamamoto, S.; Matsumura, N.; Yamaguchi, S.; Yamakido, M.; Taniyama, K.; Sasaki, N.; Schlemper, R.J. Helicobacter pylori infection and the development of gastric cancer. *N. Engl. J. Med.* **2001**, *345*, 784–789. [CrossRef]
29. Min, J.K.; Cha, J.M.; Cho, Y.K.; Kim, J.H.; Yoon, S.M.; Im, J.P.; Jung, Y.; Moon, J.S.; Kim, J.O.; Jeen, Y.T. Revision of quality indicators for the endoscopy quality improvement program of the National Cancer Screening Program in Korea. *Clin. Endosc.* **2018**, *51*, 239–252. [CrossRef]
30. Hamashima, C.; Fukao, A. Quality assurance manual of endoscopic screening for gastric cancer in Japanese communities. *Jpn. J. Clin. Oncol.* **2016**, *46*, 1053–1061. [CrossRef] [PubMed]

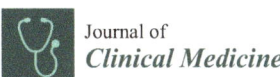

Article

Gastric Xanthelasma, Microsatellite Instability and Methylation of Tumor Suppressor Genes in the Gastric Mucosa: Correlation and Comparison as a Predictive Marker for the Development of Synchronous/Metachronous Gastric Cancer

Masashi Fukushima, Hirokazu Fukui *, Jiro Watari, Chiyomi Ito, Ken Hara, Hirotsugu Eda, Toshihiko Tomita, Tadayuki Oshima and Hiroto Miwa

Division of Gastroenterology and Hepatology, Department of Internal Medicine, Hyogo College of Medicine, Nishinomiya 663-8501, Japan; ma-fukushima@hyo-med.ac.jp (M.F.); watarij@kinentou.or.jp (J.W.); s.aurantiaca66@gmail.com (C.I.); k-hara@hyo-med.ac.jp (K.H.); eda@hyo-med.ac.jp (H.E.); tomita@hyo-med.ac.jp (T.T.); t-oshima@hyo-med.ac.jp (T.O.); miwahgi@hyo-med.ac.jp (H.M.)
* Correspondence: hfukui@hyo-med.ac.jp; Tel.: +81-798-45-6662

Citation: Fukushima, M.; Fukui, H.; Watari, J.; Ito, C.; Hara, K.; Eda, H.; Tomita, T.; Oshima, T.; Miwa, H. Gastric Xanthelasma, Microsatellite Instability and Methylation of Tumor Suppressor Genes in the Gastric Mucosa: Correlation and Comparison as a Predictive Marker for the Development of Synchronous/ Metachronous Gastric Cancer. *J. Clin. Med.* 2022, 11, 9. https://doi.org/10.3390/jcm11010009

Academic Editor: Ugo Grossi

Received: 24 November 2021
Accepted: 17 December 2021
Published: 21 December 2021

Publisher's Note: MDPI stays neutral with regard to jurisdictional claims in published maps and institutional affiliations.

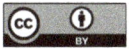

Copyright: © 2021 by the authors. Licensee MDPI, Basel, Switzerland. This article is an open access article distributed under the terms and conditions of the Creative Commons Attribution (CC BY) license (https:// creativecommons.org/licenses/by/ 4.0/).

Abstract: A predictive marker for the development of synchronous/metachronous gastric cancer (GC) would be highly desirable in order to establish an effective strategy for endoscopic surveillance. Herein, we examine the significance of gastric xanthelasma (GX) and molecular abnormalities for the prediction of synchronous/metachronous GC. Patients (n = 115) were followed up (range, 12–122; median, 55 months) in whom the presence of GX and molecular alterations, including microsatellite instability (MSI) and methylation of *human mutL homolog 1* (*hMLH1*), *cyclin-dependent kinase inhibitor 2A* (*CDKN2A*) and *adenomatous polyposis coli* (*APC*) genes, had been confirmed in non-neoplastic gastric mucosa when undergoing endoscopic submucosal dissection (ESD) for early GC. At the start of surveillance, the numbers of positive subjects were as follows: GX, 59 (51.3%); MSI, 48 (41.7%); *hMLH1*, 37 (32.2%); *CDKN2A*, 7 (6.1%); *APC*, 18 (15.7%). After ESD treatment, synchronous/metachronous GCs occurred in patients with the following positive factors: GX, 16 (27.1%); MSI, 7 (14.6%); *hMLH1*, 6 (16.2%); *CDKN2A*, 3 (42.9%); *APC*, 3 (16.7%). The presence of GX had no significant relationship to positivity for MSI or methylation of *hMLH1*, *CDKN2A* or *APC*. GX was significantly (p = 0.0059) and independently (hazard ratio, 3.275; 95% confidence interval, 1.134–9.346) predictive for the development of synchronous/metachronous GC, whereas those genetic alterations were not predictive. GX is a simple and powerful marker for predicting the development of synchronous or metachronous GC.

Keywords: gastric xanthelasma; synchronous/metachronous gastric cancer; endoscopic submucosal dissection; genetic alteration; predicting marker

1. Introduction

Gastric cancer (GC) is still a leading cause of cancer-related mortality, especially in eastern countries [1,2]. With advances in endoscopy and diagnostic strategies, a considerable number of GCs can now be detected at an early stage and be treated curatively by endoscopic submucosal dissection (ESD) [3,4]. However, after endoscopic treatment of GC, the development of synchronous and/or metachronous lesions is a concern during follow-up [5,6]. For this reason, although endoscopic surveillance is recommended, no specific strategies for assisting the frequency or risk of such lesions have yet been established. Therefore, to improve the efficiency and effectiveness of endoscopic surveillance, a predictive marker for the development of synchronous/metachronous GC would be highly desirable.

It has been accepted that irreversible accumulation of molecular abnormality occurs in precancerous conditions, i.e., atrophic gastritis and intestinal metaplasia with chronic

Helicobacter pylori (H. pylori) infection [7]. Thus, the whole of the gastric mucosa with H. pylori infection has a high potential for development of GC, which is consistent with the frequent occurrence of synchronous/metachronous GC in this situation. Interestingly, it has been shown that microsatellite instability (MSI) or methylation of tumor-suppressor genes frequently occurs in the non-neoplastic gastric mucosa of patients with GC [8–10] and that, moreover, these molecular abnormalities do not completely normalize, even after successful eradication of H. pylori [7,8,11]. These findings offer a good explanation of the relatively high frequency of GC development, even after successful eradication of H. pylori infection. In these contexts, molecular abnormalities in the gastric mucosa may be candidate markers for prediction of the development of GC [10,12,13]. We recently reported that the incidence of molecular events related to carcinogenesis was mostly observed in IM, with very few in atrophic mucosa without intestinal metaplasia [14]. On the other hand, we recently reported that gastric xanthelasma (GX), characterized by accumulation of lipid in histiocytic foam cells [15], is a useful marker for prediction of the development of GC [16,17]. In the present study, therefore, we analyzed the correlation between GX and molecular abnormalities in the gastric mucosa, especially in intestinal metaplasia, of patients with early GC and investigated its significance for prediction of synchronous/metachronous GC.

2. Materials and Methods

2.1. Patients

This was a cohort study following our previous investigation in molecular alterations in the non-neoplastic gastric mucosa of patients with early GC [8]. Written informed consent had been obtained from all patients involved in the previous study (Ethics Nos. 136 and 154), and the opt-out for this observational study (Ethics No. 0404) was announced on the website of Hyogo College of Medicine. All studies were approved by the Ethics Committee of Hyogo College of Medicine.

A total of 115 patients were investigated in this study. All patients satisfied the following criteria: 1, subjects who had undergone ESD for GCs between August 2010 and December 2013; 2, subjects who had been enrolled in the previous study [8] and examined for molecular alterations in non-neoplastic gastric mucosa when receiving ESD treatment; 3, subjects who had been followed-up for ≥ 12 months by endoscopy to examine whether synchronous or metachronous GC had occurred after ESD treatment.

In the present study, we used the criteria of the Japanese Research Society for Gastric Cancer as the histological criteria for gastric cancer. The criteria of Kimura and Takemoto, reported previously [18,19], were also adopted for the severity of gastric atrophy. Endoscopists (M.F., K.H. and H.E.), who were blinded to the data of molecular alterations and patients' clinical course, confirmed the presence of xanthomas in endoscopic examination before ESD treatment, retrospectively. At the time of ESD, the status of H. pylori infection was determined by Giemsa staining of gastric biopsy samples and the obtained serum level of anti-H. pylori antibody and then defined as positive if at least one test gave a positive result. If H. pylori had been eradicated after ESD, the status of infection was examined by urease breath test.

2.2. Analyses of MSI and Gene Methylation

Molecular alterations in the intestinal metaplasia were analyzed as described previously [8]. In brief, biopsy specimens of non-neoplastic gastric mucosa at the greater curvatures of the antrum and corpus and the lesser curvature of the angulus were embedded in paraffin blocks. Seven-micrometer-thick tissue sections were cut, samples of epithelial cells were isolated by laser microdissection, and DNA was extracted only from the goblet intestinal metaplasia glands (incomplete type) using a QIAamp DNA Micro Kit (Qiagen, Hilden, Germany).

We examined five microsatellite loci on chromosomes for MSI based on the revised Bethesda panel [20], as follows: 2p (BAT26), 4q (BAT25), 2p (D2S123), 5q (D5S346) and

17p (D17S250). The MSI status was judged as previously reported [8]. To analyze the genetic methylation status, extracted DNA was modified using sodium bisulfite with the EpiTect Plus DNA Bisulphite Kit (Qiagen, Hilden, Germany). The modified DNA was amplified using specific primer pairs for the methylated or unmethylated sequences of *human mutL homolog 1* (*hMLH1*), *cyclin-dependent kinase inhibitor 2A* (*CDKN2A*) and *adenomatous polyposis coli* (*APC*) [8]. Thereafter, the methylation status of those genes was examined by methylation-sensitive high-resolution melting analysis, as previously described [8,21]. A methylation standard curve was prepared using a set of methylated (100%) and unmethylated (0%) DNA (EpiTect PCR Control DNA Set; Qiagen, Hilden, Germany). The methylation status of each target gene was scored as low (<10%), moderate ($\geq$10% to <50%) or high ($\geq$50%). Samples with a moderate or high methylation level were considered to be methylated.

2.3. Statistical Analysis

The Statview 5.0J statistical software package (Abacus Concepts Inc., Berkeley, CA, USA) was used for all analyses in the present study. Data for age and BMI were expressed as the mean $\pm$ SD, and categorical data were presented as frequencies with proportion. Differences in age and BMI between two groups were analyzed by unpaired two-tailed *t* test or by Mann-Whitney *U*-test when the data were not parametric. Fisher's exact test was performed to investigate the relationships between groups and clinical/genetic features. Cumulative incidence of synchronous/metachronous GC development after ESD treatment was evaluated by the Kaplan-Meier method and analyzed by log-rank test. Differences at $p < 0.05$ were considered to be statistically significant.

3. Results

3.1. Relationship of GX to Clinical/Endoscopic Features in Patients with Early GC Treated by ESD

Table 1 summarizes the clinical and endoscopic features of patients with early GC treated by ESD (*n* = 115). Most of the patients (*n* = 108, 93.9%) had open-type gastric atrophy. Eighty-nine patients (77.4%) were positive for *H. pylori* infection, and 11 were negative after *H. pylori* eradication. Fifteen were negative for *H. pylori* infection without eradication, and 13 of them had atrophy, suggesting previous *H. pylori* infection.

Table 1. Comparison of clinical features between patients with and without gastric xanthelasma.

Characteristics	Total Patients (*n* = 115)	Patients with GX (*n* = 59)	Patients without GX (*n* = 56)	*p* Value
Age				
$\geq$65	97 (84.3)	52 (88.1)	45 (80.4)	0.3088
<65	18 (15.7)	7 (11.9)	11 (19.6)	
Sex				
Male	82 (71.3)	45 (76.3)	37 (66.1)	0.3027
Female	33 (28.7)	14 (23.7)	19 (33.9)	
BMI	23.0 $\pm$ 3.4	22.9 $\pm$ 3.0	23.1 $\pm$ 3.9	0.8843
Atrophy				
Open-type	108 (93.9)	57 (96.6)	51 (91.1)	0.2928
Closed-type	5 (4.4)	2 (3.4)	3 (5.3)	
None	2 (1.7)	0 (0.0)	2 (3.6)	
H. pylori				
Negative	15 (13.0)	5 (8.5)	10 (17.9)	0.2553
Era-negative	11 (9.6)	7 (11.9)	4 (7.1)	
Positive	89 (77.4)	47 (79.6)	42 (75.0)	

GX, gastric xanthelasma; BMI, body mass index.

GX was detected in 59 (51.3%) of the 115 patients investigated. None of the parameters—age, sex, BMI, severity of gastric atrophy or *H. pylori* infection status—showed a significant relationship to the prevalence of GX.

3.2. Relationship of MSI or Methylation of hMLH1, CDKN2A or APC to Clinical/Endoscopic Features in Patients with Early GC Treated by ESD

Among 115 patients with early GC who underwent ESD, 48 (41.7%) were positive for MSI (Table 2). None of the examined parameters—age, sex, BMI, severity of gastric atrophy or *H. pylori* infection status—showed a significant relationship with MSI positivity.

Methylation of the *hMLH1* gene was detected in 37 (32.2%) of the patients with early GC who underwent ESD. Positivity for *hMLH1* methylation showed no relationship with any of the above clinical/endoscopic features either.

Methylation of the *CDKN2A* and *APC* gene was detected in 7 (6.1%) and 18 (15.7%) of patients with early GC who underwent ESD, respectively. Positivity for *CDKN2A* or *APC* methylation showed no relationship with any of the above clinical/endoscopic features either.

Table 2. Comparison of clinical features between patients with and without MSI or methylation of tumor suppressor genes.

Characteristics	MSI (+) (n = 48)	MSI (−) (n = 67)	p Value	hMLH1 (+) (n = 37)	hMLH1 (−) (n = 78)	p Value	CDKN2A (+) (n = 7)	CDKN2A (−) (n = 108)	p Value	APC (+) (n = 18)	APC (−) (n = 97)	p Value
Age			0.8008			0.1003			0.3008			0.1553
≥65	40 (83.3)	57 (85.1)		28 (75.7)	69 (88.5)		5 (71.4)	92 (85.2)		13 (72.2)	84 (86.6)	
<65	8 (16.7)	10 (14.9)		9 (24.3)	9 (11.5)		2 (28.6)	16 (14.8)		5 (27.8)	13 (13.4)	
Sex			0.8356			0.1272			0.4074			0.0915
Male	35 (72.9)	47 (70.1)		30 (81.1)	52 (66.7)		4 (57.1)	78 (72.2)		16 (88.9)	66 (68.0)	
Female	13 (27.1)	20 (29.9)		7 (18.9)	26 (33.3)		3 (42.9)	30 (27.8)		2 (11.1)	31 (32.0)	
BMI	23.5 ± 3.6	22.6 ± 3.2	0.3127	22.9 ± 3.0	23.0 ± 3.6	0.8131	21.4 ± 2.3	23.1 ± 3.5	0.1226	21.9 ± 2.8	23.1 ± 3.5	0.2124
Atrophy			0.6750			0.7285			0.0284			0.3836
Open-type	44 (91.7)	64 (95.5)		35 (94.6)	73 (93.6)		6 (85.7)	102 (94.5)		16 (88.9)	92 (94.9)	
Closed-type	3 (6.2)	2 (3.0)		1 (2.7)	4 (5.1)		0 (0.0)	5 (4.6)		1 (5.55)	4 (4.1)	
None	1 (2.1)	1 (1.5)		1 (2.7)	1 (1.3)		1 (14.3)	1 (0.9)		1 (5.55)	1 (1.0)	
H. pylori			0.3368			0.8591			0.8973			0.5863
Negative	4 (8.3)	11 (16.4)		4 (10.8)	11 (14.1)		1 (14.3)	14 (12.9)		1 (5.6)	14 (14.4)	
Era-negative	6 (12.5)	5 (7.5)		4 (10.8)	7 (9.0)		1 (14.3)	10 (9.3)		2 (11.1)	9 (9.3)	
Positive	38 (79.2)	51 (76.1)		29 (78.4)	60 (76.9)		5 (71.4)	84 (77.8)		15 (83.3)	74 (76.3)	

MSI, microsatellite instability; hMLH1, human mutL homolog 1; CDKN2A, cyclin-dependent kinase inhibitor 2A; APC, adenomatous polyposis coli; BMI, body mass index.

3.3. Relationship between GX and MSI or Methylation of hMLH1, CDKN2A or APC in Patients with Early GC Treated by ESD

We next investigated the relationship between the prevalence of GX and molecular alterations in the gastric mucosa of patients with early GC (Table 3). Contrary to expectation, we found no significant correlation between the prevalence of GX and molecular alterations of MSI or methylation of *hMLH1*, *CDKN2A* or *APC*.

Table 3. Relationship between gastric xanthelasma and genetic alterations in early gastric cancer patients.

Characteristics	Patients with GX (n = 59)	Patients without GX (n = 56)	p Value
MSI			
positive	23 (39.0)	25 (44.6)	0.5744
negative	36 (61.0)	31 (55.4)	
***hMLH1* methylation**			
positive	19 (32.2)	18 (32.1)	0.9945
negative	40 (67.8)	38 (67.9)	
***CDKN2A* methylation**			
positive	3 (5.1)	4 (7.1)	0.7121
negative	56 (94.9)	52 (92.9)	
***APC* methylation**			
positive	7 (11.9)	11 (19.6)	0.3088
negative	52 (88.1)	45 (80.4)	

GX, gastric xanthelasma; MSI, microsatellite instability; *hMLH1*, human mutL homolog 1; *CDKN2A*, cyclin-dependent kinase inhibitor 2A; *APC*, adenomatous polyposis coli.

3.4. Significance of GX, MSI and Methylation of Tumor Suppressor Genes as a Predictive Marker for the Development of Synchronous/Metachronous GC

During the follow-up period, synchronous/metachronous GC was found in 21 (18.3%; 5 synchronous and 16 metachronous, respectively) of the 115 patients (Table 4). When investigating according to the prevalence of GX, 16 (27.1%) of the 59 patients with GX developed synchronous/metachronous GC after ESD treatment. On the other hand, 5 (8.9%) of 56 patients without GX had such lesions. As for the prevalence of MSI, 7 (14.6%) of 48 patients with MSI had synchronous/metachronous GC, and 14 (20.9%) of 67 patients without MSI had such lesions. In addition, 6 (16.2%) of 37 patients with *hMLH1* methylation had synchronous/metachronous GCs and 15 (19.2%) of 78 patients without *hMLH1* methylation had such lesions. Three (42.9%) of seven patients with *CDKN2A* methylation had synchronous/metachronous GCs, and 3 (16.7%) of 18 patients with *APC* methylation had such lesions.

Furthermore, we compared the cumulative incidence of synchronous/metachronous GC between GX-positive and -negative cases (Figure 1). Kaplan–Meir curves show that significantly more patients with GX developed synchronous/metachronous GC than those without GX (Figure 1). In terms of the status of MSI and methylation of *hMLH1*, *CDKN2A*, or *APC*, the Kaplan–Meir curves show no significant differences between the groups positive and negative for those genetic alterations (Figure 1).

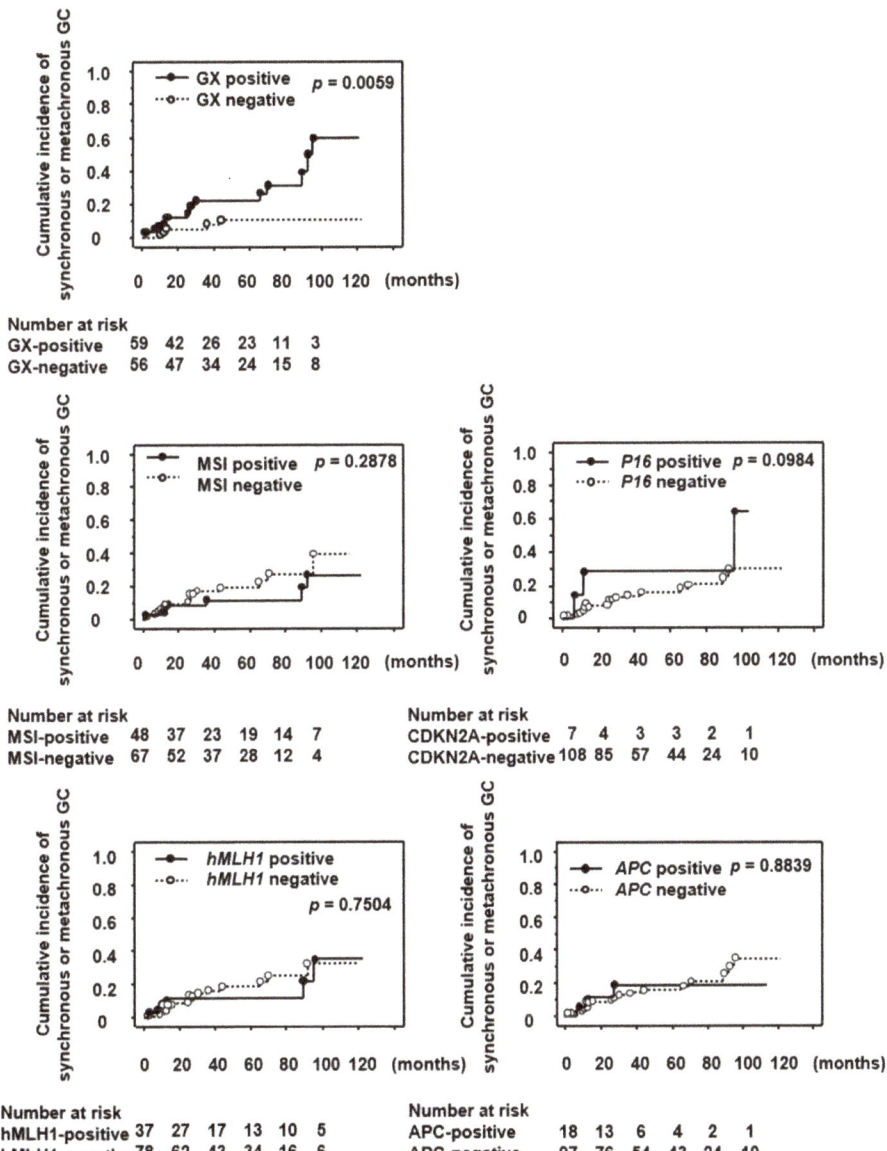

Figure 1. Cumulative incidence of synchronous/metachronous gastric cancer during endoscopic follow-up (median, 55 months; range, 12–122 months) in patients after ESD treatment. GX, gastric xanthelasma; MSI, microsatellite instability; *hMLH1, human mutL homolog 1; CDKN2A, cyclin-dependent kinase inhibitor 2A; APC, adenomatous polyposis coli.*

We next examined whether the presence of GX is an independent factor predictive of synchronous/metachronous GC development. Univariate analysis showed that GX was significantly related to the development of synchronous/metachronous GC (Table 4). Moreover, multivariate analysis clarified that the presence of GX was independently related to the development of synchronous/metachronous GC (Table 4).

Table 4. Univariate and multivariate analyses of the cumulative incidence of synchronous or metachronous gastric cancer during endoscopic follow-up in patients after ESD treatment.

Characteristics	Total with Synch or Metach GC/Total Patients	Univariate p Value	Multivariate 95% CI	p Value
Age				
≥65	18/97	0.847	1.096 (0.295–4.074)	0.892
<65	3/18		1.0	
Sex				
Male	16/82	0.790	1.828 (0.507–6.579)	0.357
Female	5/33		1.0	
GX				
Present	16/59	**0.015**	3.257 (1.134–9.346)	**0.028**
Absent	5/56		1.0	
MSI				
positive	7/48	0.468	0.711 (0.273–1.855)	0.486
Negative	14/67		1.0	
hMLH1 methylation				
Positive	6/37	0.800	0.512 (0.142–1.842)	0.305
Negative	15/78		1.0	
CDKN2A methylation				
Positive	3/7	0.113	4.673 (0.671–32.258)	0.120
Negative	18/108		1.0	
APC methylation				
Positive	3/18	0.849	1.300 (0.335–5.051)	0.705
Negative	18/97		1.0	

GX, gastric xanthelasma; MSI, microsatellite instability; hMLH1, human mutL homolog 1; CDKN2A, cyclin-dependent kinase inhibitor 2A; APC, adenomatous polyposis coli.

4. Discussion

On the basis of clinical/endoscopic features, the identification of a predictive marker for the development of synchronous/metachronous GC has long been desirable. Accumulating evidence has revealed that male sex and severe atrophy are independent risk factors for not only initial but also synchronous/metachronous GC [5,6]. In addition, we previously reported that GX is a powerful marker for prediction of the development of GC [16,17]. Moreover, in the present study, we have clarified that GX is a possible marker for prediction of the development of synchronous/metachronous GC, which is consistent with a report by Shibukawa et al. [22]. GX is characterized by accumulation of foamy histiocytes in the inflamed gastric mucosa and is thought to be the result of an inflammatory response to mucosal damage or aging [15,23]. In this regard, one might argue that gastric xanthelasma merely reflects the severity and long duration of gastric atrophy, which is a crucial risk factor for GC development. However, our previous multivariate analysis clearly indicates that GX is a factor independent of gastric atrophy for prediction of the development of GC [17]. Moreover, the present study similarly clarifies its significance as an independent predictor for synchronous/metachronous GC. It has been reported that increased release of oxygen free radicals, which cause DNA damage and play a role in the pathophysiology of various malignancies [24,25], is involved in the formation of GX [15]. Thus, it is tempting to speculate that the presence of GX may reflect the activation of oxygen free radicals and the associated promotion of genetic alterations in the gastric mucosa. In this context, we therefore investigated the relationship between the presence of GX and molecular alterations in the gastric mucosa of patients with GC.

MSI is a form of genetic instability characterized by alterations in the length of the tandem repeat sequence (termed "microsatellite") [26], owing to inactivation of mismatch repair genes, such as hMSH2 and hMLH1 [27], and it is evident that MSI and/or methylation of hMLH1 is frequent in various malignancies [28]. In addition, the methylation of tumor suppressor CDKN2A and APC is widely involved in gastrointestinal carcinogenesis by affecting cell cycle or proliferation [29–32]. In these contexts, we and others have shown that MSI and/or methylation of tumor-suppressor genes, including hMLH1, frequently occurs in the non-neoplastic gastric mucosa of patients with early GC [8,10,33] and that these molecular alterations can be potential markers for prediction of the development of GC [10,34]. In the present study, methylation of CDKN2A and APC was not very frequent in the non-neoplastic gastric mucosa, especially in intestinal metaplasia of patients with early GC and not predictive of the development of synchronous/metachronous GC, suggesting that those gene alterations may not be very critical in gastric carcinogenesis. On the other hand, it is noteworthy that H. pylori eradication is unable to normalize any molecular abnormality for MSI and hMLH1 in patients with early GC who undergo ESD [8], which supports the contention that H. pylori eradication cannot necessarily prevent the development of metachronous GC [35]. In this context, it is interesting that GX persists even after H. pylori eradication [36] and that its presence is a predictive marker for the development of synchronous/metachronous GC. We then investigated the relationship between GX and the status of MSI or hMLH1 methylation, but contrary to expectation, no significant correlations were evident. Besides these molecular alterations, considerable patterns of genetic abnormality are involved in the development of GC [37–39]. Therefore, it may be an interesting theme to identify the molecular alteration responsible for the occurrence of GX in the gastric mucosa.

We next investigated whether MSI or hMLH1 methylation in the intestinal metaplasia is predictive for the development of synchronous/metachronous GC, as such molecular alterations may be applicable to prediction of the initial development of GC [10]. However, the results suggest that neither MSI nor hMLH1 methylation is likely to predict the development of synchronous/metachronous GC in patients after ESD treatment. These results may be reasonable, as several studies have shown that MSI and/or hMLH1 methylation is not useful for prediction of the development of GC [9,40]. On the other hand, genetic researchers have continuously investigated and identified some candidate molecular markers (methylation of microRNA-34b/c and -124a3 or somatic mutation of ARID1A and MAGI1) for prediction of the development of metachronous GC [41–43]. However, since molecular alterations in GC patients are very complex and diverse [37–39], it might be difficult to select a specific genetic marker that can predict the development of synchronous/metachronous GCs.

In summary, although the molecular alteration responsible for the occurrence of GX in the gastric mucosa remains unclear, GX is a powerful marker for prediction of the development of synchronous/metachronous GC, at least compared with molecular alterations of MSI or methylation of hMLH1, CDKN2A or APC in patients with early GC. GX is very easy to detect in routine endoscopic examinations, whereas detection of molecular abnormality needs advanced equipment and technology. Thus, in clinical practice, GX may be a very useful marker for identification of patients, during follow-up surveillance, who are at high risk for development of synchronous/metachronous GC. The possibility that a powerful molecular marker might become available in the future for prediction of the development of synchronous/metachronous GC cannot be excluded. However, we believe that GX is a simple yet very effective marker in patients undergoing endoscopic surveillance for development of synchronous/metachronous GC and that the usefulness of GX should be validated in a large-scale, prospective, multi-center study.

Author Contributions: Conceptualization, M.F. and H.F.; methodology, H.F., J.W., C.I., K.H. and H.E.; validation, H.F., J.W. and C.I.; formal analysis, H.F., J.W., C.I., K.H. and H.E.; investigation,

M.F., H.F., J.W., C.I., K.H. and H.E.; resources, M.F., J.W., K.H. and H.E.; data curation, M.F., H.F., J.W., C.I., K.H. and H.E.; writing—original draft preparation, M.F. and H.F.; writing—review and editing, M.F., H.F., J.W., C.I., K.H., H.E., T.T., T.O. and H.M.; supervision, T.T., T.O. and H.M.; project administration, H.F.; funding acquisition, H.F. All authors have read and agreed to the published version of the manuscript.

Funding: This work was supported in part by Grants-in-Aid for Scientific Research 21K08016 from the Ministry of Education, Culture, Sports, Science and Technology, Japan.

Institutional Review Board Statement: The study was conducted according to the guidelines of the Declaration of Helsinki, and the collection and analyses of biomaterials and clinical records were approved by the Institutional Ethics Committee of Hyogo College of Medicine (Ethics Nos. 136, 154 and 0404).

Informed Consent Statement: Informed consent was obtained from all subjects involved in the study. The opt-out for this observational study was announced on the website of Hyogo College of Medicine.

Data Availability Statement: Any data referred to in this work will be available on request.

Acknowledgments: We thank Mayumi Yamada and Kayo Tsubota (Hyogo College of Medicine) for their technical assistance.

Conflicts of Interest: The authors declare no conflict of interest. The funders had no role in the design of the study; in the collection, analyses, or interpretation of data; in the writing of the manuscript, or in the decision to publish the results.

References

1. Kamangar, F.; Dores, G.M.; Anderson, W.F. Patterns of cancer incidence, mortality, and prevalence across five continents: Defining priorities to reduce cancer disparities in different geographic regions of the world. *J. Clin. Oncol.* **2006**, *24*, 2137–2150. [CrossRef] [PubMed]
2. Ferlay, J.; Shin, H.R.; Bray, F.; Forman, D.; Mathers, C.; Parkin, D.M. Estimates of worldwide burden of cancer in 2008: GLOBOCAN 2008. *Int. J. Cancer* **2010**, *127*, 2893–2917. [CrossRef] [PubMed]
3. Ohnita, K.; Isomoto, H.; Shikuwa, S.; Yajima, H.; Minami, H.; Matsushima, K.; Akazawa, Y.; Yamaguchi, N.; Fukuda, E.; Nishiyama, H.; et al. Early and long-term outcomes of endoscopic submucosal dissection for early gastric cancer in a large patient series. *Exp. Med.* **2014**, *7*, 594–598. [CrossRef]
4. Suzuki, H.; Oda, I.; Abe, S.; Sekiguchi, M.; Mori, G.; Nonaka, S.; Yoshinaga, S.; Saito, Y. High rate of 5-year survival among patients with early gastric cancer undergoing curative endoscopic submucosal dissection. *Gastric Cancer* **2016**, *19*, 198–205. [CrossRef]
5. Abe, S.; Oda, I.; Suzuki, H.; Nonaka, S.; Yoshinaga, S.; Nakajima, T.; Sekiguchi, M.; Mori, G.; Taniguchi, H.; Sekine, S.; et al. Long-term surveillance and treatment outcomes of metachronous gastric cancer occurring after curative endoscopic submucosal dissection. *Endoscopy* **2015**, *47*, 1113–1118. [CrossRef] [PubMed]
6. Mori, G.; Nakajima, T.; Asada, K.; Shimazu, T.; Yamamichi, N.; Maekita, T.; Yokoi, C.; Fujishiro, M.; Gotoda, T.; Ichinose, M.; et al. Incidence of and risk factors for metachronous gastric cancer after endoscopic resection and successful Helicobacter pylori eradication: Results of a large-scale, multicenter cohort study in Japan. *Gastric Cancer* **2016**, *19*, 911–918. [CrossRef]
7. Watari, J.; Chen, N.; Amenta, P.S.; Fukui, H.; Oshima, T.; Tomita, T.; Miwa, H.; Lim, K.J.; Das, K.M. Helicobacter pylori associated chronic gastritis, clinical syndromes, precancerous lesions, and pathogenesis of gastric cancer development. *World J. Gastroenterol.* **2014**, *20*, 5461–5473. [CrossRef]
8. Kawanaka, M.; Watari, J.; Kamiya, N.; Yamasaki, T.; Kondo, T.; Toyoshima, F.; Ikehara, H.; Tomita, T.; Oshima, T.; Fukui, H.; et al. Effects of Helicobacter pylori eradication on the development of metachronous gastric cancer after endoscopic treatment: Analysis of molecular alterations by a randomised controlled trial. *Br. J. Cancer* **2016**, *114*, 21–29. [CrossRef]
9. Maekita, T.; Nakazawa, K.; Mihara, M.; Nakajima, T.; Yanaoka, K.; Iguchi, M.; Arii, K.; Kaneda, A.; Tsukamoto, T.; Tatematsu, M.; et al. High levels of aberrant DNA methylation in Helicobacter pylori-infected gastric mucosae and its possible association with gastric cancer risk. *Clin. Cancer Res.* **2006**, *12*, 989–995. [CrossRef]
10. Kashiwagi, K.; Watanabe, M.; Ezaki, T.; Kanai, T.; Ishii, H.; Mukai, M.; Hibi, T. Clinical usefulness of microsatellite instability for the prediction of gastric adenoma or adenocarcinoma in patients with chronic gastritis. *Br. J. Cancer* **2000**, *82*, 1814–1818. [CrossRef]
11. Nanjo, S.; Asada, K.; Yamashita, S.; Nakajima, T.; Nakazawa, K.; Maekita, T.; Ichinose, M.; Sugiyama, T.; Ushijima, T. Identification of gastric cancer risk markers that are informative in individuals with past H. pylori. *Infect. Gastr. Cancer* **2012**, *15*, 382–388. [CrossRef] [PubMed]
12. Ando, T.; Yoshida, T.; Enomoto, S.; Asada, K.; Tatematsu, M.; Ichinose, M.; Sugiyama, T.; Ushijima, T. DNA methylation of microRNA genes in gastric mucosae of gastric cancer patients: Its possible involvement in the formation of epigenetic field defect. *Int. J. Cancer* **2009**, *124*, 2367–2374. [CrossRef] [PubMed]

13. Ushijima, T.; Hattori, N. Molecular pathways: Involvement of Helicobacter pylori-triggered inflammation in the formation of an epigenetic field defect, and its usefulness as cancer risk and exposure markers. *Clin. Cancer Res.* **2012**, *18*, 923–929. [CrossRef]
14. Michigami, Y.; Watari, J.; Ito, C.; Nakai, K.; Yamasaki, T.; Kondo, T.; Kono, T.; Tozawa, K.; Tomita, T.; Oshima, T.; et al. Long-term effects of *H. pylori* eradication on epigenetic alterations related to gastric carcinogenesis. *Sci. Rep.* **2018**, *8*, 14369. [CrossRef]
15. Kaiserling, E.; Heine, H.; Itabe, H.; Takano, T.; Remmele, W. Lipid islands in human gastric mucosa: Morphological and immunohistochemical findings. *Gastroenterology* **1996**, *110*, 369–374. [CrossRef]
16. Sekikawa, A.; Fukui, H.; Maruo, T.; Tsumura, T.; Kanesaka, T.; Okabe, Y.; Osaki, Y. Gastric xanthelasma may be a warning sign for the presence of early gastric cancer. *J. Gastroenterol. Hepatol.* **2014**, *29*, 951–956. [CrossRef] [PubMed]
17. Sekikawa, A.; Fukui, H.; Sada, R.; Fukuhara, M.; Marui, S.; Tanke, G.; Endo, M.; Ohara, Y.; Matsuda, F.; Nakajima, J.; et al. Gastric atrophy and xanthelasma are markers for predicting the development of early gastric cancer. *J. Gastroenterol.* **2016**, *51*, 35–42. [CrossRef]
18. Kimura, K.; Takemoto, T. An endoscopic recognition of the atrophic border and its significance in chronic gastritis. *Endoscopy* **1969**, *1*, 87–97. [CrossRef]
19. Kitahara, F.; Kobayashi, K.; Sato, T.; Kojima, Y.; Araki, T.; Fujino, M.A. Accuracy of screening for gastric cancer using serum pepsinogen concentration. *Gut* **1999**, *44*, 693–697. [CrossRef]
20. Umar, A.; Boland, C.R.; Terdiman, J.P.; Syngal, S.; de la Chapelle, A.; Rüschoff, J.; Fishel, R.; Lindor, N.M.; Burgart, L.J.; Hamelin, R.; et al. Revised Bethesda Guidelines for hereditary nonpolyposis colorectal cancer (Lynch syndrome) and microsatellite instability. *J. Natl. Cancer Inst.* **2004**, *96*, 261–268. [CrossRef]
21. Balic, M.; Pichler, M.; Strutz, J.; Heitzer, E.; Ausch, C.; Samonigg, H.; Cote, R.J.; Dandachi, N. High quality assessment of DNA methylation in archival tissues from colorectal cancer patients using quantitative high-resolution melting analysis. *J. Mol. Diagn.* **2009**, *11*, 102–108. [CrossRef]
22. Shibukawa, N.; Ouchi, S.; Wakamatsu, S.; Wakahara, Y.; Kaneko, A. Gastric xanthoma is a predictive marker for metachronous and synchronous gastric cancer. *World J. Gastrointest. Oncol.* **2017**, *9*, 327–332. [CrossRef] [PubMed]
23. Hori, S.; Tsutsumi, Y. Helicobacter pylori infection in gastric xanthomas: Lmmunohistochemical analysis of 145 lesions. *Pathol. Int.* **1996**, *46*, 589–593. [CrossRef]
24. Farinati, F.; Cardin, R.; Dagan, P.; Rugge, M.; Mario, F.D.; Bonvicini, P.; Naccarato, R. Oxidative DNA damage accumulation in gastric carcinogenesis. *Gut* **1998**, *42*, 351–356. [CrossRef]
25. Kountouras, J.; Chatzopoulos, D.; Zavos, C. Reactive oxygen metabolites and upper gastrointestinal diseases. *Hepatogastroenterology* **2001**, *48*, 743–751. [PubMed]
26. Mizoshita, T.; Tsukamoto, T.; Cao, X.; Otsuka, T.; Ito, S.; Takahashi, E.; Nakamura, S.; Nakamura, T.; Yamamura, Y.; Tatematsu, M. Microsatellite instability is linked to loss of *hMLH1* expression in advanced gastric cancers: Lack of a relationship with the histological type and phenotype. *Gastric Cancer* **2005**, *8*, 164–172. [CrossRef]
27. Ionov, Y.; Peinado, M.A.; Malkhosyan, S.; Shibata, D.; Perucho, M. Ubiquitous somatic mutations in simple repeated sequences reveal a new mechanism for colonic carcinogenesis. *Nature* **1993**, *363*, 558–561. [CrossRef] [PubMed]
28. Qu, Y.; Dang, S.; Hou, P. Gene methylation in gastric cancer. *Clin. Chim. Acta* **2013**, *424*, 53–65. [CrossRef] [PubMed]
29. Tsuchiya, T.; Tamura, G.; Sato, K.; Endoh, Y.; Sakata, K.; Jin, Z.; Motoyama, T.; Usuba, O.; Kimura, W.; Nishizuka, S.; et al. Distinct methylation patterns of two APC gene promoters in normal and cancerous gastric epithelia. *Oncogene* **2000**, *19*, 3642–3646. [CrossRef] [PubMed]
30. Wen, J.; Zheng, T.; Hu, K.; Zhu, C.; Guo, L.; Ye, G. Promoter methylation of tumor-related genes as a potential biomarker using blood samples for gastric cancer detection. *Oncotarget* **2017**, *8*, 77783–77793. [CrossRef] [PubMed]
31. Mizuguchi, A.; Takai, A.; Shimizu, T.; Matsumoto, T.; Kumagai, K.; Miyamoto, S.; Seno, H.; Marusawa, H. Genetic features of multicentric/multifocal intramucosal gastric carcinoma. *Int. J. Cancer* **2018**, *143*, 1923–1934. [CrossRef]
32. Zhu, L.; Li, X.; Yuan, Y.; Dong, C.; Yang, M. APC promoter methylation in gastrointestinal cancer. *Front. Oncol.* **2021**, *11*, 653222. [CrossRef] [PubMed]
33. Zaky, A.H.; Watari, J.; Tanabe, H.; Sato, R.; Moriichi, K.; Tanaka, A.; Maemoto, A.; Fujiya, M.; Ashida, T.; Kohgo, Y. Clinicopathologic implications of genetic instability in intestinal-type gastric cancer and intestinal metaplasia as a precancerous lesion: Proof of field cancerization in the stomach. *Am. J. Clin. Pathol.* **2008**, *129*, 613–621. [CrossRef] [PubMed]
34. Businello, G.; Angerilli, V.; Parente, P.; Realdon, S.; Savarino, E.; Farinati, F.; Grillo, F.; Vanoli, A.; Galuppini, F.; Paccagnella, S.; et al. Molecular landscapes of gastric pre-neoplastic and pre-invasive lesions. *Int. J. Mol. Sci.* **2021**, *22*, 9950. [CrossRef]
35. Kato, M.; Nishida, T.; Yamamoto, K.; Hayashi, S.; Kitamura, S.; Yabuta, T.; Yoshio, T.; Nakamura, T.; Komori, M.; Kawai, N.; et al. Scheduled endoscopic surveillance controls secondary cancer after curative endoscopic resection for early gastric cancer: A multicentre retrospective cohort study by Osaka University ESD study group. *Gut* **2013**, *62*, 1425–1432. [CrossRef] [PubMed]
36. Shibukawa, N.; Ouchi, S.; Wakamatsu, S.; Wakahara, Y.; Kaneko, A. Gastric xanthoma is a predictive marker for early gastric cancer detected after Helicobacter pylori eradication. *Intern. Med.* **2019**, *58*, 779–784. [CrossRef] [PubMed]
37. Cancer Genome Atlas Research Network. Comprehensive molecular characterization of gastric adenocarcinoma. *Nature* **2014**, *513*, 202–209. [CrossRef]
38. Tan, P.; Yeoh, K.-G. Genetics and molecular pathogenesis of gastric adenocarcinoma. *Gastroenterology* **2015**, *149*, 1153–1162.e3. [CrossRef] [PubMed]

39. Jacome, A.A.; Coutinho, A.K.; Lima, E.M.; Andrade, A.C.; Dos Santos, J.S. Personalized medicine in gastric cancer: Where are we and where are we going? *World J. Gastroenterol.* **2016**, *22*, 1160–1171. [CrossRef]
40. Enomoto, S.; Maekita, T.; Tsukamoto, T.; Nakajima, T.; Nakazawa, K.; Tatematsu, M.; Ichinose, M.; Ushijima, T. Lack of association between CpG island methylator phenotype in human gastric cancers and methylation in their background noncancerous gastric mucosae. *Cancer Sci.* **2007**, *98*, 1853–1861. [CrossRef]
41. Suzuki, R.; Yamamoto, E.; Nojima, M.; Maruyama, R.; Yamano, H.O.; Yoshikawa, K.; Kimura, T.; Harada, T.; Ashida, M.; Niinuma, T.; et al. Aberrant methylation of microRNA-34b/c is a predictive marker of metachronous gastric cancer risk. *J. Gastroenterol.* **2014**, *49*, 1135–1144. [CrossRef] [PubMed]
42. Asada, K.; Nakajima, T.; Shimazu, T.; Yamamichi, N.; Maekita, T.; Yokoi, C.; Oda, I.; Ando, T.; Yoshida, T.; Nanjo, S.; et al. Demonstration of the usefulness of epigenetic cancer risk prediction by a multicentre prospective cohort study. *Gut* **2015**, *64*, 388–396. [CrossRef] [PubMed]
43. Sakuta, K.; Sasaki, Y.; Abe, Y.; Sato, H.; Shoji, M.; Yaoita, T.; Yagi, M.; Mizumoto, N.; Onozato, Y.; Kon, T.; et al. Somatic alterations and mutational burden are potential predictive factors for metachronous development of early gastric cancer. *Sci. Rep.* **2020**, *10*, 22071. [CrossRef] [PubMed]

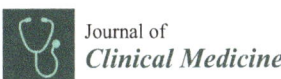

Article

Vimentin-Positive Circulating Tumor Cells as Diagnostic and Prognostic Biomarkers in Patients with Biliary Tract Cancer

Sung Yong Han [1,†], Sung Hee Park [1,†], Hyun Suk Ko [1], Aelee Jang [2], Hyung Il Seo [3], So Jeong Lee [4], Gwang Ha Kim [1] and Dong Uk Kim [1,*]

1. Division of Gastroenterology and Hepatology, Department of Internal Medicine, Biomedical Research Institute, Pusan National University Hospital, Pusan National University College of Medicine, Busan 49241, Korea; mirsaint@hanmail.net (S.Y.H.); scaletlee@hanmail.net (S.H.P.); hwtkjhs@hanmail.net (H.S.K.); doc0224@pusan.ac.kr (G.H.K.)
2. Department of Nursing, University of Ulsan, Ulsan 44610, Korea; jal0008@naver.com
3. Department of Surgery, Biomedical Research Institute, Pusan National University Hospital, Pusan National University College of Medicine, Busan 49241, Korea; seohi71@hanmail.net
4. Department of Pathology, Biomedical Research Institute, Pusan National University Hospital, Pusan National University College of Medicine, Busan 49241, Korea; gag86@naver.com
* Correspondence: amlm3@hanmail.net; Tel.: +82-51-240-7869 or +82-10-2693-9720
† Sung Yong Han and Sung Hee Park contributed equally to the work.

Abstract: Biliary tract cancer (BTC) has poor prognosis; thus, early diagnosis is important to decrease mortality. Although vimentin-positive circulating tumor cells (V-CTCs) are a good candidate for diagnostic and prognostic biomarkers, studies on the topic are limited. We aimed to evaluate the diagnostic efficacy of V-CTCs between BTC and benign biliary disease (BBD) and determine the prognostic value of V-CTCs in BTC patients. We recruited 69 participants who had BTCs and BBDs from a single tertiary referral center. We analyzed CTCs and V-CTCs in peripheral blood using the CD-PRIME^{TM} system. Seven patients were excluded due to a technical failure of CTC detection. CTCs were detected in all 62 patients. CTC count > 40/mL blood (55.8% vs. 20%, $p = 0.039$), V-CTC count > 15/mL blood (57.7% vs. 10%, $p = 0.005$), and V-CTC/CTC ratio > 40% (48.1% vs. 10%, $p = 0.025$) were significantly different between BTCs and BBDs. Two or more of these three parameters (61.5% vs. 10%, $p = 0.002$) increased the accuracy. A combination of CTC markers with CA19-9 and biopsy increased the accuracy (90.4% vs. 10%, $p = 0.000$). V-CTC > 50/mL blood was a significant factor affecting survival (140 (66.6–213.3) vs. 253 (163.9–342.1) days, $p = 0.008$). V-CTC could be a potential biomarker for early diagnosis and predicting prognosis in patients with BTC.

Keywords: biliary tract cancer; circulating tumor cell; vimentin; diagnosis; prognosis

1. Introduction

Biliary tract cancer (BTC) is a rare type of cancer that occurs in 2–3 per 100,000 persons. The incidence is more than two times higher in northeast Asia than in other countries. However, the incidence is increasing worldwide, particularly in western countries. Furthermore, the mortality rate is relatively high compared to those of other gastrointestinal malignancies, despite the development of therapeutic agents [1–5]. The poor prognosis of BTC is largely due to delayed diagnosis from late examination because of non-specific symptoms such as dyspepsia, weight loss, and abdominal discomfort in the early disease stage. Additionally, BTC tissues are paucicellular with abundant fibrous stroma, leading to false negatives in pathology and resulting in late diagnosis and poor prognosis. Therefore, an exact early diagnostic method is needed for the improvement of prognosis of BTC patients.

Circulating tumor cells (CTCs) are good candidates for diagnostic or prognostic biomarkers because they enable frequent, non-invasive analysis and provide real-time dynamics of BTC. Efficient technologies for CTC analysis have been developed since the

U.S. Food and Drug Administration approved the CellSearch system for clinical use to detect CTCs in peripheral blood in January 2004 [6–8]; however, CTC isolation and characterization remains challenging due to their rarity and heterogeneity. The use of CTCs to predict clinical outcomes is far from being applied in the real world, but these applications are being actively researched since efficient CTC enrichment is possible with recent technological advances. A centrifugal microfluidic device with fluid-assisted separation technology (FAST disc) enables label-free CTC isolation from whole blood in a size-selective manner. This system uses tangential flow filtration (TFF), which allows clog-free, ultrafast (>3 mL/min) CTC enrichment with gentle reductions in pressure (~1 kPa) for collecting a large amount of tumor cells with high viability.

CTCs are detected even in precancerous lesions by circulating along blood vessels through the epithelial to mesenchymal process [9,10]. Thus, tumor detection could be possible by detecting CTCs, especially vimentin-positive CTCs developed during the epithelial-mesenchymal transition (EMT) process in the early disease stage. Furthermore, vimentin expression in CTCs is possibly highly correlated with cancer progression rather than CTCs [11,12].

There are limited studies on using CTCs for early tumor detection and prognosis of BTC. Further, the cut-off for a positive CTC value has not yet been defined. The aim of this study was to evaluate the diagnostic efficacy of vimentin-positive circulating tumor cells (V-CTCs) in BTCs and benign biliary diseases (BBDs). Additionally, we aimed to determine the prognostic value of V-CTCs in BTC patients.

2. Materials and Methods

2.1. Patient Characteristics

We recruited 69 participants from a single tertiary referral center in South Korea between June 2018 and February 2021. The inclusion criteria for BTCs were (1) age $\geq$ 18 years; (2) BTC diagnosis based on ultrasound (US), computed tomography (CT), and magnetic resonance imaging (MRI); and (3) histological confirmation as adenocarcinoma. The inclusion criteria for BBDs were (1) age $\geq$ 18 years; (2) benign biliary diseases such as cholelithiasis and benign biliary stricture based on US, CT, and MRI; and (3) no history of other malignancies within 5 years. Blood samples were collected at the initial visit. Seven patients were excluded due to a technical failure of CTC detection. Finally, 62 patients were enrolled for the assessment of CTC number (Figure 1).

Patients were followed clinically using medical records to determine treatment regimens and responses, including surgery, disease progression, and time of death. This prospective trial was conducted at a single tertiary medical center with institutional review board approval (H-H-1801-020-062), and all patients provided written informed consent. The Clinical Research Information Service (CRIS) approved this study (KCT0003511).

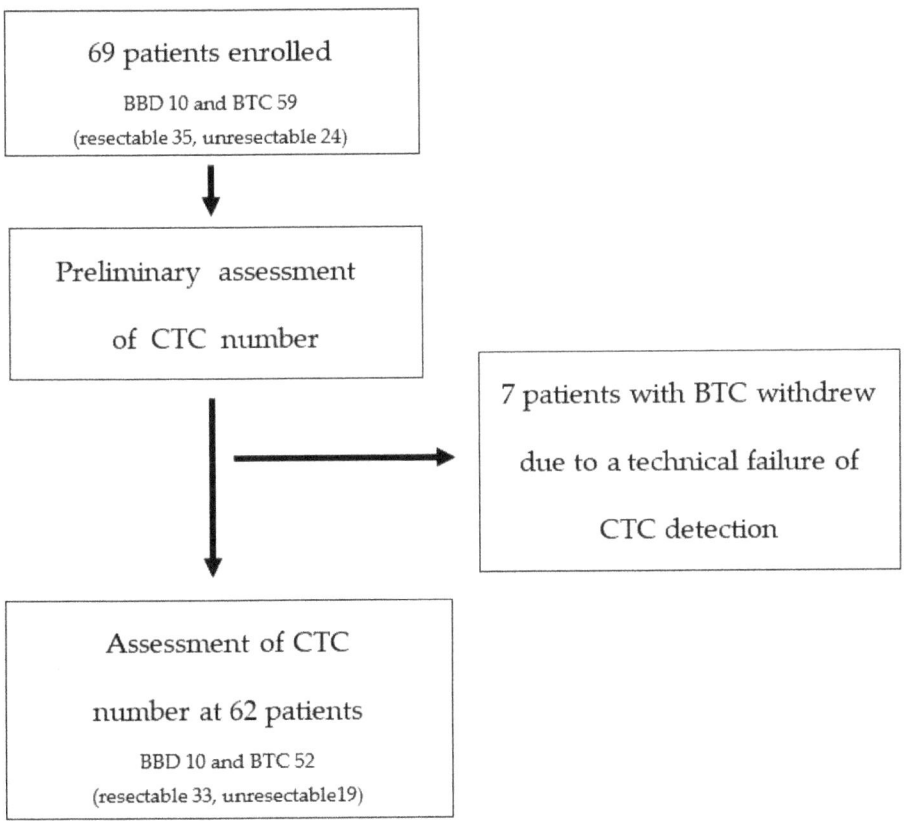

Figure 1. Flow chart of the study. BBD; benign biliary disease, BTC; biliary tract cancer, CTC; circulating tumor cell.

2.2. CTC Enumeration and Characterization

For all cases, peripheral blood samples were maintained at room temperature and pretreatment was performed within 2 h of collection. We used a CD-PRIME™ system (Clinomics, Ulsan, Korea) which is a commercialized version of the FAST disc. The system contains two parts, the CD-CTC™ Duo (disc) and a CD-OPR-1000™ (disc operating machine); we collected intact CTCs from the white buffy coat resuspended with phosphate buffered saline (PBS) in the same amount as the original blood of each BTC patient.

Immunostaining was performed to identify the isolated cells on the membrane in the filtration chamber of the FAST disc. The isolated cells were stained with fluorescence-conjugated antibodies, including FITC conjugated anti-EpCAM antibody (1:417, 9C4; BioLegend, San Diego, CA, USA), Alexa488 conjugated anti-pan-cytokeratin antibody (1:100, AE1/AE3; Invitrogen, Carlsbad, CA, USA), FITC conjugated anti-cytokeratin antibody (1:500, CAM5.2; BD Biosciences, San Diego, CA, USA), Alexa555 conjugated anti-vimentin antibody (1:125, D21H3; Cell signaling, MA, USA), and Cy5 conjugated anti-CD45 antibody (1:50, F10-89-4; Southern biotech, Birmingham, AL, USA) in PBS with 0.01% tween 20 and mounted with 4,6-diamidino-2-phenylindole (DAPI, Abcam, Cambridge, CB2, UK).

The cells were fixed in 4% paraformaldehyde for 20 min and stained with surface antibodies (CD45, EpCAM) in the dark for 20 min. Then, the cells were permeabilized with 0.01% Triton-X for 10 min and stained with intracellular antibodies (cytokeratin, pan-cytokeratin, and vimentin) in the dark for 20 min. Finally, the cells were stained with DAPI and examined under a fluorescence microscope. All staining processes were performed at room temperature, and the cells were washed with PBS in each step.

Cells were counted as CTCs if they had intact morphology (large cell with an intact nucleus; cut-off size of CTCs is 8 μm), stained positive for EpCAM, pan-cytokeratin, cytokeratin, and DAPI, and stained negative for CD45 by researchers blinded to the patient clinical status. In addition, V-CTCs were referred to positive staining for vimentin.

To validate the expression of CTCs, we spiked 100 cells of BTC cell lines such as SNU-1079, SNU-308, and SNU-1196 in 3 mL blood of healthy subjects. After the enrichment of cancer cells from spike-in blood, the cancer cells on the membrane were stained with fluorescence-conjugated antibodies and confirmed the CTCs expression marker.

2.3. Outcome Assessment

The primary study endpoint was to reveal the relationship between baseline CTC counts, V-CTC counts, V-CTC proportion, and the pathologic BTC diagnosis. The secondary endpoints were to find correlations between baseline V-CTC counts, progression free survival (PFS), and overall survival (OS).

The patients were followed for disease progression by imaging and laboratory testing. PFS was defined as the relapsed time from the time of pathologic diagnosis, and was assessed by peripheral blood sample collection, CT, MRI, and positron emission tomography (CA19-9) imaging. OS was defined as the time elapsed from the time of pathologic diagnosis until death.

2.4. Statistical Analysis

Statistical analysis was performed using IBM SPSS statistical software, version 21.0 (IBM Corp, Armonk, NY, USA). Descriptive statistics are presented as frequencies and percentages for categorical variables and as means ± standard deviations for continuous variables. Two or three-sample comparisons were performed using the Student's t-tests and ANOVA test for normally distributed variables. Wilcoxon rank sum tests and Kruskal–Wallis tests were used for non-parametric comparisons. A two-sided p-value of <0.05 was used to indicate statistical significance in all analyses. Differences in OS were plotted using Kaplan–Meier survival plots and tested using log-rank tests. The optimal cut-off value for CTC counts was determined using receiver operating characteristic (ROC) curves and the area under the curve (AUC) values were calculated. To evaluate the factors affecting the prognosis, COX regression analysis was performed, with factors known as prognostic markers and CTC markers as variables.

3. Results

3.1. Patient Characteristics

A total of 62 patients were enrolled for the assessment of CTC markers. Of them, 10 were diagnosed with BBDs and 52 were diagnosed with BTC (8 with gallbladder cancer (GB), 12 with intrahepatic cholangiocarcinoma (IHCC), 21 with extrahepatic cholangiocarcinoma (EHCC), and 11 with perihilar cholangiocarcinoma (PHCC)). Table 1 shows the characteristics of patients with benign, resectable, and unresectable BTC. All epidemiologic factors except smoking status were the same between patients. The mean age of patients with BBDs (50% male) was 66.1 years and that of patients with BTCs (61.5% male) was 69.2 years. The alanine transaminase ALT (28.6 vs. 119.9%, $p = 0.026$), alkaline phosphatase (ALP) (139.9 vs. 326.7, $p = 0.035$), and total bilirubin (0.81 vs. 5.76, $p = 0.048$) levels were significantly different between the BBD and BTC groups, respectively. These factors are markers of biliary obstruction. The CEA (3.0 vs. 3.9 vs. 11.1, $p = 0.021$) and CA19-9 (16.0 vs. 434.3 vs. 1165.1, $p = 0.040$) levels were also significantly different between BBD, resectable BTC, and unresectable BTC groups.

Table 1. Patient characteristics and CTC counts/v-CTC proportion.

	Benign Biliary Disease n = 10	Biliary Tract Cancer n = 52		p-Value
		Resectable n = 33	Unresectable n = 19	
Sex male, (%)	5 (50)	32 (61.5)		0.504
		20 (60.6)	12 (63.2)	0.536
Age	66.1 ± 8.2	69.2 ± 10.8		0.393
		71.4 ± 9.7	65.4 ± 11.8	0.095
Diagnosis	IHD stone/CBD stone/benign biliary stricture 3 (30)/3 (30)/4 (40)	GB/IHCC/EHCC/PHCC 8 (15.4)/12 (23.1)/21 (40.4)/11 (21.2)		
		5 (15.2)/4 (12.1)/18 (54.5)/6 (18.2)	3 (15.8)/8 (42.1)/3 (15.8)/5 (26.3)	
Hepatitis HBV/HCV	0 (0)/0 (0)	3 (5.8)/1 (1.9)		0.402
		1 (3.0)/0 (0)	2 (10.5)/1 (5.3)	0.058
LC	1 (10)	1 (1.9)		0.191
		1 (3.0)	0 (0)	0.171
Hypertension	3 (30)	17 (32.7)		0.870
		14 (42.4)	3 (15.8)	0.245
Diabetes	1 (10)	10 (19.2)		0.492
		8 (24.2)	2 (10.5)	0.771
Smoking none/current/ex-	9 (90)/1 (10)/0 (0)	40 (76.9)/8 (15.4)/4 (7.7)		0.301
		29 (87.9)/3 (33.3)/1 (3.0)	11 (57.9)/5 (26.3)/3 (15.8)	0.012 *
Alcoholic	5 (50)	14 (26.9)		0.152
		8 (24.2)	6 (31.6)	0.477
Dyslipidemia	0 (0)	5 (9.6)		0.314
		3 (9.1)	2 (10.5)	0.382
BMI	23.8 ± 1.7	22.8 ± 3.0		0.283
		23.4 ± 3.0	21.6 ± 2.8	
		Laboratory Findings		
WBC	6068.0 ± 1797.6	7492.1 ± 3739.5		0.246
		7504.2 ± 4093.8	7471.1 ± 3134.6	0.512
NLR	2.59 ± 1.86	4.06 ± 4.27		0.290
		4.26 ± 5.12	3.73 ± 2.22	0.519
Hb	12.7 ± 1.2	12.4 ± 1.7		0.718
		12.6 ± 1.74	12.1 ± 1.74	0.536
PLT (k)	221.6 ± 47.6	270.3 ± 85.3		0.086
		276.3 ± 82.5	259.9 ± 91.4	0.181
ALT	28.6 ± 21.0	119.9 ± 125.0		0.026 *
		140.5 ± 132.5	84.0 ± 104.5	0.020 *
ALP	139.9 ± 163.9	326.7 ± 263.1		0.035 *
		367.9 ± 293.7	255.1 ± 184.9	0.032 *
Total Bilirubin	0.81 ± 3.44	5.76 ± 7.70		0.048 *
		5.60 ± 7.40	6.04 ± 8.38	0.140
Albumin	4.29 ± 0.43	4.01 ± 0.54		0.128
		4.10 ± 0.45	3.84 ± 0.65	0.075

Table 1. Cont.

	Benign Biliary Disease n = 10	Biliary Tract Cancer n = 52		p-Value
		Resectable n = 33	Unresectable n = 19	
PNI	50.9 ± 5.4	47.6 ± 6.5		0.134
		48.6 ± 5.6	46.0 ± 7.8	0.118
BUN	11.6 ± 3.6	14.4 ± 5.2		0.108
		15.2 ± 4.9	13.0 ± 5.5	0.092
Creatinine	0.72 ± 0.10	0.79 ± 0.21		0.325
		0.83 ± 0.20	0.72 ± 0.22	0.105
C-related protein	1.52 ± 1.57	2.54 ± 3.86		0.421
		2.16 ± 3.65	3.19 ± 4.22	0.446
CEA	3.0 ± 1.2	6.5 ± 9.8		0.430
		3.9 ± 2.8	11.1 ± 15.0	0.021 *
CA19-9	16.0 ± 9.5	701.3 ± 1240.2		0.185
		434.3 ± 930.8	1165.1 ± 1568.3	0.040 *

IHD (intrahepatic duct), CBD (common bile duct), GB (gallbladder), IHCC (intrahepatic cholangiocarcinoma), EHCC (extrahepatic cholangiocarcinoma), HBV (hepatitis B virus), HCV (hepatitis C virus), LC (liver cirrhosis), NLR (neutrophil/lymphocyte ratio), PNI (prognostic nutrition index) *: p-value < 0.05.

3.2. CTC Counts in BTC and BBD

Figure 2 shows the results of CTC and V-CTC analysis in patients with unresectable and resectable BTC and patients with BBD. Though the CTC and V-CTC counts differed between the BTC and BBD groups, this difference was not significant, whereas the V-CTC/total CTC count ratio (VCR) showed a statistically significant difference between the groups (35.7% vs. 23.8%, respectively, p = 0.048). There were no statistically significant differences in CTC count, V-CTC count, and VCR between patients with resectable and unresectable BTC (Figure 3). The CTC count, V-CTC count, and VCR cut-off values, determined via ROC curve analysis, were 40/mL blood, 15/mL blood, and 40%, respectively (Supplementary Figure S1.) When CTCs were analyzed using these cut-off values, significant difference across all three parameters were found between the BTC and BBD groups (CTC > 40: 55.8% vs. 20%, p = 0.039; V-CTC > 15: 57.7% vs. 10%, p = 0.005; VCR > 40%: 48.1% vs. 10%, p = 0.025, respectively). Analyzing any two of the three parameters in combination precipitated a more statistically significant difference between the BTC and BBD groups (61.5% vs. 10%, p = 0.002) than using any one parameter alone (p = 0.002). Notably, when patients showed two of three parameters plus biopsy results or elevated CA19-9 levels, the sensitivity and specificity of discrimination between BBD and BTC increased (90.4% vs. 10%, p < 0.001). (Table 2).

Table 2. CTC count and sensitivity and specificity of each parameter between benign and biliary tract cancer.

	Benign Biliary Disease n = 10	Biliary Tract Cancer n = 52		p-Value
		Resectable n = 33	Unresectable n = 19	
CTC count	30.9 ± 16.7	125.7 ± 259.8		0.256
		145.8 ± 320.2	90.7 ± 82.9	0.386
CTC count > 40	2 (20)	29 (55.8)		0.039 *
		18 (54.5)	11 (57.9)	0.090
V-CTC	8.6 ± 7.3	39.8 ± 89.6		0.278
		45.6 ± 110.3	29.8 ± 30.4	0.449
V-CTC > 15	1 (10)	30 (57.7)		0.005 *
		17 (51.5)	13 (68.4)	0.004 *

Table 2. Cont.

	Benign Biliary Disease $n = 10$	Biliary Tract Cancer $n = 52$		p-Value
		Resectable $n = 33$	Unresectable $n = 19$	
VCR (%)	23.8 ± 11.8	35.7 ± 17.9		0.048 *
		36.2 ± 17.7	34.9 ± 18.6	0.139
VCR > 40% (%)	1 (10)	25 (48.1)		0.025 *
		15 (45.5)	10 (52.6)	0.045 *
Over two of three parameters (1)	1 (10)	32 (61.5)		0.002 *
		19 (68.4)	13 (68.4)	0.005 *
(1) and/or biopsy	1 (10)	47 (90.4)		<0.001 *
		29 (87.9)	18 (94.7)	<0.001 *
(1) and/or CA19-9	1 (10)	47 (90.4)		<0.001 *
		28 (84.8)	19 (100)	<0.001 *
	AUC	Sensitivity		Specificity
Over two of three parameters (1)	0.758	61.5%		90%
Biopsy	0.885	78%		100%
CA19-9 > UNL	0.846	60.6%		100%
(1) and/or biopsy (+)	0.902	90.4%		90%
(1) and/or CA19-9 > UNL	0.902	90.4%		90%

BTC, biliary tract cancer; V-CTC, Vimentin + CTC; VCR, vimentin/CTC ratio; Three parameter (CTC count > 40, V-CTC > 15, VCR > 40%), Biopsy (+): malignancy was proven by biopsy, UNL: upper normal limit, AUC: area under curve, *: p-value < 0.05.

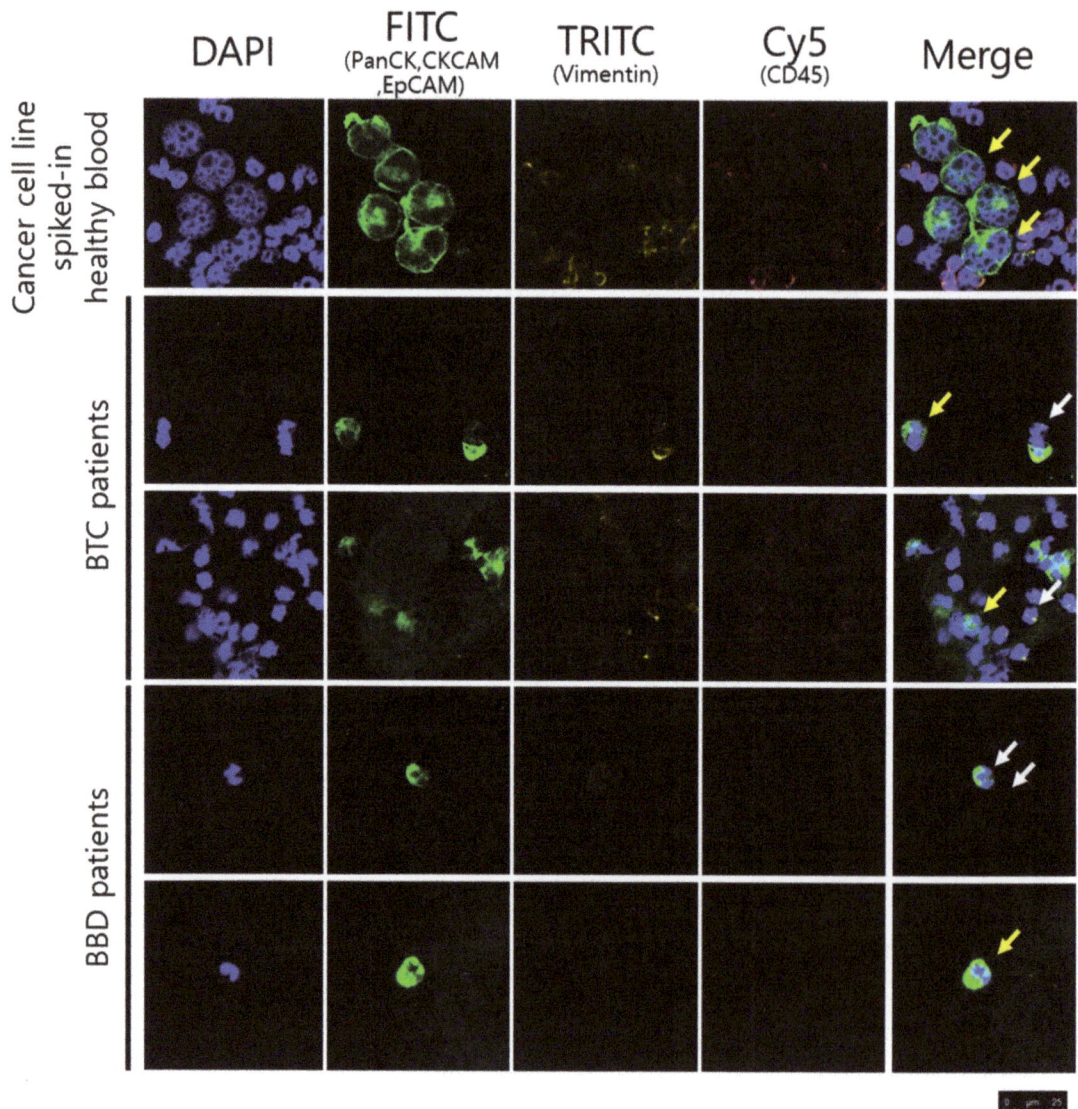

Figure 2. The yellow arrows indicate CTCs (PanCK+/CKCAM+/EpCAM+/CD45-) and white arrows indicate V-CTCs (PanCK+/CKCAM+/EpCAM+/CD45-, vimentin+) in BTC and BBD patients.

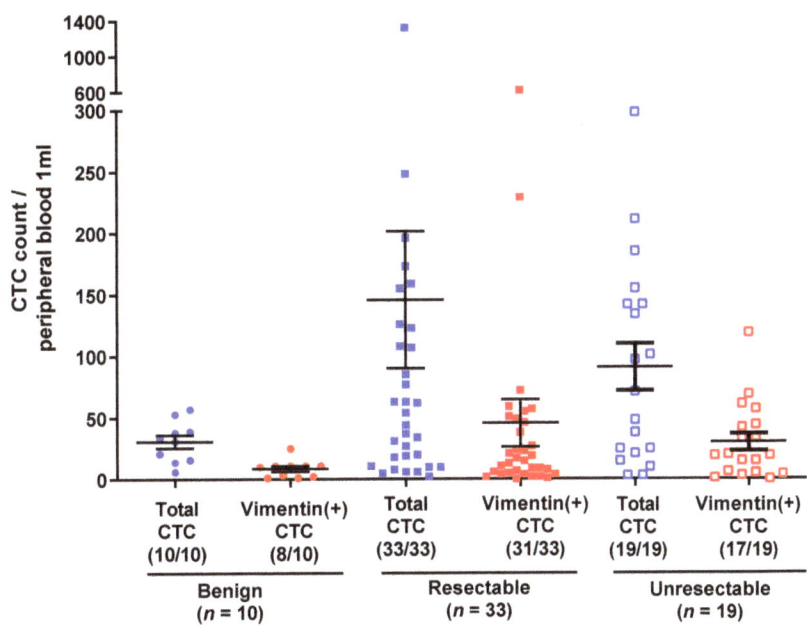

Figure 3. CTC counts and V-CTC counts in patients with biliary disease.

3.3. Subgroup Analysis: Benign vs. Resectable Biliary Tract Cancer

Table 3 shows the CTC counts of the BBD and resectable BTC groups. The indicators used to distinguish the BTC and BBD groups were applied between resectable BTC and BBDs. CTC count > 40/mL blood (54.5% vs. 20%, $p = 0.002$), V-CTC count > 15/mL blood (51.5% vs. 10%, $p < 0.001$), and VCR > 40% (45.5% vs. 10%, $p = 0.000$) were used to differentiate the two groups. Using two of the three parameters in combination (57.6% vs. 10%, $p = 0.007$) also yielded statistically significant results. Further, using a combination of these parameters, patient biopsy results, and elevated CA19-9 level data also increased the sensitivity and specificity of discriminating between BBDs and resectable BTC (Table 3).

Table 3. CTC count and sensitivity and specificity of each parameter between benign and resectable biliary tract cancer.

	Benign Biliary Disease $n = 10$	Resectable BTC $n = 33$	p-Value
CTC count	30.9 ± 16.7	145.8 ± 320.1	0.194
CTC count > 40	2 (20)	18 (54.5)	0.002 *
V-CTC	8.6 ± 7.3	45.6 ± 110.3	0.087
V-CTC >15	1 (10)	17 (51.5)	<0.001 *
VCR	23.8 ± 11.8	36.18 ± 17.7	0.031 *
VCR > 40%	1 (10)	15 (45.5)	<0.001 *
Over two of three parameter (1)	1 (10)	19 (57.6)	0.007 *
(1) and/or biopsy	1 (10)	29 (87.9)	<0.001 *
(1) and/or CA19-9	1 (10)	28 (84.8)	<0.001 *

Table 3. *Cont.*

	Benign Biliary Disease $n = 10$	Resectable BTC $n = 33$	*p*-Value
	AUC	Sensitivity	Specificity
Over two of three parameter (1)	0.738	57.6%	90%
(1) and/or biopsy	0.889	87.9%	90%
(1) and/or CA19-9	0.874	84.8%	90%

BTC, biliary tract cancer; V-CTC, Vimentin + CTC; VCR, vimentin/CTC ratio; Three parameter (CTC count > 40, V-CTC > 15, VCR > 40%) AUC: area under curve, *: *p*-value < 0.05.

3.4. Association of the CTC Count with Prognosis

In the prognostic analysis of patients with BTC using their neutrophil/lymphocyte ratio (NLR), CA19-9 level, CTC count, V-CTC count, and VCR data, V-CTC counts > 50/mL blood was found to be the most significant (Table 4.) This cut-off value of V-CTC count was determined by ROC curve analysis, under or over 250 days (mean OS = 257 ± 184 days, AUC = 0.615, sensitivity = 32.1%, specificity = 87.5%). There was no significant difference in the baseline characteristics between the groups according to V-CTC counts of 50/mL blood (Table 5). Other non-significantly different prognostic markers included the NLR. Figure 4 shows the Kaplan–Meier survival analysis. Patients BTC with V-CTC count > 50/mL blood showed a poorer prognosis than other patients with BTC (median survival: 140 (66.6–213.3) vs. 253 (163.9–342.1) days, p = 0.008). In patients with resectable BTC, the prognosis was significantly different between patients with V-CTC count >50/mL blood and V-CTC count < 50/mL blood (median survival: 167 (97.7–236.3) vs. 311 (254.8–367.2) days, p = 0.004). The median survival of the V-CTC count > 50 and count < 50 groups in subgroup analysis according to the location of the cancer was 170 (0–345.3) vs. 95 (0–224.6) days for IHCC (p = 0.076), 307 (267.8–346.2) vs. 218 (117.1–318.9) days for EHCC (p = 0.072), and 324 (6.8–443.1) vs. 138 days for GB cancer (p = 0.353), which was similar to the result obtained with the total number of patients, though the number of patients in each subgroup was too low to obtain meaningful results. The PHCC group showed similar median survival between the >50 and <50 V-CTC count groups (293 (141.1–444.9) vs. 245 days, p = 0.835) (Supplementary Table S1.) However, PFS was not significantly different between the groups in accordance with any CTC marker, except CA19-9 level (CA19-9 < 40 vs. >40: 284 (168.5–399.5) vs. 163 (152.5–217.4) days, p = 0.011, respectively) (Supplementary Table S2).

Table 4. Prognostic factor analysis via Cox regression analysis.

	Univariable Analysis		Multivariable Analysis	
	HR (95%CI)	*p*-Value	HR (95%CI)	*p*-Value
V-CTC > 50	2.042 (1.006–4.146)	0.048 *	2.172 (1.064–4.433)	0.033 *
CTC count > 40	1.665 (0.927–2.989)	0.088	1.427 (0.717–2.841)	0.311
VCR > 40%	1.154 (0.660–2.016)	0.615	1.030 (0.583–1.820)	0.919
CA19-9 > UNL	1.622 (0.881–2.988)	0.121	1.705 (0.924–3.148)	0.088
NLR > 3.5	1.149 (0.637–2.073)	0.645	1.716 (0.885–3.327)	0.110

HR, Hazard ratio; CI, confidence interval; CTC, circulating tumor cells; V-CTC, Vimentin + CTC; VCR, vimentin/CTC rate; UNL, upper normal limit; NLR, neutrophil-lymphocyte ratio, *: *p*-value < 0.05.

Table 5. Baseline characteristics according to V-CTC level.

	V-CTC Over 50 (n = 11)	V-CTC Under 50 (n = 41)	p-Value
Sex male, (%)	5 (45.5)	27 (65.9)	0.225
Age	73.1 ± 12.2	68.1 ± 10.3	0.179
Diagnosis GB/IHCC/EHCC/PHCC	1 (9.1)/3 (27.3)/5 (45.5)/2 (18.2)	7 (17.1)/9 (22.0)/16 (39.0)/9 (22.0)	0.839
hepatitis HBV/HCV	0 (0)/1 (9.1)	3 (7.3)/0 (0)	0.376
Liver cirrhosis	0 (0)	1 (2.4)	0.609
Hypertension	6 (54.5)	11 (26.8)	0.085
Diabetes	3 (27.3)	7 (17.1)	0.456
smoking none/current/ex-	8 (72.7)/3 (27.3)/0 (0)	32 (78.0)/5 (12.2)/4 (9.8)	0.833
alcoholic	3 (27.3)	11 (26.8)	0.977
Dyslipidemia	2 (18.2)	3 (7.3)	0.287
BMI	22.4 ± 2.6	22.9 ± 3.2	0.617
Pathology well-/moder-/poor	0 (0)/2 (18.2)/2 (18.2)	4 (9.8)/17 (41.5)/7 (17.1)	0.031 *
Metastatic	3 (27.3)	9 (22.0)	0.716
Operable	7 (63.6)	26 (63.4)	0.989
Palliative Chemotherapy	2 (18.2)	11 (26.8)	0.565
Op and no recurrence	3 (27.3)	16 (39.0)	0.320
Laboratory Findings			
WBC	6503.6 ± 1789.0	7757.3 ± 4085.1	0.328
NLR	3.2 ± 1.3	4.3 ± 4.8	0.444
Hb	11.9 ± 0.9	12.6 ± 1.9	0.292
PLT (k)	241.6 ± 91.2	278.0 ± 83.1	0.213
ALT	124.5 ± 117.8	118.6 ± 128.3	0.890
ALP	349.8 ± 328.0	320.5 ± 247.3	0.746
Total bilirubin	7.81 ± 8.97	5.21 ± 7.34	0.323
Albumin	3.93 ± 0.61	4.03 ± 0.53	0.609
PNI	46.7 ± 7.8	47.9 ± 6.2	0.618
BUN	16.7 ± 5.8	13.8 ± 4.9	0.095
Creatinine	0.86 ± 0.23	0.77 ± 0.21	0.250
C-related protein	2.0 ± 2.1	2.7 ± 4.2	0.632
CEA	11.1 ± 18.9	5.2 ± 4.6	0.082
CA19-9	654.5 ± 1198.6	713.9 ± 1265.3	0.889

GB (gallbladder), IHCC (intrahepatic cholangiocarcinoma), EHCC (extrahepatic cholangiocarcinoma), PHCC (perihilar cholangiocarcinoma), HBV (hepatitis B virus), HCV (hepatitis C virus), LC (liver cirrhosis), NLR (neutrophil/lymphocyte ratio), PNI (prognostic nutrition index), *: p-value < 0.05.

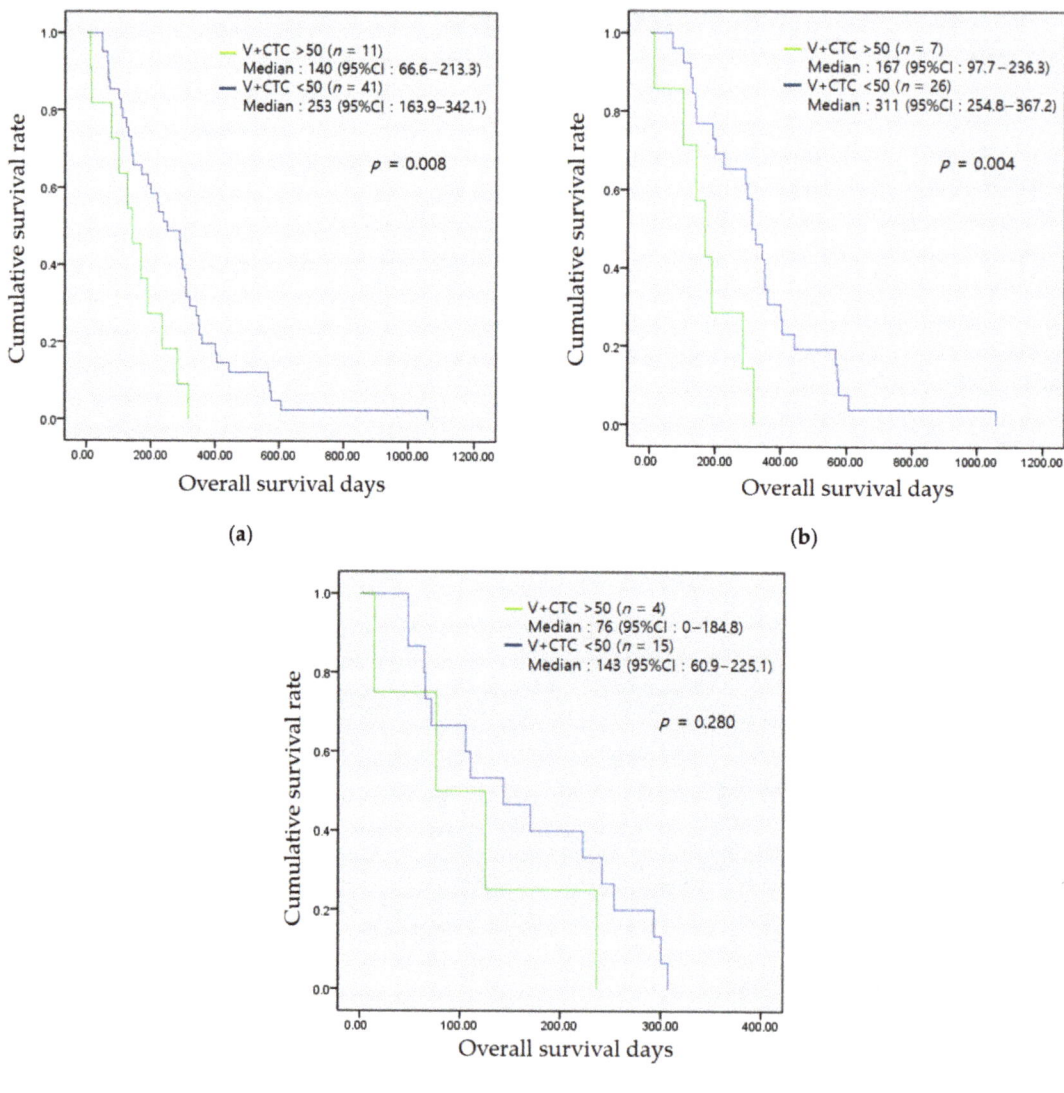

Figure 4. Kaplan–Meier overall survival in total (**a**), resectable (**b**) and unresectable (**c**) biliary tract cancer patients.

3.5. Technical Failure of CTC Detection in Patients with Biliary Tract Cancers

CTC detection failed in 7 of the 69 patients with BTC enrolled in this study, all of whom were in the advanced disease stage. In all seven patients, large amounts of amorphous necrotic matrices made it impossible to count the CTCs accurately. Further, all seven patients showed more frequent metastasis (71.4% vs. 23.1%, $p = 0.007$), significantly lower platelet counts (187k vs. 270k, $p = 0.017$), higher NLR (18.7 vs. 4.1, $p < 0.001$), and higher CA19-9 levels (4475 vs. 701, $p < 0.001$) than patients with detectable CTCs (Supplementary Table S3).

4. Discussion

The estimation of V-CTCs is a potential diagnostic approach for BTC, in addition to evaluating CA 19-9 levels, radiologic imaging, and core or forceps biopsy. Since the CTC markers have low diagnostic accuracy when used independently, we used the CTC markers in combination. Though evaluation using a combination of CTC markers improves accuracy, diagnosing BTC based on CTC markers alone is difficult. Thus, combining the results of this estimation with those obtained by traditional method, such as biopsy and CA19-9 level assessment, can facilitate accurate BTC diagnosis. Furthermore, the V-CTC count was related to OS, especially that of patients with resectable BTC. In multivariate analysis including CA19-9 levels, which is a well-known prognostic factor of BTC, the only significant prognostic factor was a V-CTC count > 50. However, additional studies are needed to support this result.

Efforts towards early diagnosis and prognosis prediction are constantly being made in cancer research. Recently, with the advent of precision medicine, interest in the use of target markers to provide personalized treatment, based on the systemic biology of cancer, has increased. However, there are no minimally invasive methods currently available to accurately diagnose early-stage cancer or predict cancer progression. Recently, studies have been conducted to analyze CTCs, circulating tumor DNA (ctDNA), and extracellular vesicles derived from tumors. Beyond aiding in early cancer diagnosis and prognosis determination, these circulating tumor markers form the basis of many key aspects of precision medicine, including determining actionable targets, monitoring treatment response and resistance, and selecting therapeutics.

There are two important steps in the assessment of CTCs. First, cell enrichment is performed using biological and physical properties. Then, protein-based techniques are used for positive CTC selection. This selection relies on the detection of specific markers by antibodies. However, the expression of epithelial markers such as EpCAM and pan-cytokeratin can be reduced during EMT, which can result in false negatives. Thus, mesenchymal markers, such as N-cadherin and vimentin, should be used [13]. The proportion of true mesenchymal phenotype of CTCs would be very limited because the EMT is a dynamic process when entering the circulation [14,15]. Another way to enrich CTCs is to distinguish CTCs based on their physical properties.

There are many challenges in the assessment of CTCs. The reproducibility of these assessments is difficult since the detected CTC subpopulations may vary across experiments. Additionally, CTCs are large and can be trapped in peripheral blood vessels. CTCs also undergo apoptosis 1–2 h after entering the bloodstream, which may result in low levels of CTCs being detected. Another challenge is the discrimination of CTCs from normal circulating cells. In a study involving patients with benign colonic disease, 11–19% of the patients had epithelial cells that were considered CTCs [16]. For this reason, CTC detection methods usually use epithelial cell adhesion molecules (EpCAMs), which may lead to an underestimation of CTC counts [17].

In this study, we used a platform comprising a centrifugal microfluidic device with a fluid-assisted separation filter membrane (FAST disc) to collect CTCs. The FAST disc enabled label-free CTC isolation from whole blood in a size-selective manner via tangential flow filtration (TFF). This system allowed a clog-free, ultrafast (>3 mL/min) CTC enrichment with gentle pressure drops (~1 kPa) for high viability. Since only gentle pressure was used, cells of various sizes were captured on the membrane, thus facilitating the counting of intact CTCs and allowing for the collection of a large number of tumor cells with high viability. Using vimentin to identify cells in the EMT process increased CTC counts [18,19]. In our study, high counts of CTCs, especially V-CTCs, were found even in patients with BBDs, indicating that the EMT process may also occur in BBDs.

A novel platform to diagnose BTC and predict its prognosis is required for several reasons. Patients with BTC usually present with non-specific symptoms, such as dyspepsia, weight loss, and abdominal discomfort in the early disease stage. A positive BTC diagnosis is usually only made in the later stages of the disease when overt symptoms, such as jaundice, are present. Imaging by US, CT, and MRI is effective for detecting masses in the biliary tract. However, due to the low incidence of the disease, these methods are not cost-effective for BTC diagnosis. The pathologic diagnosis of BTC is difficult due to various anatomical factors, such as the deep location of the liver, the superficial spread of the bile duct, and the complex blood vessel distribution around the tumor. Although liver core biopsy, forceps biopsy through endoscopic retrograde cholangiopancreatography (ERCP), and brush cytology through ERCP are currently available techniques, they are both invasive and unsuitable for obtaining a sufficiently large cell for pathologic diagnosis because BTC tissues are paucicellular within abundant stroma. However, it is not always possible to obtain tissue samples from primary or metastatic sites. Even if tissue samples are obtained at the time of initial diagnosis, it is not certain that they can be obtained at recurrence or during tumor progression. Therefore, we aimed to develop a method for detecting high-risk groups by screening images during early BTC diagnosis.

In early BTC research, CTCs were detected using CEA-nested RT-PCR in the nucleated cell fraction. The detection rate of CEA-mRNA was 47.8–52.5% (21 of 40 patients with biliary-pancreatic cancers), which was relatively lower than that reported in a recent study [20,21].

Through analysis using the CellSearch system, low counts of CTCs were found in patients with BTC. The detection rate of CTCs in 3 of 13 BTCs is 23.1% [22]. The 12-month survival rates of the patients in the CTC-positive and CTC-negative groups were 25% and 50%, respectively. In another study [23], 88 patients (17%) were positive for CTCs with more than two, which was an independent predictor of survival. Although CTC detection is rare, assessing CTC counts may be useful for predicting the mortality risk of BTC. However, in a recent study evaluating the therapeutic efficacy of cediranib, no relationship between CTC count detection and survival was found. Furthermore, the benefits of cediranib treatment could not be predicted by the combined analysis of baseline and cycle 3 CTC count [24].

A new marker was evaluated for the detection of more CTCs in patients with BTC. In nonconventional CTCs (ncCTCs) lacking epithelial and leukocyte markers, the positive identification of CTCs increased from 19% to 83% [25]. ncCTCs are also correlated with disease-specific survival. Using a novel glycosaminoglycan, SCH45, CTCs were detected in 65 patients with advanced BTC. Furthermore, SCH45-based CTC counts were correlated with the prognosis of patients with BTC receiving chemotherapy [26]. Ninety percent of patients with pancreatic biliary cancers expressed pan-cytokeratin or V-CTCs, which increased the diagnostic accuracy of pancreatic biliary cancers [27].

We excluded seven patients in whom CTCs were not detected from the analysis. In all seven patients, only large amounts of amorphous necrotic matrices were found. These patients had a high ratio of metastasis, high levels of CA19-9, and a higher NLR compared to the other patients. Since CTCs were mostly not detected in patients with advanced cancers, the non-detection of CTCs with extensive necrotic materials may indicate an advanced cancer stage.

There are several limitations to this study. First, this study was conducted with a small number of patients with BTC and BBDs. Second, the patients with BBDs presented with active inflammation. Although blood was drawn immediately after the infection was controlled, the active inflammation may have affected the detection of epithelial cells in circulation. Third, we did not obtain follow-up blood samples to assess the dynamics of CTCs during therapy.

Many researchers have worked to identify the best biomarkers for diagnosing early-stage BTC. However, this is made difficult by the anatomical and histological characteristics of BTC. The combined assessment of circulating tumor markers and CA 19-9 levels, radiological imaging, and core or forceps biopsy may be helpful in discriminating CTCs between early-stage BTC and BBDs, and in determining future prognosis in patients with resectable BTCs. Although there are still limitations to early BTC diagnosis using V-CTCs, further studies may provide a framework for realizing precision medicine by conducting liquid biopsies using CTCs in a complementary manner.

Supplementary Materials: The following are available online at https://www.mdpi.com/article/10.3390/jcm10194435/s1, Table S1: prognostic value according to V-CTC level in subgroup analysis, Table S2: comparison of PFS according to CTC marker and CA19-9 in 35 patients who underwent curative surgery or palliative chemotherapy, Table S3: Baseline characteristics between BTC patients with CTC detected and those without CTC detection, Figure S1: ROC curves of CTC, V-CTC, and VCR.

Author Contributions: S.Y.H. and S.H.P. contributed equally to the work. Study concept and design; D.U.K.; Data acquisition; S.Y.H., S.H.P., A.J., S.J.L.; Data analysis and interpretation; S.Y.H., S.H.P., H.S.K.; Drafting of the manuscript; S.Y.H., S.H.P., H.I.S., D.U.K.; Critical revision of the manuscript; G.H.K., D.U.K. All authors have read and agreed to the published version of the manuscript.

Funding: This research was supported by a grant of the Korea Health Technology R&D Project through the Korea Health Industry Development Institute (KHIDI), funded by the Ministry of Health & Welfare, Republic of Korea (grant number: HI19C0521).

Institutional Review Board Statement: Approved by Institutional Review Board of Pusan National University Hospital (H-H-1801-020-062). The clinical research information service (CRIS) approved the study (KCT0003511).

Informed Consent Statement: Informed consent was obtained from all subjects involved in the study.

Data Availability Statement: All relevant data contained within the article and supplementary materials.

Conflicts of Interest: The authors declare no conflict of interest.

References

1. Banales, J.M.; Marin, J.J.; Lamarca, A.; Rodrigues, P.M.; Khan, S.A.; Roberts, L.R.; Cardinale, V.; Carpino, G.; Andersen, J.B.; Braconi, C. Cholangiocarcinoma 2020: The next horizon in mechanisms and management. *Nat. Rev. Gastroenterol. Hepatol.* **2020**, *17*, 557–588. [CrossRef] [PubMed]
2. Florio, A.A.; Ferlay, J.; Znaor, A.; Ruggieri, D.; Alvarez, C.S.; Laversanne, M.; Bray, F.; McGlynn, K.A.; Petrick, J.L. Global trends in intrahepatic and extrahepatic cholangiocarcinoma incidence from 1993 to 2012. *Cancer* **2020**, *126*, 2666–2678. [CrossRef] [PubMed]
3. Kim, D.; Konyn, P.; Cholankeril, G.; Bonham, C.A.; Ahmed, A. Trends in the Mortality of Biliary Tract Cancers Based on Their Anatomical Site in the United States From 2009 to 2018. *Am. Coll. Gastroenterol.* **2021**, *116*, 1053–1062. [CrossRef] [PubMed]
4. Petrick, J.L.; Yang, B.; Altekruse, S.F.; Van Dyke, A.L.; Koshiol, J.; Graubard, B.I.; McGlynn, K.A. Risk factors for intrahepatic and extrahepatic cholangiocarcinoma in the United States: A population-based study in SEER-Medicare. *PLoS ONE* **2017**, *12*, e0186643. [CrossRef]
5. Van Dyke, A.L.; Shiels, M.S.; Jones, G.S.; Pfeiffer, R.M.; Petrick, J.L.; Beebe-Dimmer, J.L.; Koshiol, J. Biliary tract cancer incidence and trends in the United States by demographic group, 1999–2013. *Cancer* **2019**, *125*, 1489–1498. [CrossRef] [PubMed]
6. Uenishi, T.; Kubo, S.; Yamamoto, T.; Shuto, T.; Ogawa, M.; Tanaka, H.; Tanaka, S.; Kaneda, K.; Hirohashi, K. Cytokeratin 19 expression in hepatocellular carcinoma predicts early postoperative recurrence. *Cancer Sci.* **2003**, *94*, 851–857. [CrossRef] [PubMed]
7. Gabriel, M.T.; Calleja, L.R.; Chalopin, A.; Ory, B.; Heymann, D. Circulating tumor cells: A review of non–EpCAM-based approaches for cell enrichment and isolation. *Clin. Chem.* **2016**, *62*, 571–581. [CrossRef] [PubMed]
8. Millner, L.M.; Linder, M.W.; Valdes, R. Circulating tumor cells: A review of present methods and the need to identify heterogeneous phenotypes. *Ann. Clin. Lab. Sci.* **2013**, *43*, 295–304.
9. Onuigbo, W.B. An index of the fate of circulating cancer cells. *Lancet* **1963**, *282*, 828–831. [CrossRef]
10. Robinson, K.; McGrath, R.; McGrew, E. Circulating cancer cells in patients with lung tumors. *Surgery* **1963**, *53*, 630–636.
11. Xie, X.; Wang, L.; Wang, X.; Fan, W.-H.; Qin, Y.; Lin, X.; Xie, Z.; Liu, M.; Ouyang, M.; Li, S. Evaluation of cell surface vimentin positive circulating tumor cells as a diagnostic biomarker for lung cancer. *Front. Oncol.* **2021**, *11*, 1712.
12. Satelli, A.; Li, S. Vimentin in cancer and its potential as a molecular target for cancer therapy. *Cell. Mol. Life Sci.* **2011**, *68*, 3033–3046. [CrossRef]
13. Pantel, K.; Alix-Panabières, C. Liquid biopsy and minimal residual disease—Latest advances and implications for cure. *Nat. Rev. Clin. Oncol.* **2019**, *16*, 409–424. [CrossRef]
14. Semaan, A.; Bernard, V.; Kim, D.U.; Lee, J.J.; Huang, J.; Kamyabi, N.; Stephens, B.M.; Qiao, W.; Varadhachary, G.R.; Katz, M.H. Characterisation of circulating tumour cell phenotypes identifies a partial-EMT sub-population for clinical stratification of pancreatic cancer. *Br. J. Cancer* **2021**, *124*, 1970–1977. [CrossRef]
15. De Craene, B.; Berx, G. Regulatory networks defining EMT during cancer initiation and progression. *Nat. Rev. Cancer* **2013**, *13*, 97–110. [CrossRef] [PubMed]

16. Pantel, K.; Denève, E.; Nocca, D.; Coffy, A.; Vendrell, J.-P.; Maudelonde, T.; Riethdorf, S.; Alix-Panabières, C. Circulating epithelial cells in patients with benign colon diseases. *Clin. Chem.* **2012**, *58*, 936–940. [CrossRef] [PubMed]
17. Grover, P.; Cummins, A.; Price, T.; Roberts-Thomson, I.; Hardingham, J. Circulating tumour cells: The evolving concept and the inadequacy of their enrichment by EpCAM-based methodology for basic and clinical cancer research. *Ann. Oncol.* **2014**, *25*, 1506–1516. [CrossRef]
18. Wei, T.; Zhang, X.; Zhang, Q.; Yang, J.; Chen, Q.; Wang, J.; Li, X.; Chen, J.; Ma, T.; Li, G. Vimentin-positive circulating tumor cells as a biomarker for diagnosis and treatment monitoring in patients with pancreatic cancer. *Cancer Lett.* **2019**, *452*, 237–243. [CrossRef]
19. Gao, Y.; Fan, W.-H.; Song, Z.; Lou, H.; Kang, X. Comparison of circulating tumor cell (CTC) detection rates with epithelial cell adhesion molecule (EpCAM) and cell surface vimentin (CSV) antibodies in different solid tumors: A retrospective study. *PeerJ* **2021**, *9*, e10777. [CrossRef]
20. Miyazono, F.; Takao, S.; Natsugoe, S.; Uchikura, K.; Kijima, F.; Aridome, K.; Shinchi, H.; Aikou, T. Molecular detection of circulating cancer cells during surgery in patients with biliary-pancreatic cancer. *Am. J. Surg.* **1999**, *177*, 475–479. [CrossRef]
21. Uchikura, K.; Takao, S.; Nakajo, A.; Miyazono, F.; Nakashima, S.; Tokuda, K.; Matsumoto, M.; Shinchi, H.; Natsugoe, S.; Aikou, T. Intraoperative molecular detection of circulating tumor cells by reverse transcription-polymerase chain reaction in patients with biliary-pancreatic cancer is associated with hematogenous metastasis. *Ann. Surg. Oncol.* **2002**, *9*, 364–370. [CrossRef]
22. Al Ustwani, O.; Iancu, D.; Yacoub, R.; Iyer, R. Detection of circulating tumor cells in cancers of biliary origin. *J. Gastrointest. Oncol.* **2012**, *3*, 97. [CrossRef] [PubMed]
23. Yang, J.D.; Campion, M.B.; Liu, M.C.; Chaiteerakij, R.; Giama, N.H.; Ahmed Mohammed, H.; Zhang, X.; Hu, C.; Campion, V.L.; Jen, J. Circulating tumor cells are associated with poor overall survival in patients with cholangiocarcinoma. *Hepatology* **2016**, *63*, 148–158. [CrossRef] [PubMed]
24. Backen, A.C.; Lopes, A.; Wasan, H.; Palmer, D.H.; Duggan, M.; Cunningham, D.; Anthoney, A.; Corrie, P.G.; Madhusudan, S.; Maraveyas, A. Circulating biomarkers during treatment in patients with advanced biliary tract cancer receiving cediranib in the UK ABC-03 trial. *Br. J. Cancer* **2018**, *119*, 27–35. [CrossRef] [PubMed]
25. Reduzzi, C.; Vismara, M.; Silvestri, M.; Celio, L.; Niger, M.; Peverelli, G.; De Braud, F.; Daidone, M.G.; Cappelletti, V. A novel circulating tumor cell subpopulation for treatment monitoring and molecular characterization in biliary tract cancer. *Int. J. Cancer* **2020**, *146*, 3495–3503. [CrossRef] [PubMed]
26. Gopinathan, P.; Chiang, N.J.; Bandaru, A.; Sinha, A.; Huang, W.Y.; Hung, S.C.; Shan, Y.S.; Lee, G.B. Exploring circulating tumor cells in cholangiocarcinoma using a novel glycosaminoglycan probe on a microfluidic platform. *Adv. Healthc. Mater.* **2020**, *9*, 1901875. [CrossRef] [PubMed]
27. Konno, N.; Suzuki, R.; Takagi, T.; Sugimoto, M.; Asama, H.; Sato, Y.; Irie, H.; Hikichi, T.; Ohira, H. Clinical utility of a newly developed microfluidic device for detecting circulating tumor cells in the blood of patients with pancreatico-biliary malignancies. *J. Hepato-Biliary-Pancreat. Sci.* **2021**, *28*, 115–124. [CrossRef]

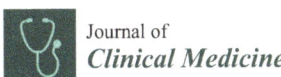

Article

Clinical Limitations of Tissue Annexin A2 Level as a Predictor of Postoperative Overall Survival in Patients with Hepatocellular Carcinoma

Shu-Wei Huang [1,2], Yen-Chin Chen [3], Yang-Hsiang Lin [2,*] and Chau-Ting Yeh [2,*]

1. Department of Gastroenterology and Hepatology, New Taipei Municipal Tucheng Hospital, New Taipei 236, Taiwan; huangshuwei@gmail.com
2. Liver Research Center, Chang Gung Memorial Hospital, Linkou, Taoyuan 333, Taiwan
3. Graduate Institute of Clinical Medicine, Chang Gung University, Taoyuan 333, Taiwan; sunnychen168@gmail.com
* Correspondence: yhlin0621@cgmh.org.tw (Y.-H.L.); chautingy@gmail.com (C.-T.Y.); Tel.: +886-3328-1200 (ext. 7785) (Y.-H.L.); +886-3328-1200 (ext. 8129) (C.-T.Y.); Fax: +886-3328-2824 (C.-T.Y.)

Abstract: Hepatocellular carcinoma (HCC) is the second common cause of cancer-related death in Taiwan. Tumor recurrence is frequently observed in HCC patients receiving surgical resection, resulting in unsatisfactory overall survival (OS). Therefore, it is pivotal to identify effective prognostic makers, so that intensive surveillance or adjuvant treatments can be applied to predictively unfavorable patients. Previous studies indicated that Annexin A2 (ANXA2) was an effective prognostic marker in several cancers, including HCC. However, the prognostic value of ANXA2 in Taiwanese HCC patients remains unclear, where a great proportion of patients had chronic hepatitis B with liver cirrhosis. Here, ANXA2 was highly expressed in HCC tissues compared with para-neoplastic noncancerous tissues. Furthermore, high ANXA2 expression in HCC tissues independently predicted shorter OS. In subgroup analysis, however, ANXA2 expression could not effectively predict OS in the following subgroups: female, age > 65 years old, Child–Pugh classification B, hepatitis B virus surface antigen negative or anti-hepatitis C antibody positive, alcoholism, tumor number >1, presence of micro- or macrovascular invasion, absence of capsule, non-cirrhosis and high alpha-fetoprotein. In conclusion, ANXA2 expression in HCC tissues could predict postoperative OS. However, the predictive value was limited in patients with specific clinical conditions.

Keywords: hepatocellular carcinoma; annexin A2; prognostic marker; survival outcome

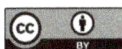

1. Introduction

Hepatocellular carcinoma (HCC) is the second most common cause of cancer-related death in Taiwan [1]. Infection with hepatitis B virus (HBV) and hepatitis C virus (HCV) can lead to chronic hepatitis, liver fibrosis, cirrhosis and eventually HCC [2]. Despite the improvement in the treatment of chronic viral hepatitis and the successful implantation of neonatal vaccination program against HBV, HCC is still a severe public health concern in Taiwan [3]. Surgical treatment is considered one of the most efficient therapies for early-stage HCC. However, incidence of tumor recurrence and distant metastasis remains high in HCC patients receiving surgical resection, resulting in unsatisfactory clinical outcomes. Several biomarkers such as alpha-fetoprotein (AFP) were used for diagnosis and outcome prediction in HCC patients. However, approximately 40% HCC patients still presented with normal levels of AFP, suggesting that the diagnostic and prognostic role of AFP in HCC patients is still limited [4,5]. Therefore, it is very important to identify new prognostic makers for these patients, so that more intensive surveillance and/or adjuvant treatments, if available, could be applied to unfavorable patients.

Annexin A2 (ANXA2) belongs to annexin family and is responsible for regulating cell growth, cell–cell junctions and apoptosis [6–8]. ANXA2 has been reported to act as an early-stage HCC biomarker [9]. Another study [10] reported that ANXA2 was overexpressed in hepatoma cells compared to normal cells. Depletion of ANXA2 repressed cell proliferation and enhanced 5-fluorouracil-mediated effects via suppression of β-catenin and cyclin D1 expression. Yang et al. [11] demonstrated that ANXA2 enhanced liver fibrosis through regulation of the von Willebrand factor (vWF) in vitro and in vivo. These findings suggest that ANXA2 plays an oncogenic role in HCC progression. However, another study [12] indicated that expression levels of ANXA2 in HCC tissue and serum specimens were not correlated well with clinical outcomes, suggesting that ANXA2 was not a good prognostic maker for HCC patients with HBV-related liver cirrhosis. Accordingly, the predictive value of ANXA2 in Taiwanese HCC patients needed to be determined, where a great proportion of HCC was HBV-related, arising from a cirrhotic background.

In this study, ANXA2 expression levels were determined by Western blot followed by densitometry-based quantification. The clinical correlation between ANXA2 expression and postoperative outcomes was analyzed in Taiwanese HCC patients.

2. Materials and Methods

2.1. Patients and Basic Clinical Data

This was a retrospective longitudinal cohort study. From 1996 to 2006, a total of 148 paired HCC specimens (cancerous and para-neoplastic noncancerous tissues) obtained from surgical resection of HCC in LinKou Chang Gung Memorial Hospital were retrieved (cohort 1) and subjected to ANXA2 expression analysis by Western blot. Samples providing sufficient amounts of protein for Western blot analysis were randomly selected from the tissue bank. Only those with written informed consent from patients were included. The clinicopathological data were collected, including age, gender, tumor number, tumor size, histological grading, microvascular invasion, macrovascular invasion, capsule, microsatellite distribution, liver cirrhosis, Child–Pugh classification of liver function, ascites, alpha-fetoprotein (AFP), albumin, bilirubin, prothrombin time (PT), aspartate transaminase (AST), alanine transaminase (ALT), HBV surface antigen (HBsAg), anti-HCV antibody and alcoholism (Table 1). Meanwhile, longitudinal data of recurrence-free survival (RFS) and overall survival (OS) were collected and calculated for survival outcome analysis. RFS was calculated as the period from the time of operation to the time of tumor recurrence or metastasis. OS was calculated as the period from the time of operation to the time of death. The time-point when a patient was lost to follow up was censored. In addition, expression levels of ANXA2 in online available datasets (TCGA, cohort 2 and GSE14520, (cohort 3) were analyzed to further confirm its prognostic value in patients with HCC [13].

2.2. Western Blot Analysis

The procedure of Western blot analysis was described in the previous study [14]. Cells were collected and lysed with RIPA buffer (BIOTOOLS Co., Ltd., Taipei, Taiwan, TAAR-ZBZ5) containing protease inhibitors (Merck Millipore, Temecula, CA, USA, #539134). Protein concentrations of these samples were determined using the Bradford assay. Protein samples (60 μg) were loaded and separated by SDS-PAGE. The voltage (V) at stacking gel and resolution gel was 60–80 and 120–150 V, respectively. After loading dye reached the end of the gel, the gel was transferred to 0.45 μm PVDF membrane. The blocking buffer was added to the membrane for 1 h at room temperature. The membrane was incubated with specific antibody against ANXA2 (BD Biosciences, Franklin Lakes, NJ, USA) overnight at 4 °C. In addition, β-actin (Sigma-Aldrich, St Louis, MO, USA) was also visualized and used as loading control. The signal intensity of ANXA2 and β-actin was calculated by Image Gauge software (Fujifilm, Tokyo, Japan).

Table 1. Basic clinicopathological factors of patients with or without liver cirrhosis (cohort 1).

Variable	All Patients	Non-Cirrhosis	Cirrhosis	p
Patient number	148	80	68	
Gender				
Female	36(24.3%)	20(25.0%)	16(23.5%)	0.835
Male	112(75.7%)	60(75.0%)	52(76.5%)	
Age (years)	56.0 ± 14.9	54.2 ± 16.1	58.1 ± 13.2	0.106
Child–Pugh Classification				
A	127(85.8%)	70(87.5%)	57(83.8%)	0.523
B	21(14.2%)	10(12.5%)	11(16.2%)	
Ascites				
No	136(91.9%)	74(92.5%)	62(91.2%)	0.769
Yes	12(8.1%)	6(7.5%)	6(8.8%)	
HBsAg				
Negative	46(31.1%)	24(30.0%)	22(32.4%)	0.758
Positive	102(68.9%)	56(70.0%)	46(67.6%)	
Anti-HCV Ab				
Negative	107(72.3%)	68(85.0%)	39(57.4%)	<0.001 *
Positive	41(27.7%)	12(15.0%)	29(42.6%)	
Alcohol consumption				
No	104(70.3%)	59(73.8%)	45(66.2%)	0.315
Yes	44(29.7%)	21(26.3%)	23(33.8%)	
Tumor status				
Tumor number				
1	95(64.2%)	51(63.8%)	44(64.7%)	0.904
≥2	53(35.8%)	29(36.3%)	24(35.3%)	
Tumor size (cm)	6.9 ± 4.8	8.5 ± 5.1	5.1 ± 3.6	<0.001 *
Histological grading				
1–2	47(31.8%)	22(27.5%)	25(36.8%)	0.228
3–4	101(68.2%)	58(72.5%)	43(63.2%)	
Microvascular invasion				
No	103(69.6%)	54(67.5%)	49(72.1%)	0.548
Yes	45(30.4%)	26(32.5%)	19(27.9%)	
Macrovascular invasion				
No	136(91.9%)	74(92.5%)	62(91.2%)	0.769
Yes	12(8.1%)	6(7.5%)	6(8.8%)	
Capsule				
No	37(25.0%)	22(27.5%)	15(22.1%)	0.446
Yes	111(75.0%)	58(72.5%)	53(77.9%)	
Microsatellite distribution				
No	123(83.1%)	63(78.8%)	60(88.2%)	0.125
Yes	25(16.9%)	17(21.3%)	8(11.8%)	
Annexin A2 expression				
<0.8 (Low)	96(64.9%)	62(77.5%)	34(50.0%)	<0.001 *
≥0.8 (High)	52(35.1%)	18(22.5%)	34(50.0%)	
Laboratory data				
AFP (ng/mL)	14.9(1.5-327.500)	6.5(2.9–327.500)	22.0(1.5–89,637.7)	0.642
Albumin (g/dL)	3.7 ± 0.7	3.8 ± 0.7	3.7 ± 0.6	0.427
Bilirubin (mg/dL)	1.3 ± 1.7	1.4 ± 2.1	1.2 ± 1.0	0.550
Prothrombin time (sec)	12.4 ± 1.5	12.1 ± 1.5	12.7 ± 1.5	0.042 *
AST (U/L)	94.6 ± 118.8	111.7 ± 151.0	74.5 ± 57.7	0.044 *
ALT (U/L)	77.0 ± 96.8	87.9 ± 120.5	64.2 ± 56.0	0.119
Creatinine (mg/dL)	1.2 ± 1.4	1.3 ± 1.8	1.1 ± 0.7	0.428

Abbreviations: AST, aspartate aminotransferase; ALT, alanine aminotransferase; AFP, α-fetoprotein; HBsAg, hepatitis B surface antigen; Anti-HCV Ab, anti-hepatitis C virus antibody. * $p < 0.05$.

2.3. Statistical Analysis

The univariate analysis, multivariate analysis, Kaplan–Meier survival curve and forest plot analysis were performed using SPSS version 20 (SPSS Inc., Chicago, IL, USA). p values < 0.05 were considered significant (* $p < 0.05$).

3. Results

3.1. Elevated ANXA2 Expression Is Negatively Correlated with Clinical Outcomes

A total of 148 HCC patients receiving surgical resection were included. Of them, 80 (54%) patients were non-cirrhotic, and 68 (46%) of patients were cirrhotic. The basic clinical data were listed in Table 1. Compared with the non-cirrhosis group, the liver cirrhosis group had higher anti-HCV-positive rate, smaller tumor size, higher proportion of high ANXA2 expression, longer PT prolongation and lower AST level. To investigate whether ANXA2 acted as a prognostic biomarker, the expression levels of ANXA2 in HCC specimens were determined by Western blot followed by densitometry semi-quantification. The cancerous to non-cancerous (T/N) ratios of ANXA2 were calculated and the minimal p value method was applied to determine the cut off [15]. We found that ANXA2 expression was highly expressed in HCC tissues compared to noncancerous tissues (Figure 1A, $p < 0.001$). We retrieved the longitudinal data of RFS and OS to analyze whether AXNA2 expression (calculated as T/N ratio) was associated with prognosis in HCC. Kaplan–Meier plot with log-rank analysis showed that there was no significant association between AXNA2 expression (the T/N ratio) and RFS ($p > 0.05$). However, patients with high ANXA2 expression (T/N ratio ≥ 0.8) had a significantly shorter OS compared to those with low ANXA2 expression (Figure 1B). Similar results were observed in datasets available online (TCGA, cohort 2 and GSE14520, cohort 3) (Figure S1A,B). These findings clearly support that ANXA2 acts as a prognostic maker in patients with HCC. Notably, ANXA2 expression was positively correlated with cirrhosis, AST, anti-HCV antibody and the presence of capsule (Table 2). Taken together, ANXA2 might serve as a prognostic factor for HCC patients receiving surgical treatment.

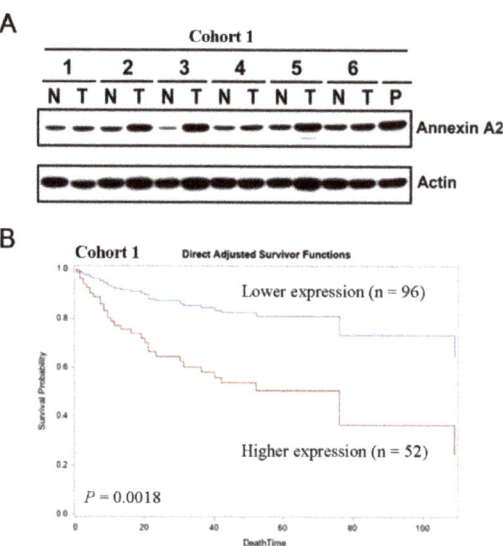

Figure 1. ANXA2 is clinically relevant in HCC. (**A**) Protein levels of ANXA2 in tumor tissues (T) and non-tumor tissues (N) were determined by Western blotting. P: positive control. (**B**) Kaplan–Meier survival curves with log-rank test stratified by high ANXA2 expression (higher T/N ratio ≥ 0.8) and low ANXA2 expression.

Table 2. Clinicopathological correlations of ANXA2 in HCC specimens (cohort 1).

Parameters	HCC Samples (n = 148)	Mean ± SE	p [a]
Gender			
Male	112	0.6116 ± 0.0475	0.8186
Female	36	0.6583 ± 0.1143	
Age (years)			
≤65	100	0.6470 ± 0.0623	0.8222
>65	48	0.5729 ± 0.0518	
Cirrhosis			
No	80	0.4913 ± 0.0505	0.0003 *
Yes	68	0.7779 ± 0.0748	
Child–Pugh classification			
A	127	0.6213 ± 0.0505	0.6987
B	21	0.6333 ± 0.0942	
Ascites			
No	136	0.6191 ± 0.0483	0.4494
Yes	12	0.6667 ± 0.1157	
HBsAg			
Negative	46	0.7087 ± 0.0917	0.1533
Positive	102	0.5843 ± 0.0509	
Anti-HCV Ab			
Negative	107	0.5514 ± 0.0488	0.0039 *
Positive	41	0.8098 ± 0.0976	
Alcohol consumption			
No	104	0.6115 ± 0.0483	0.5390
Yes	44	0.6667 ± 0.1157	
Tumor number			
1	95	0.6316 ± 0.0579	0.8248
≥2	53	0.6500 ± 0.0730	
Tumor size			
≤5 cm	72	0.6528 ± 0.0544	0.2919
>5 cm	76	0.5947 ± 0.0826	
Histological grading			
1–2	47	0.6500 ± 0.0951	0.7070
3–4	101	0.6083 ± 0.0475	
Microvascular invasion			
No	103	0.6291 ± 0.0535	0.5899
Yes	45	0.6089 ± 0.0858	
Macrovascular invasion			
No	136	0.6154 ± 0.0482	0.2173
Yes	12	0.7083 ± 0.1202	
Capsule			
No	37	0.4378 ± 0.0647	0.0069 *
Yes	111	0.6847 ± 0.0553	
Microsatellite distribution			
No	123	0.6235 ± 0.0513	0.6822
Yes	25	0.6200 ± 0.0923	
AFP			
Normal	75	0.5533 ± 0.0414	0.6768
>ULN	73	0.6945 ± 0.0809	
Albumin			
Normal	93	0.6290 ± 0.0550	0.5360
≤LLN	55	0.6127 ± 0.0793	
Bilirubin			
Normal	115	0.6130 ± 0.0506	0.7281
>ULN	33	0.6575 ± 0.1017	
Prothrombin time			
Prolonged ≤ 4 s	137	0.6255 ± 0.0480	0.9589
Prolonged > 4 s	11	0.5909 ± 0.1254	

Table 2. *Cont.*

Parameters	HCC Samples (n = 148)	Mean ± SE	p [a]
AST			
Normal	45	0.4311 ± 0.0490	0.0048 *
>ULN	103	0.7068 ± 0.0597	
ALT			
Normal	60	0.5800 ± 0.0742	0.2407
>ULN	88	0.6523 ± 0.0571	
Creatinine			
Normal	117	0.5820 ± 0.0424	0.3514
> ULN	31	0.7774 ± 0.1438	

[a]: Mann–Whitney U test (for two groups). * $p < 0.05$. Abbreviations: SE, standard error; ULN, upper limit of normal; LLN, lower limit of normal; AST, aspartate aminotransferase; ALT, alanine aminotransferase; AFP, α-fetoprotein; HBsAg, hepatitis B surface antigen; Anti-HCV Ab, anti-hepatitis C virus antibody.

3.2. Clinicopathological Predictors for RFS and OS

To identify the clinicopathological predictors for RFS and OS, univariate and multivariate Cox proportional hazard analysis was performed and is shown in Tables 3 and 4. For RFS, presence of ascites, tumor number ≥ 2, presence of microvascular invasion and microsatellite distribution of tumors, high Annexin A2 expression, AFP and AST > upper limit of normal were associated with RFS by univariate analysis. Multivariate analysis showed that the presence of ascites, tumor number ≥ 2 and AST > upper limit of normal were the independent predictors for RFS (Table 3). For OS, age > 65 years, Child–Pugh liver function classification B, the presence of ascites, microvascular invasion, high ANXA2 expression, AFP, bilirubin and AST > upper limit of normal were associated with short OS in the univariate Cox proportional analysis. Multivariate analysis showed that Child–Pugh liver function classification B, presence of ascites and high AXNA2 expression were the independent predictors for OS (Table 4).

Table 3. Analysis of factors that influenced RFS of all patients (cohort 1).

			RFS					
			Univariate Analysis			Multivariate Analysis		
Parameters	n	HR	95% CI	p	HR	95% CI	p
Gender								
Female	36							
Male	112	1.263	0.760–2.098	0.3668			
Age (years)								
≤65	100							
>65	48	0.785	0.491–1.256	0.3125			
Cirrhosis								
No	80							
Yes	68	1.466	0.967–2.223	0.0717			
Child–Pugh classification								
A	127							
B	21	1.345	0.714–2.535	0.3587			
Ascites								
No	136							
Yes	12	3.301	1.715–6.352	<0.001 *	2.274	1.156–4.472	0.0173 *
HBsAg								
Negative	46							
Positive	102	1.113	0.701–1.767	0.6507			
Anti-HCV Ab								
Negative	107							
Positive	41	1.180	0.736–1.891	0.4923			
Alcohol consumption								
No	104							
Yes	44	1.205	0.775–1.873	0.4069			

Table 3. Cont.

Parameters	n	RFS					
		Univariate Analysis			Multivariate Analysis		
		HR	95% CI	p	HR	95% CI	p
Tumor status							
Tumor number							
1	95						
≥2	53	3.240	2.097–5.005	<0.0001 *	2.649	1.571–4.467	0.0003 *
Tumor size (cm)							
≤5	72						
>5	76	1.475	0.968–2.247	0.0706			
Histological grading							
1–2	47						
3–4	101	1.217	0.760–1.950	0.4133			
Microvascular invasion							
No	103						
Yes	45	2.514	1.623–3.895	<0.0001 *	1.489	0.878–2.523	0.1394
Macrovascular invasion thrombosis							
No	136						
Yes	12	1.516	0.760–3.028	0.2379			
Capsule							
No	37						
Yes	111	0.778	0.486–1.245	0.2954			
Microsatellite distribution							
No	123						
Yes	25	2.300	1.391–3.803	0.0012 *	0.881	0.468–1.661	0.6962
Annexin A2 expression							
<0.8 (Low)	96						
≥0.8 (High)	52	1.726	1.120–2.659	0.0133 *	1.459	0.934–2.279	0.0969
Laboratory data							
AFP							
Normal	75						
>ULN	73	1.903	1.248–2.900	0.0028 *	1.544	0.994–2.399	0.0531
Albumin							
Normal	93						
≤LLN	55	0.769	0.497–1.189	0.2369			
Bilirubin							
Normal	115						
>ULN	33	1.384	0.847–2.261	0.1951			
Prothrombin time							
Prolonged ≤ 4 s	137						
Prolonged > 4 s	11	1.289	0.619–2.686	0.4981			
AST							
Normal	45						
>ULN	103	1.846	1.132–3.010	0.0141 *	1.719	1.027–2.880	0.0394 *
ALT							
Normal	60						
>ULN	88	1.304	0.852–1.995	0.2210			
Creatinine							
Normal	117						
>ULN	31	0.898	0.515–1.568	0.7057			

* $p < 0.05$. Abbreviations: RFS, recurrence-free survival; HR, hazard ratio; CI, confidence interval; ULN, upper limit of normal; LLN, lower limit of normal; AST, aspartate aminotransferase; ALT, alanine aminotransferase; AFP, α-fetoprotein; HBsAg, hepatitis B surface antigen; Anti-HCV Ab, anti-hepatitis C virus antibody.

Table 4. Analysis of factors that influenced OS of all patients (cohort 1).

			OS					
			Univariate Analysis			Multivariate Analysis		
Parameters	n	HR	95% CI	p	HR	95% CI	p
---	---	---	---	---	---	---	---
Gender							
Female	36						
Male	112	1.826	0.701–4.755	0.2175			
Age (years)							
≤65	100						
>65	48	0.345	0.121–0.986	0.0470 *	0.494	0.160–1.527	0.2204
Cirrhosis							
No	80						
Yes	68	1.357	0.677–2.720	0.3891			
Child–Pugh classification							
A	127						
B	21	4.894	2.345–10.215	<0.001 *	3.687	1.484–9.159	0.0050 *
Ascites							
No	136						
Yes	12	4.241	1.812–9.926	<0.001 *	3.361	1.328–8.507	0.0105 *
HBsAg							
Negative	46						
Positive	102	1.003	0.463–2.171	0.9949			
Anti-HCV Ab							
Negative	107						
Positive	41	1.026	0.460–2.287	0.9509			
Alcohol consumption							
No	104						
Yes	44	1.723	0.856–3.468	0.1275			
Tumor status							
Tumor number							
1	95						
≥2	53	1.666	0.807–3.439	0.1679			
Tumor size (cm)							
≤5	72						
>5	76	1.731	0.834–3.592	0.1410			
Histological grading							
1–2	47						
3–4	101	1.108	0.506–2.429	0.7974			
Microvascular Invasion							
No	103						
Yes	45	2.796	1.356–5.765	0.0053 *	1.921	0.873–4.227	0.1045
Macrovascular invasion thrombosis							
No	136						
Yes	12	2.488	0.953–6.495	0.0627			
Capsule							
No	37						
Yes	111	0.811	0.363–1.811	0.6097			
Microsatellite distribution							
No	123						
Yes	25	2.172	0.964–4.893	0.0612			
Annexin A2 expression							
<0.8 (Low)	96						
≥0.8 (High)	52	3.210	1.542–6.684	0.0018 *	2.497	1.109–5.619	0.0270 *
Laboratory data							
AFP							
Normal	75						
>ULN	73	2.292	1.102–4.766	0.0264 *	1.381	0.603–3.162	0.4446

Table 4. Cont.

Parameters	n	OS Univariate Analysis HR	95% CI	p	OS Multivariate Analysis HR	95% CI	p
Albumin							
Normal	93	0.515	0.257-1.036	0.0626			
≤LLN	55						
Bilirubin							
Normal	115						
>ULN	33	2.186	1.033-4.627	0.0410 *	1.077	0.457–2.538	0.8659
Prothrombin time							
Prolonged ≤ 4 s	137						
Prolonged > 4 s	11	2.031	0.773–5.340	0.1508			
AST							
Normal	45						
>ULN	103	3.362	1.179–9.586	0.0233 *	1.955	0.630–6.062	0.2458
ALT							
Normal	60						
>ULN	88	1.063	0.524-2.154	0.8662			
Creatinine							
Normal	117						
>ULN	31	0.683	0.263-1.776	0.4346			

* $p < 0.05$. Abbreviations: OS, overall survival; HR, hazard ratio; CI, confidence interval; ULN, upper limit of normal; LLN, lower limit of normal; AST, aspartate aminotransferase; ALT, alanine aminotransferase; AFP, α-fetoprotein; HBsAg, hepatitis B surface antigen; Anti-HCV Ab, anti-hepatitis C virus antibody.

3.3. ANXA2 Expression Levels in HCC Tissues Are an Effective Prognosis Predictor in Specific Clinical Subgroups of HCC

In addition, we studied the predictive role of high AXNA2 expression in various clinical subgroups using Cox proportional hazard method (Figure 2). The ANXA2 expression was associated with OS when all HCC patients were included for assessment In addition, it was also associated with OS in the following subgroups: male (HR = 2.772, 95% CI 1.254–6.130, $p = 0.0118$), age ≤ 65 (HR = 2.943, 95% CI 1.361–6.367, $p = 0.0051$), Child–Pugh liver function classification A (HR = 3.324, 95% CI 1.354–8.159, $p = 0.0087$), no ascites (HR = 2.705, 95% CI 1.182–6.188, $p = 0.0185$), HBsAg-positive (HR = 3.269, 95% CI 1.375–7.771, $p = 0.0073$), anti-HCV Ab negative (HR = 3.796, 95% CI 1.635–8.813, $p = 0.0019$), no alcohol consumption (HR = 3.398, 95% CI 1.314–8.787, $p = 0.0116$), tumor number =1 (HR = 6.027, 95% CI 2.109–17.223, $p = 0.0008$), tumor size ≤ 5 cm (HR = 6.241, 95% CI 1.321–29.490, $p = 0.0208$), tumor size > 5 cm (HR = 2.860, 95% CI 1.185–6.900, $p = 0.0194$), histological grading 1–2 (HR = 6.057, 95% CI 1.211–30.285, $p = 0.0283$) and 3–4 (HR = 2.592, 95% CI 1.116–6.021, $p = 0.0267$), no microvascular invasion (HR = 3.772, 95% CI 1.365–10.422, $p = 0.0105$), no macrovascular invasion (HR = 2.983, 95% CI 1.367–6.506, $p = 0.006$), presence of capsule (HR = 3.877, 95% CI 1.649–9.117, $p = 0.0019$), no microsatellite distribution (HR = 3.338, 95% CI 1.422–7.836, $p = 0.0056$), presence of cirrhosis (HR = 5.220, 95% CI 1.464–18.610, $p = 0.0061$), normal AFP (HR = 7.756, 95% CI 1.600–37.603, $p = 0.011$), Albumin ≤ LLN (HR = 3.262, 95% CI 1.106–9.623, $p = 0.0322$), normal bilirubin (HR = 3.585, 95% CI 1.478–8.699, $p = 0.0048$), Prothrombin time ≤ 4 s (HR = 3.519, 95% CI 1.592–7.782, $p = 0.0019$), AST > ULN (HR = 3.095, 95% CI 1.373–6.977, $p = 0.0064$), ALT normal (HR = 4.599, 95% CI 1.518–13.933, $p = 0.007$) and >ULN (HR = 2.841, 95% CI 1.045–7.720, $p = 0.0407$) and creatinine normal (HR = 3.098, 95% CI 1.388–6.915, $p = 0.0058$). In contrast, the association was not present in the following subgroups ($p > 0.05$ for all): female, age > 65 years, Child–Pugh classification B, presence of ascites, HBsAg negative, anti-HCV-positive, alcoholism; tumor number ≥ 2, micro- or macrovascular invasion, microsatellite distribution of tumors, non-cirrhosis, AFP or bilirubin > upper limit of normal, PT prolongation > 4 s, normal AST or creatinine > upper limit of normal.

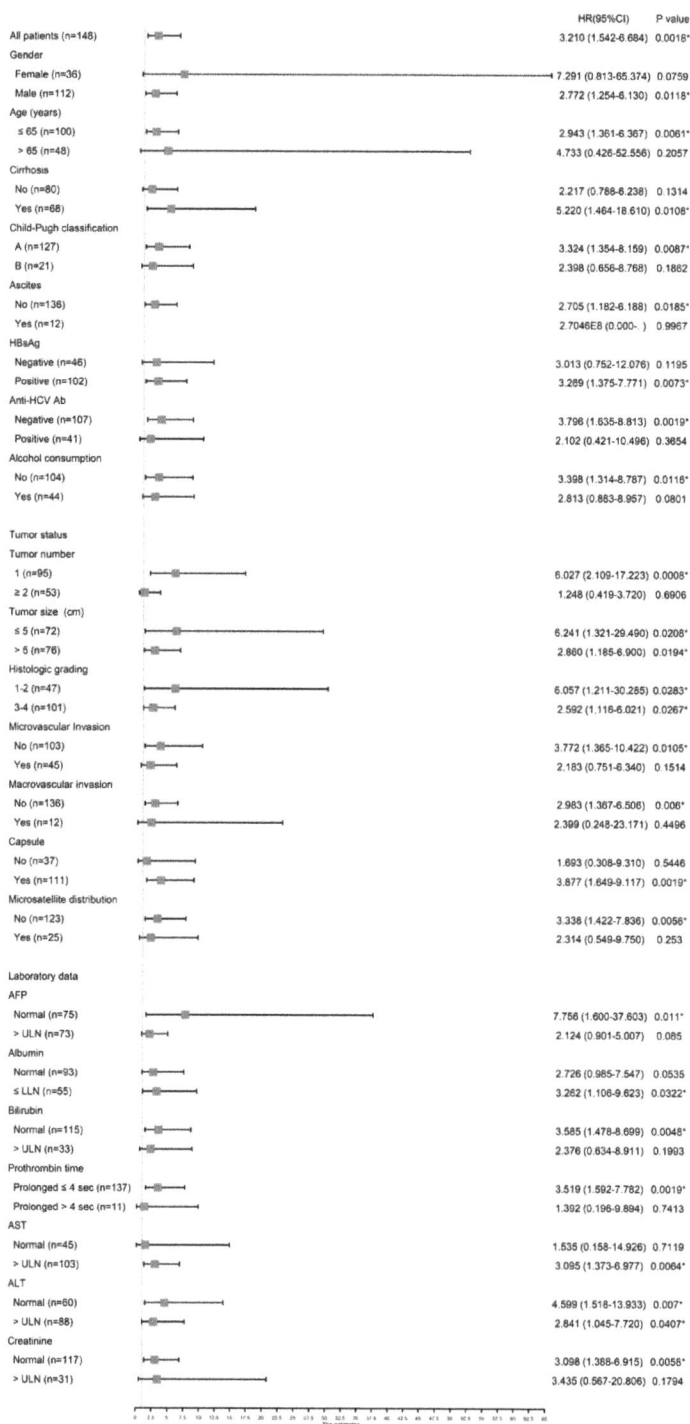

Figure 2. Forest plot of HRs for the associations between high AXNA2 expression and OS in various clinical subgroups. The subgroup-specific HR (95% CI) is shown by the green box (black lines). Statistically significant differences ($p < 0.05$) are indicated by a single asterisk "*".

Taken together, these findings suggest that high expression of ANXA2 in HCC cancerous parts could predict shorter OS in HCC patients receiving surgical treatment. However, in patients with more advanced stage of HCC or poorer liver function, non-cirrhosis patients or HBsAg-negative patients, the predictive value diminished.

4. Discussion

Previously, ANXA2 was identified as an independent prognostic marker in several cancer types, including laryngeal cancer [16], breast cancer [17], ovarian cancer [18] and endometrial cancer [19]. A similar predictive role of ANXA2 in HCC development has also been reported [9]. In the current study, we found that high expression of ANXA2 in HCC tissues was associated with a significantly shorter OS, indicating that ANXA2 was a predictor for unfavorable prognosis in liver cancer. Carbon tetrachloride (CCl_4) treatment induces liver fibrosis, which mimics the sequel of chronic virus infection. Long-term CCl_4 treatment renders fibrotic liver-to-liver cirrhosis, as a pre-malignant stage of HCC development [20]. Yang and co-workers demonstrated that ANXA2 levels were induced upon CCl_4 treatment in Sprague Dawley rats compared to those in the control group [11]. Our results showed that ANXA2 expression was increased in patients with liver cirrhosis compared to those with non-cirrhosis (Table 2). Another report demonstrated that serum ANXA2 levels in chronic hepatitis B patients were significantly higher than those in the normal group [21]. On the other hand, a previous investigation indicated that ANXA2 functioned as a modulator in HCV assembly but not in HCV replication or viron release [22]. Our study revealed that ANXA2 expression was higher in the HCV-positive group compared to the HCV-negative group, suggesting ANXA2 expression was regulated by HCV infection through a yet unknown mechanism. However, in subgroup analysis, ANXA2 higher expression was not correlated with survival outcome in HCV-positive patients. Taken together, the evidence suggested that ANXA2 may be involved in early-stage HCC development, i.e., liver fibrosis to cirrhosis progression.

In contrast, Liu et al. indicated that ANXA2 expression in serum or HCC tissues were not significantly correlated with survival outcomes [12]. In an Egypt study, ANXA2 expression was lower in cirrhotic group than those in control group in HCC tissues [23]. These controversial results for ANXA2 on survival outcomes of HCC may be explained as follows: First, most of our specimens analyzed in this study were from cirrhotic or HBV-related patients. Second, in this study, ANXA2 expression in HCC tissues was detected by Western blot analysis followed by densitometry quantification. In contrast, an early study had assayed the serum levels of ANXA2 by ELISA. The detection method (Western blot vs. ELISA) and quantitative criteria may lead to different results. Third, these studies were performed in different countries; thereby, the geographic/ethnic issue may also have caused the inconsistent results. Fourth, a previous study reported that ANXA2 could be secreted to the extracellular environment upon interferon-γ treatment [24], suggesting that hepatitis activities might play a role. The intracellular and extracellular ANXA2 proteins also exert different functions [25]. We believe that these are possible reasons for the inconsistencies.

Zhang and co-workers demonstrated that knockdown of ANXA2 in hepatoma cell lines reduced cell migration and invasion [26]. Mechanistically, ANXA2 interacted with CD147 and regulated CD147 localization, thereby inducing matrix metallopoateinase 2 (MMP2) expression. Furthermore, knockdown of ANXA2 in a hepatoma cell line, MHCC97-H, repressed cell growth and invasive ability [27]. Oncogenic roles of transgelin-2 in HCC have been demonstrated, and its high expression is associated with ANXA2, which, in turn, promotes tumor metastasis through the NFκB pathway [28]. Another investigation indicated that ANXA2 was involved in immune escape of HCC via modulation of immune cells such as regulatory T cells, natural killer cells and dendritic cells [29]. In addition to HCC, the ANXA2-mediated immunosuppression phenotypes were observed in nasopharyngeal carcinoma cells [30] and renal cell carcinoma [31]. Another study revealed that expression levels of ANXA2 in liver tissues were upregulated in a thioacetamide (TAA)-induced cirrhotic rat model [32]. The authors found that immuno-related factors such as transforming growth factor beta and interleukin were increased in TAA-treated rats, suggesting ANXA2 might be involved in the immune response pathway. A long non-coding RNA, named lung cancer-associated transcript 1 (LUCAT1), induced cell growth and metastasis of hepatoma cell lines in vitro and in vivo [33]. LUCAT1 associated with ANXA2 was identified by an RNA pull-down assay, leading to inhibition of ANXA2 phosphorylation and induction of MMP9 activation. Recently, circular RNA (circRNA) has been found responsible for regulating cancer progression [34]. The expression levels of circ_0021093 were upregulated in HCC specimens, and a higher level of circ_0021093 was correlated with poor survival outcomes [35]. Depletion of circ_0021093 reduced cell proliferation, migration and invasion by modulating miR-432. Moreover, ANXA2 is a direct targeted gene of miR-432. These findings indicated that the circ_0021093/miR-432/ANXA2 axis was another important pathway regulating HCC progression. This evidence supported that ANXA2 played an oncogenic role in liver cancer.

5. Conclusions

In conclusion, we showed that ANXA2 was a prognostic marker for HCC patients receiving surgical treatment. However, the predictive value diminished in several clinical subgroups such as those with more advanced stage of HCC or poorer liver function, as well as non-cirrhosis and HBsAg-negative patients.

Supplementary Materials: The following are available online at https://www.mdpi.com/article/10.3390/jcm10184158/s1, Figure S1: Elevated ANXA2 expression was correlated with poor prognosis in patients with HCC in online available dataset analysis.

Author Contributions: Y.-H.L. and C.-T.Y. designed and supervised the study; S.-W.H., Y.-C.C., Y.-H.L. and C.-T.Y. drafted the manuscript; S.-W.H. and Y.-C.C. performed the experiments; S.-W.H., Y.-C.C., Y.-H.L. and C.-T.Y. interpreted the data; S.-W.H., Y.-C.C., Y.-H.L. and C.-T.Y. collected and analyzed the clinical data. All authors have read and agreed to the published version of the manuscript.

Funding: This work was supported by grants from Chang Gung Memorial Hospital, Taiwan (CMRPG3K1551 to YHL).

Institutional Review Board Statement: This study was approved by the Institutional Review Board of Chang Gung Medical Center (IRB: 201900957B0). The experiments conformed to the ethical guidelines of the 1975 Declaration of Helsinki.

Informed Consent Statement: Informed consent was obtained from patients, prior to their participation in the study.

Data Availability Statement: The available datasets can be analyzed and download from Gene Expression Profiling Interactive Analysis (http://gepia.cancer-pku.cn/, accessed on 1 September 2021, Beijing, China) and Gene Expression Omnibus (GEO; http://www.ncbi.nlm.nih.gov/geo, accessed on 1 September 2021, Bethesda MD, USA) with accession numbers GSE14520, respectively.

Acknowledgments: The authors appreciate the technical and administrative support provided by all members of the Liver Research Center in Chang Gung Memorial Hospital, Taoyuan, Taiwan.

Conflicts of Interest: The authors have no conflict to disclose.

References

1. Kim, E.; Viatour, P. Hepatocellular carcinoma: Old friends and new tricks. *Exp. Mol. Med.* **2020**, *52*, 1898–1907. [CrossRef]
2. Elpek, G.O. Molecular pathways in viral hepatitis-associated liver carcinogenesis: An update. *World J. Clin. Cases* **2021**, *9*, 4890–4917. [CrossRef]
3. Chiang, C.J.; Yang, Y.W.; You, S.L.; Lai, M.S.; Chen, C.J. Thirty-year outcomes of the national hepatitis B immunization program in Taiwan. *JAMA* **2013**, *310*, 974–976. [CrossRef] [PubMed]
4. Park, S.J.; Jang, J.Y.; Jeong, S.W.; Cho, Y.K.; Lee, S.H.; Kim, S.G.; Cha, S.W.; Kim, Y.S.; Cho, Y.D.; Kim, H.S.; et al. Usefulness of AFP, AFP-L3, and PIVKA-II, and their combinations in diagnosing hepatocellular carcinoma. *Medicine* **2017**, *96*, e5811. [CrossRef]

5. Chan, M.Y.; She, W.H.; Dai, W.C.; Tsang, S.H.Y.; Chok, K.S.H.; Chan, A.C.Y.; Fung, J.; Lo, C.M.; Cheung, T.T. Prognostic value of preoperative alpha-fetoprotein (AFP) level in patients receiving curative hepatectomy—An analysis of 1182 patients in Hong Kong. *Transl. Gastroenterol. Hepatol.* **2019**, *4*, 52. [CrossRef] [PubMed]
6. Chen, L.; Lin, L.; Xian, N.; Zheng, Z. Annexin A2 regulates glioma cell proliferation through the STAT3cyclin D1 pathway. *Oncol. Rep.* **2019**, *42*, 399–413.
7. Lee, D.B.; Jamgotchian, N.; Allen, S.G.; Kan, F.W.; Hale, I.L. Annexin A2 heterotetramer: Role in tight junction assembly. *Am. J. Physiol.-Ren. Physiol.* **2004**, *287*, F481–F491. [CrossRef] [PubMed]
8. Jiang, S.L.; Pan, D.Y.; Gu, C.; Qin, H.F.; Zhao, S.H. Annexin A2 silencing enhances apoptosis of human umbilical vein endothelial cells in vitro. *Asian Pac. J. Trop. Med.* **2015**, *8*, 952–957. [CrossRef] [PubMed]
9. Sun, Y.; Gao, G.; Cai, J.; Wang, Y.; Qu, X.; He, L.; Liu, F.; Zhang, Y.; Lin, K.; Ma, S.; et al. Annexin A2 is a discriminative serological candidate in early hepatocellular carcinoma. *Carcinogenesis* **2013**, *34*, 595–604. [CrossRef] [PubMed]
10. Wang, C.; Guo, Y.; Wang, J.; Min, Z. Annexin A2 knockdown inhibits hepatoma cell growth and sensitizes hepatoma cells to 5-fluorouracil by regulating beta-catenin and cyclin D1 expression. *Mol. Med. Rep.* **2015**, *11*, 2147–2152. [CrossRef] [PubMed]
11. Yang, M.; Wang, C.; Li, S.; Xv, X.; She, S.; Ran, X.; Li, S.; Hu, H.; Hu, P.; Zhang, D.; et al. Annexin A2 promotes liver fibrosis by mediating von Willebrand factor secretion. *Dig. Liver Dis.* **2017**, *49*, 780–788. [CrossRef]
12. Liu, Z.; Ling, Q.; Wang, J.; Xie, H.; Xu, X.; Zheng, S. Annexin A2 is not a good biomarker for hepatocellular carcinoma in cirrhosis. *Oncol. Lett.* **2013**, *6*, 125–129. [CrossRef]
13. Roessler, S.; Jia, H.L.; Budhu, A.; Forgues, M.; Ye, Q.H.; Lee, J.S.; Thorgeirsson, S.S.; Sun, Z.; Tang, Z.Y.; Qin, L.X.; et al. A unique metastasis gene signature enables prediction of tumor relapse in early-stage hepatocellular carcinoma patients. *Cancer Res.* **2010**, *70*, 10202–10212. [CrossRef] [PubMed]
14. Lin, Y.H.; Wu, M.H.; Liu, Y.C.; Lyu, P.C.; Yeh, C.T.; Lin, K.H. LINC01348 suppresses hepatocellular carcinoma metastasis through inhibition of SF3B3-mediated EZH2 pre-mRNA splicing. *Oncogene* **2021**, *40*, 4675–4685. [CrossRef] [PubMed]
15. Mazumdar, M.; Glassman, J.R. Categorizing a prognostic variable: Review of methods, code for easy implementation and applications to decision-making about cancer treatments. *Stat. Med.* **2000**, *19*, 113–132. [CrossRef]
16. Luo, S.; Xie, C.; Wu, P.; He, J.; Tang, Y.; Xu, J.; Zhao, S. Annexin A2 is an independent prognostic biomarker for evaluating the malignant progression of laryngeal cancer. *Exp. Ther. Med.* **2017**, *14*, 6113–6118. [CrossRef]
17. Zhang, F.; Zhang, H.; Wang, Z.; Yu, M.; Tian, R.; Ji, W.; Yang, Y.; Niu, R. P-glycoprotein associates with Anxa2 and promotes invasion in multidrug resistant breast cancer cells. *Biochem. Pharm.* **2014**, *87*, 292–302. [CrossRef]
18. Lokman, N.A.; Pyragius, C.E.; Ruszkiewicz, A.; Oehler, M.K.; Ricciardelli, C. Annexin A2 and S100A10 are independent predictors of serous ovarian cancer outcome. *Transl. Res.* **2016**, *171*, 83–95.e2. [CrossRef]
19. Alonso-Alconada, L.; Santacana, M.; Garcia-Sanz, P.; Muinelo-Romay, L.; Colas, E.; Mirantes, C.; Monge, M.; Cueva, J.; Oliva, E.; Soslow, R.A.; et al. Annexin-A2 as predictor biomarker of recurrent disease in endometrial cancer. *Int. J. Cancer* **2015**, *136*, 1863–1873. [CrossRef]
20. Scholten, D.; Trebicka, J.; Liedtke, C.; Weiskirchen, R. The carbon tetrachloride model in mice. *Lab. Anim.* **2015**, *49* (Suppl. 1), 4–11. [CrossRef]
21. Kolgelier, S.; Demir, N.A.; Inkaya, A.C.; Sumer, S.; Ozcimen, S.; Demir, L.S.; Pehlivan, F.S.; Arslan, M.; Arpaci, A. Serum Levels of Annexin A2 as a Candidate Biomarker for Hepatic Fibrosis in Patients with Chronic Hepatitis B. *Hepat. Mon.* **2015**, *15*, e30655. [CrossRef]
22. Backes, P.; Quinkert, D.; Reiss, S.; Binder, M.; Zayas, M.; Rescher, U.; Gerke, V.; Bartenschlager, R.; Lohmann, V. Role of annexin A2 in the production of infectious hepatitis C virus particles. *J. Virol.* **2010**, *84*, 5775–5789. [CrossRef] [PubMed]
23. Shaker, M.K.; Abdel Fattah, H.I.; Sabbour, G.S.; Montasser, I.F.; Abdelhakam, S.M.; El Hadidy, E.; Yousry, R.; El Dorry, A.K. Annexin A2 as a biomarker for hepatocellular carcinoma in Egyptian patients. *World J. Hepatol.* **2017**, *9*, 469–476. [CrossRef] [PubMed]
24. Chen, Y.D.; Fang, Y.T.; Cheng, Y.L.; Lin, C.F.; Hsu, L.J.; Wang, S.Y.; Anderson, R.; Chang, C.P.; Lin, Y.S. Exophagy of annexin A2 via RAB11, RAB8A and RAB27A in IFN-gamma-stimulated lung epithelial cells. *Sci. Rep.* **2017**, *7*, 5676. [CrossRef]
25. Hitchcock, J.K.; Katz, A.A.; Schafer, G. Dynamic reciprocity: The role of annexin A2 in tissue integrity. *J. Cell Commun. Signal.* **2014**, *8*, 125–133. [CrossRef]
26. Zhang, W.; Zhao, P.; Xu, X.L.; Cai, L.; Song, Z.S.; Cao, D.Y.; Tao, K.S.; Zhou, W.P.; Chen, Z.N.; Dou, K.F. Annexin A2 promotes the migration and invasion of human hepatocellular carcinoma cells in vitro by regulating the shedding of CD147-harboring microvesicles from tumor cells. *PLoS ONE* **2013**, *8*, e67268.
27. Dong, Z.; Yao, M.; Zhang, H.; Wang, L.; Huang, H.; Yan, M.; Wu, W.; Yao, D. Inhibition of Annexin A2 gene transcription is a promising molecular target for hepatoma cell proliferation and metastasis. *Oncol. Lett.* **2014**, *7*, 28–34. [CrossRef]
28. Shi, J.; Ren, M.; She, X.; Zhang, Z.; Zhao, Y.; Han, Y.; Lu, D.; Lyu, L. Transgelin-2 contributes to proliferation and progression of hepatocellular carcinoma via regulating Annexin A2. *Biochem. Biophys. Res. Commun.* **2020**, *523*, 632–638. [CrossRef]
29. Qiu, L.W.; Liu, Y.F.; Cao, X.Q.; Wang, Y.; Cui, X.H.; Ye, X.; Huang, S.W.; Xie, H.J.; Zhang, H.J. Annexin A2 promotion of hepatocellular carcinoma tumorigenesis via the immune microenvironment. *World J. Gastroenterol.* **2020**, *26*, 2126–2137. [CrossRef]
30. Chen, C.Y.; Lin, Y.S.; Chen, C.H.; Chen, Y.J. Annexin A2-mediated cancer progression and therapeutic resistance in nasopharyngeal carcinoma. *J. Biomed. Sci.* **2018**, *25*, 30. [CrossRef] [PubMed]

31. Aarli, A.; Skeie Jensen, T.; Kristoffersen, E.K.; Bakke, A.; Ulvestad, E. Inhibition of phytohaemagglutinin-induced lymphoproliferation by soluble annexin II in sera from patients with renal cell carcinoma. *APMIS* **1997**, *105*, 699–704. [CrossRef] [PubMed]
32. An, J.H.; Seong, J.; Oh, H.; Kim, W.; Han, K.H.; Paik, Y.H. Protein expression profiles in a rat cirrhotic model induced by thioacetamide. *Korean J. Hepatol.* **2006**, *12*, 93–102. [PubMed]
33. Lou, Y.; Yu, Y.; Xu, X.; Zhou, S.; Shen, H.; Fan, T.; Wu, D.; Yin, J.; Li, G. Long non-coding RNA LUCAT1 promotes tumourigenesis by inhibiting ANXA2 phosphorylation in hepatocellular carcinoma. *J. Cell. Mol. Med.* **2019**, *23*, 1873–1884. [CrossRef]
34. Cheng, D.; Wang, J.; Dong, Z.; Li, X. Cancer-related circular RNA: Diverse biological functions. *Cancer Cell Int.* **2021**, *21*, 11. [CrossRef] [PubMed]
35. Wang, Y.; Xu, W.; Zu, M.; Xu, H. Circular RNA circ_0021093 regulates miR-432/Annexin A2 pathway to promote hepatocellular carcinoma progression. *Anticancer Drugs* **2021**, *32*, 484–495. [CrossRef]

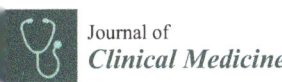

Article

Metabolic Effects of Gastrectomy and Duodenal Bypass in Early Gastric Cancer Patients with T2DM: A Prospective Single-Center Cohort Study

Young Ki Lee [1,†], Eun Kyung Lee [1,2,†], You Jin Lee [1,*], Bang Wool Eom [3], Hong Man Yoon [2,3], Young-Il Kim [2,3], Soo Jeong Cho [3], Jong Yeul Lee [3], Chan Gyoo Kim [3], Sun-Young Kong [2,4], Min Kyong Yoo [5], Yul Hwangbo [1,6], Young-Woo Kim [3], Il Ju Choi [3,6], Hak Jin Kim [7], Mi Hyang Kwak [7] and Keun Won Ryu [3,*]

1. Division of Endocrinology and Metabolism, Department of Internal Medicine, National Cancer Center, Goyang 10408, Korea; yklee@ncc.re.kr (Y.K.L.); eklee@ncc.re.kr (E.K.L.); yulhwangbo@ncc.re.kr (Y.H.)
2. Department of Cancer Biomedical Science, National Cancer Center Graduate School of Cancer Science and Policy, National Cancer Center, Goyang 10408, Korea; red10000@ncc.re.kr (H.M.Y.); 11996@ncc.re.kr (Y.-I.K.); ksy@ncc.re.kr (S.-Y.K.)
3. Center for Gastric Cancer, National Cancer Center, Goyang 10408, Korea; kneeling79@ncc.re.kr (B.W.E.); crystal5@snu.ac.kr (S.J.C.); jylee@ncc.re.kr (J.Y.L.); glse@ncc.re.kr (C.G.K.); youngwookim@ncc.re.kr (Y.-W.K.); cij1224@ncc.re.kr (I.J.C.)
4. Department of Laboratory Medicine, National Cancer Center, Goyang 10408, Korea
5. Department of Clinical Nutrition, National Cancer Center, Goyang 10408, Korea; mkyoo52@ncc.re.kr
6. Department of Cancer Control and Population Health, National Cancer Center Graduate School of Cancer Science and Policy, National Cancer Center, Goyang 10408, Korea
7. Division of Cardiology, Department of Internal Medicine, National Cancer Center, Goyang 10408, Korea; drkhj@ncc.re.kr (H.J.K.); cardiokmh@ncc.re.kr (M.H.K.)
* Correspondence: eulee@ncc.re.kr (Y.J.L.); docryu@ncc.re.kr (K.W.R.); Tel.: +82-31-920-1644 (Y.J.L.); +82-31-920-1628 (K.W.R.)
† Young Ki Lee and Eun Kyung Lee contributed equally to this work.

Abstract: We evaluated the metabolic effects of gastrectomies and endoscopic submucosal dissections (ESDs) in early gastric cancer (EGC) patients with type 2 diabetes mellitus (T2DM). Forty-one EGC patients with T2DM undergoing gastrectomy or ESD were prospectively evaluated. Metabolic parameters in the patients who underwent gastrectomy with and without a duodenal bypass (groups 1 and 2, $n = 24$ and $n = 5$, respectively) were compared with those in patients who underwent ESD (control, $n = 12$). After 1 year, the proportions of improved/equivocal/worsened glycemic control were 62.5%/29.2%/8.3% in group 1, 40.0%/60.0%/0.0% in group 2, and 16.7%/50.0%/33.3% in the controls, respectively ($p = 0.046$). The multivariable ordered logistic regression analysis results showed that both groups had better 1-year glycemic control. Groups 1 and 2 showed a significant reduction in postprandial glucose (−97.9 and −67.8 mg/dL), body mass index (−2.1 and −2.3 kg/m^2), and glycosylated hemoglobin (group 1 only, −0.5% point) (all $p < 0.05$). Furthermore, improvements in group 1 were more prominent when preoperative leptin levels were high (p for interaction < 0.05). Metabolic improvements in both groups were also observed for insulin resistance, leptin, plasminogen activator inhibitor-1, and resistin. Gastrectomy improved glycemic control and various metabolic parameters in EGC patients with T2DM. Patients with high leptin levels may experience greater metabolic benefits from gastrectomy with duodenal bypass.

Keywords: gastrectomy; endoscopic submucosal dissection; early gastric cancer; type 2 diabetes mellitus; glycemic control; insulin resistance

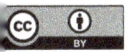

1. Introduction

Gastric cancer is the most frequently diagnosed cancer in Korea and has the fifth-highest incidence among newly diagnosed cancer cases worldwide [1,2]. While the incidence of gastric cancer has steadily decreased, the number of gastric cancer survivors has increased due to early diagnosis and improved treatment techniques [1–3]. In Korea, the 5-year survival rate of gastric cancer has dramatically improved from 43.9% in 1993–1995 to 76.5% in 2013–2017, and the number of gastric cancer survivors reached about 300,000 in 2017 [1].

Type 2 diabetes mellitus (T2DM) is one of the most common comorbidities that determine overall mortality, non-cancer mortality, and quality of life in cancer survivors [4–6]. The prevalence of T2DM has been increasing worldwide, and it reached 13.8% in 2018 in Korea [7,8]. Patients with T2DM are at a higher risk for gastric cancer development, and the incidence of T2DM increases after gastric cancer development [9,10]. Therefore, proper management of T2DM is an important issue in many gastric cancer patients.

Gastrectomy and endoscopic submucosal dissection (ESD) are two curative treatment modalities for early gastric cancer (EGC) that show comparable overall and disease-specific survival [11]. Interestingly, gastrectomy performed as bariatric surgery improves glycemic control in morbidly obese patients with T2DM [12–14]. Moreover, studies have reported improvement in T2DM in gastric cancer patients after gastrectomy [15–18]. This evidence suggests that gastrectomy may have additional benefits over ESD in improving glycemic control in EGC patients with T2DM. However, to date, no study has compared the effects of gastrectomy with those of ESD on glycemic control in gastric cancer patients with T2DM using laboratory results.

This study aimed to prospectively examine the metabolic effects of gastrectomy with or without the duodenal bypass and compare the findings with those for ESD in EGC patients with T2DM. We also aimed to explore preoperative conditions in which the metabolic advantage of gastrectomy over ESD increases to identify patients who would benefit the most from gastrectomy.

2. Materials and Methods

2.1. Study Subjects and Protocols

This nonrandomized, controlled, prospective cohort study initially recruited 62 eligible EGC patients with T2DM who were scheduled to undergo ESD or gastrectomy between April 2012 and December 2014 at the National Cancer Center in Korea (clinicaltrials.gov accesed on 14 July 2014, identifier: NCT01643811). The enrollment criteria were as follows: (1) histologically proven primary gastric adenocarcinoma; (2) in clinical stage Ia or Ib examined with endoscopy, endoscopic ultrasound, and computed tomography; (3) aged 20–80 years; (4) performance status of 0 or 1 on the Eastern Cooperative Oncology Group scale; (5) diagnosis of T2DM; (6) plan to undergo gastrectomy or ESD; and (7) provision of written informed consent. The exclusion criteria were as follows: (1) having a high risk regarding the operation, such as severe heart disease or respiratory disease; (2) being pregnant or planning for pregnancy; (3) having experienced previous abdominal surgery or radiation therapy; or (4) having a proven more advanced disease than pathological stage II requiring adjuvant chemotherapy.

All treatment options were chosen at the discretion of each surgeon. We categorized all patients into three groups according to the intervention: (1) gastrectomy with duodenal bypass group (total and subtotal gastrectomy with Roux-en-Y gastrojejunostomy, and subtotal gastrectomy with loop gastrojejunostomy), (2) gastrectomy without bypass group (subtotal gastrectomy with gastroduodenostomy), and (3) ESD group (the control). Each preoperative and follow-up (3 and 12 months after treatment) examination included measurements of the patient's height and body weight, along with blood tests (glycosylated hemoglobin (HbA1c), fasting blood glucose (FBG), 2-hour postprandial glucose (PP2), metabolic hormones, and adipokines). After the follow-up examination at 12 months, the patients were followed up regularly in a routine care setting. The protocol and data were approved by the institutional review board of the National Cancer Center (IRB No. NCCNCS-12-563) and all patients provided written informed consent.

2.2. Identification and Management Protocols for T2DM

Patients who had previously received antidiabetic drugs were classified as having diabetes. Among patients with no previous history of diabetes, DM was defined based on the result of preoperative evaluation according to the American Diabetes Association criteria: FBG $\geq$ 126 mg/dL, random glucose $\geq$ 200 mg/dL, or HbA1c $\geq$ 6.5% [19]. During a follow-up after 1 year, the diabetes medications were titrated by endocrinologists to achieve HbA1c < 7.0%.

2.3. Metabolic Hormones and Adipokines Measurement

Patient blood samples (fasting and postprandial) were stored in a $-70\ ^\circ$C deep freezer and used for the measurement of metabolic hormones and adipokines using Bio-Plex Pro™ Diabetes Assay Panels (Luminex, Austin, TX, USA). Insulin, glucagon, ghrelin, gastric inhibitory polypeptide (GIP), glucagon-like peptide-1 (GLP-1), leptin, plasminogen activator inhibitor-1 (PAI-1), resistin, and visfatin levels were assessed. The homeostasis model of insulin resistance (HOMA-IR) was calculated using the following formula: fasting insulin (IU/mL) $\times$ FBG (mg/dL)/405.

2.4. Glycemic Control Status Assessment

Glycemic control status was assessed at the 1-year visit. Glycemic control status was considered to be "improved" if patients had lower HbA1c with medication with a dose equal to or lower than the baseline and "worsened" if patients had higher HbA1c with medication with a dose equal to or higher than the baseline. Other cases excluded from the "improved" and "worsened" categories were defined as "equivocal".

2.5. Long-Term Outcomes

The composite event was recorded until 3 February 2021, and it included the recurrence of gastric cancer, myocardial infarction, stroke, coronary revascularization, and all-cause death.

2.6. Statistical Analysis

Continuous values were presented as means with standard deviations or medians with interquartile ranges. Categorical values were presented as frequencies and percentages. Baseline characteristics, according to intervention groups, were compared via an analysis of variance followed by a Bonferroni post hoc test, a Kruskal–Wallis test followed by Dunn's post hoc test, or Fisher's exact test, according to the variable type.

The association between the types of the intervention and glycemic control status (the order of "improved", "equivocal", and "worsened") at the 1-year visit was assessed using the ordered logistic regression analysis. Demographic characteristics and baseline metabolic parameters were considered as potential confounders, and the final multivariable model was adjusted for statistically significant potential confounders through a stepwise selection method. The associations are presented as odds ratios (ORs) with 95% confidence intervals (CIs).

Each metabolic parameter (HbA1c, FBG, PP2, BMI, and HOMA-IR) and levels of metabolic hormones and adipokines during the 1-year follow-up period were compared between the groups of gastrectomy with duodenal bypass patients, gastrectomy without duodenal bypass patients, and ESD patients using the linear mixed model. HOMA-IR, metabolic hormones, and adipokines levels were log-transformed to improve the normality. The differences between groups were adjusted for age, sex, time from the baseline, and the baseline measurements of each assessed variable. The difference between the groups in log-transformed levels of metabolic hormones and adipokines was exponentially transformed and interpreted as a ratio of hormone levels between the groups on the basis of the following equation:

difference between groups in log(measurements) = log(measurements in the gastrectomy group) − log(measurements in the ESD group) = log(measurements in the gastrectomy group/measurements in the ESD group) = log(a ratio of measurements between groups).

Additionally, the changes in each measurement at the 3-month and 1-year visits, relative to the baseline levels, were assessed using a paired t-test, and p-values were adjusted using Dunnett's method for multiple comparisons between two visit points and the baseline.

For long-term outcomes, the Kaplan–Meier method was used to generate survival curves, while the log-rank test was performed to evaluate differences in composite event-free survival according to the types of the interventions.

2.7. Assessment of Effect Modification

Whether the effects of gastrectomy on the 1-year glycemic control status (with ESD as the control) were altered by the baseline metabolic characteristics was explored using the interaction terms, which were defined as the product of the type of interventions and the levels of each parameter. The significance of the effect modification was tested by entering each interaction term into the multivariable ordered logistic regression model for the 1-year glycemic control status.

Patient subgroups were classified based on the median values of the significant effect modifiers detected in the preceding test. Stratified analyses for changes in metabolic parameters were performed according to the subgroups using the linear mixed models. The significance of the heterogeneity according to the subgroups was tested by entering the product of the type of interventions and subgroups into the linear mixed models.

All statistical analyses were performed using SAS 9.4 (SAS Institute Inc., Cary, NC, USA). Analysis items with $p < 0.05$ were considered to be statistically significant.

3. Results

3.1. Patient Baseline Characteristics

A total of 62 EGC patients with T2DM were initially enrolled and underwent either gastrectomy or ESD (Figure 1). Among them, 21 patients were excluded due to withdrawal of agreement ($n = 18$), failure to follow-up ($n = 2$), and advancement of the disease beyond pathological stage II ($n = 1$). Finally, a total of 41 patients were included in the 1-year outcome analysis. The number of patients was 24, 5, and 12 in the gastrectomy with duodenal bypass, gastrectomy without duodenal bypass, and ESD groups, respectively. The gastrectomy with duodenal bypass group consisted of patients who underwent a total ($n = 5$) and subtotal ($n = 9$) gastrectomy with Roux-en-Y gastrojejunostomy and patients who underwent subtotal gastrectomy with loop gastrojejunostomy ($n = 10$).

The patient baseline characteristics are presented in Table 1. There were no significant differences in age, sex, duration of diabetes, HbA1c, FBG, PP2, and HOMA-IR between the groups. The mean BMI values were different between the groups (24.1, 21.9, and 26.1 kg/m^2 in gastrectomy with duodenal bypass, without bypass, and ESD groups, respectively, $p = 0.022$), and the gastrectomy without duodenal bypass group had a lower BMI than did the ESD group (adjusted $p = 0.024$). The levels of metabolic hormones and adipokines were similar between the groups, except for fasting and postprandial PAI-1 levels; the postprandial PAI-1 levels were lower in the gastrectomy without duodenal bypass group than in the ESD group (adjusted $p = 0.015$). Most patients (40 of 41) did not use insulin; the gastrectomy with duodenal bypass group included one patient who took insulin.

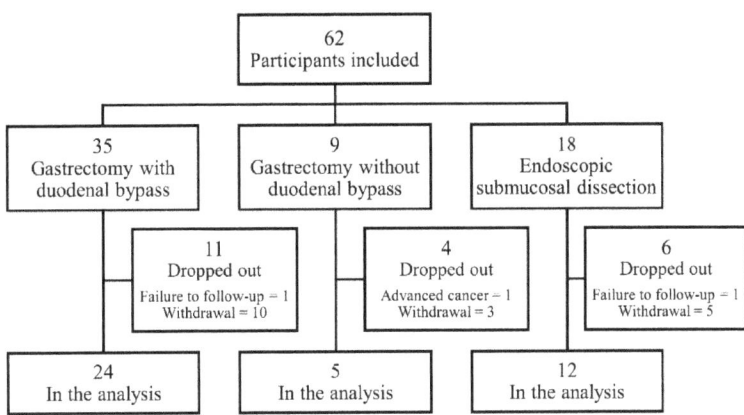

Figure 1. Flow chart of the study.

Table 1. Baseline characteristics of patients included in the analysis.

Baseline Characteristics	Total (n = 41)	Gastrectomy with Duodenal Bypass (n = 24)	Gastrectomy without Duodenal Bypass (n = 5)	Endoscopic Submucosal Dissection (n = 12)	p-Value
Age (years)	62.4 ± 8.4	61.6 ± 9.0	63.8 ± 10.9	63.3 ± 6.3	0.800
Female sex	8 (19.5%)	4 (16.7%)	3 (60.0%)	1 (8.3%)	0.054
DM duration (years)	6.8 ± 6.1	6.1 ± 5.7	6.2 ± 3.9	8.6 ± 7.5	0.489
BMI (kg/m^2)	24.5 ± 3.1	24.1 ± 2.6	21.9 ± 1.7 *	26.1 ± 3.6	**0.022**
HbA1c (%)	7.3 ± 1.6	7.5 ± 1.8	6.8 ± 1.5	7.1 ± 0.9	0.579
Fasting glucose (mg/dL)	132.5 ± 43.7	141.2 ± 53.3	120.8 ± 18.8	120.2 ± 22.3	0.332
Postprandial 2-hour glucose (mg/dL)	292.4 ± 97.8	301.2 ± 105.2	318.8 ± 140.5	262.9 ± 52.5	0.474
HOMA-IR	1.7 (1.1–3.8)	2.5 (1.2–3.8)	1.0 (0.9–1.5)	1.7 (1.3–4.3)	0.169
Fasting					
Ghrelin (pg/mL)	501.8 (242.1–935.8)	460.6 (234.7–968.5)	941.5 (152.5–1457.0)	520.5 (372.5–873.8)	0.937
GIP (pg/mL)	211.3 (123.1–261.5)	235.4 (170.6–295.9)	211.2 (118.6–224.7)	144.7 (113.7–204.7)	0.097
GLP-1 (pg/mL)	191.8 (102.9–259.5)	222.5 (134.3–261.8)	129.8 (93.4–538.9)	186.6 (72.9–232.4)	0.657
Glucagon (pg/mL)	124.0 (75.7–258.4)	144.2 (78.7–263.3)	84.8 (79.6–385.3)	85.1 (69.6–121.4)	0.182
Leptin (ng/mL)	2.1 (1.1–3.9)	2.1 (1.1–4.0)	1.2 (0.7–5.8)	2.4 (0.9–3.0)	0.932
PAI-1 (ng/mL)	47.6 (37.5–72.6)	43.5 (35.8–66.9)	35.2 (28.6–71.7)	53.8 (47.6–149.0)	**0.036**
Resistin (ng/mL)	5.4 (3.0–8.8)	5.1 (2.6–8.0)	5.1 (3.5–10.6)	5.9 (3.2–9.5)	0.570
Visfatin (ng/mL)	2.7 (1.1–5.8)	2.7 (0.8–4.6)	4.1 (1.5–9.4)	2.3 (1.3–6.8)	0.406
Postprandial 2 h					
Ghrelin (pg/mL)	444.3 (278.3–774.5)	370.7 (273.3–751.5)	693.9 (123.3–1173.3)	505.2 (374.4–779.3)	0.789
GIP (pg/mL)	355.1 (299.8–474.2)	367.4 (297.0–551.3)	427.3 (368.6–496.8)	314.6 (260.0–445.4)	0.418
GLP-1 (pg/mL)	222.3 (127.5–276.9)	229.4 (147.2–291.8)	206.6 (162.1–530.3)	205.6 (85.5–266.6)	0.624
Glucagon (pg/mL)	127.2 (74.8–245.3)	172.7 (83.8–251.3)	110.1 (82.8–382.7)	91.2 (70.8–139.0)	0.453
Leptin (ng/mL)	1.8 (0.9–3.3)	1.7 (0.9–3.4)	1.1 (0.7–5.4)	1.8 (0.9–2.6)	0.972
PAI-1 (ng/mL)	45.1 (33.7–69.0)	47.5 (31.1–66.1)	33.7 (25.6–37.1) *	61.0 (43.2–222.9)	**0.016**
Resistin (ng/mL)	4.5 (2.5–6.5)	4.9 (2.7–6.0)	3.9 (2.5–5.8)	3.8 (2.4–9.4)	0.867
Visfatin (ng/mL)	2.0 (1.0–5.8)	1.9 (0.9–5.2)	2.1 (1.6–4.4)	2.2 (0.9–9.7)	0.762

Data are presented as mean ± standard deviation, median (interquartile range), or frequency (%). Significant p-values ($p < 0.05$) are in boldface type. * Significant difference from the ESD group in the post hoc analysis (adjusted $p < 0.05$). DM, diabetes mellitus; BMI, body mass index; HbA1c, hemoglobin A1c; HOMA-IR, homeostasis model assessment of insulin resistance; ESD, endoscopic submucosal dissection; GIP, gastric inhibitory polypeptide; GLP-1, glucagon-like peptide-1; PAI-1, plasminogen activator inhibitor-1.

3.2. Glycemic Control Status at the 1-Year Visit

After 1 year of follow-up, the glycemic control status was different according to the type of intervention (Supplementary Figure S1 online); the proportions of improved/equivocal/worsened glycemic control were 62.5%/29.2%/8.3% in the gastrectomy with duodenal bypass group, 40.0%/60.0%/0.0% in the gastrectomy without duodenal bypass group, and 16.7%/50.0%/33.3% in the ESD group, respectively ($p = 0.046$).

The independent effect of each type of surgery on the 1-year glycemic control status was assessed using ordered logistic regression analysis (Table 2). In the univariable analysis, gastrectomy with duodenal bypass was associated with a better glycemic control status than was an ESD (OR = 7.93, 95% CI = 1.81–34.70). In the final multivariable model, the effects of gastrectomy were adjusted for the baseline HOMA-IR, which was the only significant variable among potential confounders, including age, sex, DM duration, BMI, and HbA1c. In this final model, both gastrectomy with duodenal bypass (OR = 8.68, 95% CI = 1.81–41.63) and gastrectomy without duodenal bypass (OR = 10.60, 95% CI = 1.10–102.35) were associated with a better glycemic control status than was ESD. These estimates for ORs were similar in the full multivariable model that included all potential confounding variables.

Table 2. The effects of gastrectomy with or without duodenal bypass on the probability of better glycemic control at the 1-year visit.

Variables	Univariable Model		Full Multivariable Model		Final Multivariable Model [1]	
	OR (95% CI)	*p*-Value	OR (95% CI)	*p*-Value	OR (95% CI)	*p*-Value
Type of the intervention						
ESD	1	Reference	1	Reference	1	Reference
Gastrectomy with duodenal bypass	**7.93 (1.81–34.70)**	**0.006**	**11.94 (2.03–70.26)**	**0.006**	**8.68 (1.81–41.63)**	**0.007**
Gastrectomy without duodenal bypass	4.27 (0.55–33.37)	0.166	12.02 (0.74–193.91)	0.080	**10.60 (1.10–102.35)**	**0.041**
Age (years)	0.98 (0.92–1.06)	0.658	0.99 (0.90–1.09)	0.890		
Female sex	2.05 (0.44–9.54)	0.359	1.98 (0.24–16.18)	0.525		
DM duration (years)	0.92 (0.84–1.02)	0.119	0.97 (0.85–1.11)	0.658		
BMI (kg/m^2)	1.06 (0.87–1.29)	0.557	1.15 (0.87–1.53)	0.323		
HbA1c (%)	0.90 (0.62–1.30)	0.562	0.79 (0.48–1.31)	0.362		
HOMA-IR	**1.65 (1.07–2.54)**	**0.024**	**1.96 (1.08–3.55)**	**0.027**	**1.88 (1.16–3.07)**	**0.011**

The association between each baseline characteristic, including the type of the intervention and better glycemic control (the order of "improved", "equivocal", and "worsened") at the 1-year visit is presented as an OR and its CI estimated using ordered logistic regression analysis. [1] Variables included in the final multivariable model were selected through a stepwise selection method. This model, including only significant variables, was chosen as the final model for parsimoniousness. Significant values ($p < 0.05$) are in boldface type. OR, odds ratio; CI, confidence interval; ESD, endoscopic submucosal dissection; DM, diabetes mellitus; BMI, body mass index; HbA1c, hemoglobin A1c; HOMA-IR, homeostasis model assessment of insulin resistance.

3.3. Changes in Metabolic Parameters after Gastrectomy

To investigate the effect of surgery on the metabolic parameters (HbA1c, FBG, PP2, BMI, and HOMA-IR), we compared each measurement during the follow-up period between the groups (Table 3). Compared with the ESD group, the gastrectomy with duodenal bypass group showed significantly lower HbA1c (−0.5% point), PP2 (−97.9 mg/dL), BMI (−2.1 kg/m^2), and log10-transformed HOMA-IR (−0.21) (all $p < 0.05$). The gastrectomy without duodenal bypass group showed similar patterns of metabolic improvements in PP2 (−67.8 mg/dL), BMI (−2.3 kg/m^2), and log10-transformed HOMA-IR (−0.31) (all $p < 0.05$), but the improvement in HbA1c was not significant (−0.5% point, $p = 0.184$). The improvement in FBG was not significant in either of the gastrectomy groups, with or without duodenal bypass.

Metabolic parameters at the 3-month and 1-year visits were also compared with the baseline levels (Table 3 and Supplementary Figure S2 online). Compared with the preoperative levels, HbA1c, PP2, and BMI showed significant improvements in the gastrectomy with duodenal bypass group, while only BMI showed a significant improvement in the gastrectomy without duodenal bypass group. In contrast, the ESD group showed significant worsening in the FBG levels (+23.8 mg/dL at the 1-year visit, $p = 0.024$).

Table 3. Metabolic parameters during the 1-year follow-up period.

Metabolic Parameters	Groups	Difference from the Control Group [1]		Change from the Baseline [2]			
				3-Month Visit		1-Year Visit	
		Estimates	p-Value	Mean ± SD	p-Value	Mean ± SD	p-Value
HbA1c (%)	ESD	0	Ref	−0.3 ± 1.2	0.885	−0.1 ± 1.5	>0.999
	Group 1	−0.5	**0.028**	−1.1 ± 1.6	**0.007**	−0.9 ± 1.7	**0.045**
	Group 2	−0.5	0.184	−0.5 ± 1.1	0.640	0.0 ± 1.3	>0.999
Fasting glucose (mg/dL)	ESD	0	Ref	17.4 ± 27.1	0.095	23.8 ± 27.4	**0.024**
	Group 1	−11.1	0.328	−12.2 ± 71.8	0.831	0.2 ± 54.5	>0.999
	Group 2	−0.6	0.971	19.2 ± 33.2	0.532	9.0 ± 21.6	0.808
Postprandial 2 h glucose (mg/dL)	ESD	0	Ref	−17.2 ± 49.4	0.551	13.6 ± 50.2	0.828
	Group 1	−97.9	**<0.001**	−151.1 ± 103.8	**<0.001**	−99.0 ± 109.0	**0.001**
	Group 2	−67.8	**0.044**	−121.4 ± 123.5	0.186	−117.0 ± 113.2	0.261
BMI (kg/m^2)	ESD	0	Ref	−0.2 ± 1.3	>0.999	−0.4 ± 1.9	0.983
	Group 1	−2.1	**<0.001**	−2.2 ± 1.8	**<0.001**	−1.6 ± 1.9	**0.002**
	Group 2	−2.3	**0.001**	−2.0 ± 0.4	**0.001**	−1.5 ± 0.8	0.062
Log(HOMA-IR)	ESD	0	Ref	0.00 ± 0.31	>0.999	0.01 ± 0.30	>0.999
	Group 1	−0.21	**0.019**	−0.21 ± 0.44	0.064	−0.28 ± 0.58	0.067
	Group 2	−0.31	**0.036**	−0.10 ± 0.41	>0.999	0.01 ± 0.11	>0.999

[1] During the 1-year follow-up period, each metabolic parameter in the gastrectomy with duodenal bypass group (group 1) and the gastrectomy without duodenal bypass group (group 2) was compared with each respective parameter in the control group using a linear mixed model. The estimates and p-values were adjusted for age, sex, time from the baseline, and the baseline measurements of each assessed variable. [2] Statistical significance of the change in each variable at each visit, relative to the baseline value, was assessed using a paired t-test. The p-values were adjusted using Dunnett's method for multiple comparisons between two visit points and the baseline. Significant values ($p < 0.05$) are in boldface type. SD, standard deviation; HbA1c, hemoglobin A1c; ESD, endoscopic submucosal dissection; Ref, reference value; BMI, body mass index; Log, log10-transformed; HOMA-IR, homeostasis model assessment of insulin resistance.

3.4. Changes in Metabolic Hormones and Adipokines after Gastrectomy

Metabolic hormone and adipokine levels in the gastrectomy groups during the follow-up period were compared with those in the ESD group (Figure 2 and Supplementary Table S1 online). The gastrectomy with duodenal bypass group showed a significant reduction in fasting leptin, postprandial leptin, and fasting PAI-1 levels (reduced to 61.1%, 67.5%, and 60.1% of those in the ESD group, respectively, all $p < 0.05$). The gastrectomy without duodenal bypass group showed a similar magnitude of reduction in fasting leptin, postprandial leptin, and fasting PAI-1 levels (reduced to 60.5%, 54.4%, and 53.3% of those in the ESD group, respectively), but the reduction in leptin levels was not statistically significant. Fasting resistin levels were reduced only in the gastrectomy without duodenal bypass group (reduced to 63.8% of those in the ESD group, $p = 0.040$). Ghrelin, GIP, GLP-1, glucagon, visfatin, postprandial PAI-1, and postprandial resistin levels after gastrectomy were not different from those in the ESD groups.

3.5. Factors Influencing the Metabolic Effects of Gastrectomy with Duodenal Bypass

We explored the influence of preoperative metabolic characteristics on the improvement of the 1-year glycemic control status in patients treated using gastrectomy with duodenal bypass (Supplementary Table S2 online). Due to a small number of cases, potential effect modifiers for gastrectomy without duodenal bypass were not explored. In this exploratory analysis, the beneficial effect of gastrectomy with duodenal bypass was more prominent in patients with higher preoperative fasting or postprandial leptin levels (p for interaction = 0.011 and 0.009, respectively) but was attenuated in those with higher preoperative fasting PAI-1 levels (p for interaction = 0.013). The effect of gastrectomy with duodenal bypass on the 1-year glycemic control status was not changed by the preoperative BMI, HbA1c, FBG, PP2, HOMA-IR, other metabolic hormones, or adipokines levels.

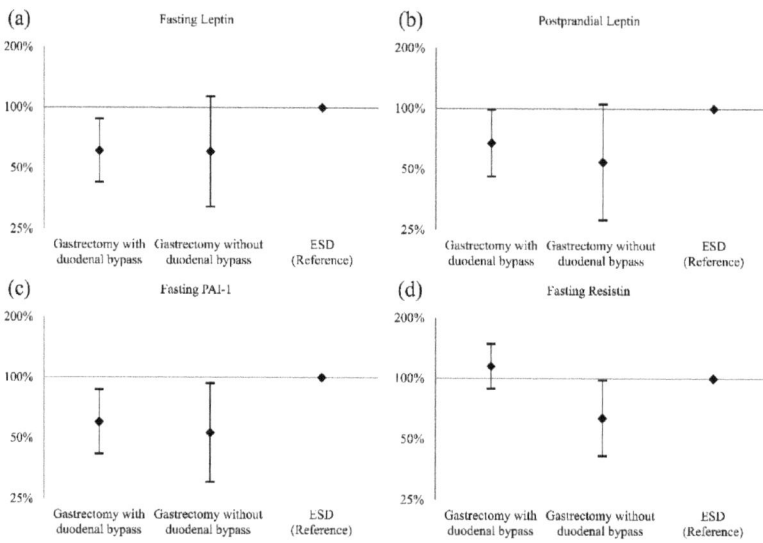

Figure 2. The ratios of metabolic hormone and adipokine levels after gastrectomy and after ESD (the reference). (**a**) Fasting leptin, (**b**) postprandial leptin, (**c**) fasting PAI-1, and (**d**) fasting resistin. The ratios and 95% confidence intervals were estimated using linear mixed models for log-transformed hormone levels, with adjustments for age, sex, time from the baseline, and the baseline measurements of each assessed variable. ESD, endoscopic submucosal dissection; PAI-1, plasminogen activator inhibitor-1.

Next, patient subgroups were classified according to the median values of the preoperative fasting leptin (2.1 ng/mL), postprandial leptin (1.8 ng/mL), and fasting PAI-1 (47.6 ng/mL) levels (Table 4). In the stratified analyses, those with high fasting leptin levels showed a greater decrease in PP2 (-127.1 vs. -72.3 mg/dL, p for interaction = 0.017) and BMI (-3.1 vs. -1.2 kg/m^2, p for interaction = 0.018) than did those with lower fasting leptin levels, after gastrectomy with duodenal bypass. Similarly, patients with high postprandial leptin levels showed a greater decrease in PP2 (-133.5 vs. -72.4 mg/dL, p for interaction = 0.017) and BMI (-3.0 vs. -1.2 kg/m^2, p for interaction = 0.010) than did those with lower postprandial leptin levels. However, the metabolic improvement after gastrectomy with duodenal bypass was not different, according to fasting PAI-1 levels.

3.6. Long-Term Outcomes

During the postoperative follow-up period (median, 5.7 years; interquartile range, 4.9–6.9), one case each of recurrence (ESD group), stroke (gastrectomy without duodenal bypass group), and coronary revascularization (ESD group), and three cases of death from other malignancies (gastrectomy with duodenal bypass group; one biliary cancer and two hematologic malignancies) were recorded (Supplementary Figure S3 online). There was no difference in the composite event-free survival rate between groups ($p = 0.647$).

Table 4. Changes in the metabolic parameters after gastrectomy with duodenal bypass compared with ESD as a reference in the subgroups classified by preoperative fasting leptin, postprandial leptin, and fasting PAI-1 levels.

Metabolic Parameters	Subgroups by Preoperative Fasting Leptin						Subgroups by Preoperative Postprandial Leptin						Subgroups by Preoperative Fasting PAI-1					
	High (≥2.1 ng/mL)		Low (<2.1 ng/mL)		p for Interaction [1]		High (≥1.8 ng/mL)		Low (<1.8 ng/mL)		p for Interaction [1]		High (≥47.6 ng/mL)		Low (<47.6 ng/mL)		p for Interaction [1]
	Effects	p-Value	Effects	p-Value			Effects	p-Value	Effects	p-Value			Effects	p-Value	Effects	p-Value	
HbA1c (%)	−0.6	0.016	−0.4	0.342	0.182		−0.6	0.011	−0.5	0.229	0.290		−0.3	0.505	−1.1	0.009	0.510
Fasting glucose (mg/dL)	−22.3	0.068	6.9	0.718	0.255		−20.2	0.065	2.6	0.896	0.381		−7.9	0.641	−6.5	0.741	0.574
Postprandial 2-h glucose (mg/dL)	−127.1	<0.001	−72.3	0.050	0.017		−133.5	<0.001	−72.4	0.046	0.017		−80.5	0.005	−100.3	0.002	0.375
BMI (kg/m^2)	−3.1	<0.001	−1.2	0.090	0.018		−3.0	<0.001	−1.2	0.075	0.010		−1.7	0.004	−3.4	<0.001	0.147
Log(HOMA-IR)	−0.9	0.001	−0.1	0.743	0.223		−0.9	0.002	−0.1	0.696	0.224		−0.3	0.322	−0.9	0.015	0.266

The effects of gastrectomy with duodenal bypass on each metabolic parameter during the follow-up period, relative to the effects of ESD (the control), were estimated using a linear mixed model in the subgroups that were classified by preoperative fasting leptin, postprandial leptin, and fasting PAI-1 levels. The estimates and p-values were adjusted for gastrectomy without duodenal bypass, age, sex, time from the baseline, and the baseline measurements of each assessed metabolic parameter. [1] Significance of the differences in the effects of gastrectomy with duodenal bypass according to the subgroups was tested by entering the product of "gastrectomy with duodenal bypass" and the subgroups into the linear mixed models. Significant values (p < 0.05 and p for interaction <0.05) are in boldface type. ESD, endoscopic submucosal dissection; PAI-1, plasminogen activator inhibitor-1; HbA1c, hemoglobin A1c; BMI, body mass index; Log, log10-transformed; HOMA-IR, homeostasis model assessment of insulin resistance.

4. Discussion

This single-center prospective controlled cohort study compared standard curative treatment modalities for EGC in patients with T2DM in terms of metabolic effects. EGC patients with T2DM who underwent gastrectomy, with or without duodenal bypass, showed improvement in glycemic control status more frequently than did those who underwent ESD at 1 year postoperatively. The metabolic improvement by gastrectomy was significant in terms of the PP2, HbA1c, and BMI, as well as some metabolic hormones and adipokines, such as leptin and PAI-1. In particular, the patients with higher preoperative leptin levels experienced a greater metabolic benefit from gastrectomy with duodenal bypass versus ESD than did those with lower leptin levels; in this subgroup, the probability for better 1-year glycemic control status was much higher and the degree of improvement in PP2 and BMI was more pronounced.

It is well established in meta-analyses of randomized controlled trials (RCTs) that gastrectomy, performed as bariatric surgery, is excellent at improving or alleviating serum glucose in obese T2DM patients compared to medical therapy [20,21]. In the meta-analysis by Pack et al., both Roux-en-Y gastric bypass and sleeve gastrectomy showed higher remission rates than did standard medical therapy at 1 to 2 years post operation (risk ratios for remission = 9.13 and 11.15, respectively), and this superiority was maintained until 5 years post operation [21]. Bariatric surgery reduced the microvascular and macrovascular diabetic complications and improved the related mortality [22–24]. Although most studies included patients with BMI > 35 kg/m^2, meta-analyses of selected RCTs and non-randomized studies showed that bariatric surgery was similarly effective in T2DM patients with BMI < 30~35 kg/m^2 [25–27].

Gastrectomy to treat gastric cancer is technically similar to bariatric surgery; therefore, it was expected to have metabolic benefits in gastric cancer patients with T2DM. Several studies have discussed improvement in glycemic control and weight reduction after gastrectomy in gastric cancer patients [15–18,28,29]. However, no studies have compared gastrectomy to non-surgical treatment in gastric cancer patients, except for our previous epidemiological study [18]. This absence of an appropriate control group is an important limitation that can distort the estimate of the effect of gastrectomy in existing observational studies. Previously, we analyzed the Korean National Health Insurance System claims database and showed that, compared with endoscopic resection, total gastrectomy decreased the requirement for antidiabetic medications in gastric cancer patients [18]. However, due to the lack of biochemical data, the improvement of disease control could only be assessed with drug discontinuation [18]. In the current study, we regularly evaluated antidiabetic medications; biochemical data, including serum glucose and HbA1c levels; and anthropometric parameters. Consequently, we showed that the glycemic control status and BMI in EGC patients with T2DM who underwent gastrectomy were significantly improved relative to those in patients who underwent ESD.

In this study, patients who underwent gastrectomy with duodenal bypass had lower leptin and PAI-1 levels than did those who underwent ESD. The improvement in metabolic hormones and adipokines levels after gastrectomy has been demonstrated in studies on bariatric surgery, and Askarpour et al. reported in their recent meta-analysis that bariatric surgery reduced serum leptin, PAI-1, and chemerin levels [30]. A decrease in leptin levels after gastrectomy was also reported in gastric cancer patients, although the control group with non-surgical treatment was limited [15]. Leptin is a satiety hormone that is secreted mainly by the adipocytes [31]. It decreases body weight by suppressing appetite and promoting energy expenditure in physiologic conditions, but hyperleptinemia is observed in patients with obesity and T2DM due to leptin resistance [31,32]. Hyperleptinemia is associated with insulin resistance and micro- and macrovascular diabetic complications, and leptin-mediated hypertension was suggested as one of the mechanisms of developing cardiovascular diseases [32–34]. PAI-1 is an inflammatory adipokine that is associated with T2DM, diabetic nephropathy, and cardiovascular diseases [35,36]. Thus, reductions in leptin and PAI-1 levels after gastrectomy in ECG patients with T2DM might predict or mediate a reduction in risk for diabetic complications.

Another notable finding in this study was that higher preoperative leptin levels played a predictive role for a greater metabolic benefit from gastrectomy with duodenal bypass versus ESD. Such a predictive role has not been widely investigated, but there are a few recent studies on this topic [15,37]. In an RCT that included 40 patients that compared the glycemic control effects of gastric cancer surgery according to surgery type, patients who experienced improvement or remission of diabetes at 12 months after surgery had higher preoperative leptin levels than those who did not [15]. In contrast, in a cohort study on 38 obese patients (mean BMI = 47.3 kg/m^2) with diabetes who underwent bariatric surgery, those with higher than mean preoperative leptin levels (27.3 ng/mL) had higher glucose levels at 3 months post operation [37]. However, this leptin level was approximately 13 times higher than that measured in our study (2.1 ng/mL) due to differences in study populations (obesity vs. EGC) [37]. Since an improvement in hyperleptinemia is one of the remarkable effects of gastrectomy [30], the metabolic benefit from gastrectomy might be less prominent in those without hyperleptinemia. Our results suggest that choosing gastrectomy with duodenal bypass over ESD might be particularly advantageous in EGC patients with T2DM with high leptin levels.

This study had some limitations. The small sample size of this study led to underpowered results, and results on gastrectomy without duodenal bypass may not be reliable due to the small number of patients included. In addition, given the exploratory nature of the study, statistical adjustment for multiplicity was not conducted for multiple outcomes. Therefore, the possibility cannot be excluded that some of the statistically significant results in this study appeared by chance and, thus, they should be interpreted with caution based on the existing scientific knowledge. Because this was a nonrandomized observational study, the results may have been influenced by unmeasured confounders, although most of the measured potential confounders did not differ significantly between groups and were additionally controlled in multivariable analyses. The high dropout rate (33.9%) might serve as a source of bias via differential dropout, although the dropout rates were similar between groups, and the most common reason for dropout was the withdrawal of consent rather than medical problems or failure to follow-up. Furthermore, we could not confirm the difference in the long-term cardiovascular outcome, which could be dependent on diabetes control, due to the small number of events. Studies with a larger sample size are warranted to overcome these limitations and to validate our results.

In summary, our study suggests that gastrectomy has an advantage over ESD in terms of better diabetes management and weight reduction in EGC patients with T2DM and that this advantage can be more prominent in those with higher leptin levels. Metabolic benefits from gastrectomy should be considered in treatment decisions in these patients.

Supplementary Materials: The following are available online at https://www.mdpi.com/article/10.3390/jcm10174008/s1: Supplementary Table S1. Changes in the metabolic hormone levels (log10-transformed); Supplementary Table S2. Changes in the effects of gastrectomy with duodenal bypass according to the candidate effect modifiers on the probability of better 1-year glycemic control at the 1-year visit; Supplementary Figure S1. Glycemic control status at the 1-year visit according to the type of intervention. ESD, endoscopic submucosal dissection; Supplementary Figure S2. Changes in the metabolic parameters from the baseline values; Supplementary Figure S3. Kaplan–Meier curves for composite events (recurrence of gastric cancer, myocardial infarction, stroke, coronary revascularization, and all-cause death) according to the type of intervention.

Author Contributions: Writing—original draft, formal analysis, Y.K.L.; conceptualization, methodology, formal analysis, E.K.L. and Y.J.L.; data curation, writing—review and editing, B.W.E., H.M.Y., Y.-I.K., S.J.C., J.Y.L., C.G.K., M.K.Y., Y.-W.K. and I.J.C.; writing—review and editing, S.-Y.K., Y.H., H.J.K. and M.H.K.; conceptualization, methodology, data curation, supervision, K.W.R. All authors read and agreed to the published version of the manuscript.

Funding: This work was supported by research grants NCC1210552-3 (PI: Keun Won Ryu), NCC1510 740-1 (PI: Mi Hyang Kwak), and NCC1410650-1 (PI: Eun Kyung Lee) from the National Cancer Center, Republic of Korea.

Institutional Review Board Statement: The study was conducted according to the guidelines of the Declaration of Helsinki, and the protocol and data were approved by the institutional review board of the National Cancer Center (IRB No. NCCNCS-12-563).

Informed Consent Statement: Informed consent was obtained from all subjects involved in the study.

Data Availability Statement: The datasets generated for this study are available on reasonable request to the corresponding author. The data are not publicly available due to privacy reasons.

Conflicts of Interest: The authors declare that there are no conflict of interest. The funding sources were not involved in study design, data collection, analysis, interpretation of data, or the decision to submit the paper for publication.

References

1. Hong, S.; Won, Y.J.; Park, Y.R.; Jung, K.W.; Kong, H.J.; Lee, E.S. Cancer statistics in korea: Incidence, mortality, survival, and prevalence in 2017. *Cancer Res. Treat.* **2020**, *52*, 335–350. [CrossRef]
2. Bray, F.; Ferlay, J.; Soerjomataram, I.; Siegel, R.L.; Torre, L.A.; Jemal, A. Global cancer statistics 2018: Globocan estimates of incidence and mortality worldwide for 36 cancers in 185 countries. *CA Cancer J. Clin.* **2018**, *68*, 394–424. [CrossRef] [PubMed]
3. Jun, J.K.; Choi, K.S.; Lee, H.Y.; Suh, M.; Park, B.; Song, S.H.; Jung, K.W.; Lee, C.W.; Choi, I.J.; Park, E.C.; et al. Effectiveness of the korean national cancer screening program in reducing gastric cancer mortality. *Gastroenterology* **2017**, *152*, 1319–1328.e7. [CrossRef] [PubMed]
4. Edwards, B.K.; Noone, A.M.; Mariotto, A.B.; Simard, E.P.; Boscoe, F.P.; Henley, S.J.; Jemal, A.; Cho, H.; Anderson, R.N.; Kohler, B.A.; et al. Annual report to the nation on the status of cancer, 1975–2010, featuring prevalence of comorbidity and impact on survival among persons with lung, colorectal, breast, or prostate cancer. *Cancer* **2014**, *120*, 1290–1314. [CrossRef] [PubMed]
5. Van Gelder, T.; Mulhern, B.; Schoormans, D.; Husson, O.; Lourenço, R.D.A. Assessing health-related quality of life in cancer survivors: Factors impacting on eortc qlu-c10d-derived utility values. *Qual. Life Res.* **2020**, *29*, 1483–1494. [CrossRef]
6. Sarfati, D.; Gurney, J.; Lim, B.T.; Bagheri, N.; Simpson, A.; Koea, J.; Dennett, E. Identifying important comorbidity among cancer populations using administrative data: Prevalence and impact on survival. *Asia Pac. J. Clin. Oncol.* **2016**, *12*, e47–e56. [CrossRef]
7. Cho, N.H.; Shaw, J.E.; Karuranga, S.; Huang, Y.; Fernandes, J.D.d.R.; Ohlrogge, A.W.; Malanda, B. Idf diabetes atlas: Global estimates of diabetes prevalence for 2017 and projections for 2045. *Diabetes Res. Clin. Pract.* **2018**, *138*, 271–281. [CrossRef]
8. Jung, C.H.; Son, J.W.; Kang, S.; Kim, W.J.; Kim, H.S.; Kim, H.S.; Seo, M.; Shin, H.J.; Lee, S.S.; Jeong, S.J.; et al. Diabetes fact sheets in korea, 2020: An appraisal of current status. *Diabetes Metab. J.* **2021**, *45*, 1–10. [CrossRef]
9. Hwangbo, Y.; Kang, D.; Kang, M.; Kim, S.; Lee, E.K.; Kim, Y.A.; Chang, Y.J.; Choi, K.S.; Jung, S.Y.; Woo, S.M.; et al. Incidence of diabetes after cancer development: A korean national cohort study. *JAMA Oncol.* **2018**, *4*, 1099–1105. [CrossRef]
10. Yoon, J.M.; Son, K.Y.; Eom, C.S.; Durrance, D.; Park, S.M. Pre-existing diabetes mellitus increases the risk of gastric cancer: A meta-analysis. *World J. Gastroenterol.* **2013**, *19*, 936–945. [CrossRef]
11. Guideline Committee of the Korean Gastric Cancer Association (KGCA); Development Working Group and Review Panel. Korean practice guideline for gastric cancer 2018: An evidence-based, multi-disciplinary approach. *J. Gastric Cancer* **2019**, *19*, 1–48. [CrossRef] [PubMed]
12. Ikramuddin, S.; Korner, J.; Lee, W.J.; Connett, J.E.; Inabnet, W.B.; Billington, C.J.; Thomas, A.J.; Leslie, D.B.; Chong, K.; Jeffery, R.W.; et al. Roux-en-y gastric bypass vs. intensive medical management for the control of type 2 diabetes, hypertension, and hyperlipidemia: The diabetes surgery study randomized clinical trial. *JAMA* **2013**, *309*, 2240–2249. [CrossRef]
13. Schauer, P.R.; Kashyap, S.R.; Wolski, K.; Brethauer, S.A.; Kirwan, J.P.; Pothier, C.E.; Thomas, S.; Abood, B.; Nissen, S.E.; Bhatt, D.L. Bariatric surgery versus intensive medical therapy in obese patients with diabetes. *N. Engl. J. Med.* **2012**, *366*, 1567–1576. [CrossRef] [PubMed]
14. Schauer, P.R.; Bhatt, D.L.; Kirwan, J.P.; Wolski, K.; Brethauer, S.A.; Navaneethan, S.D.; Aminian, A.; Pothier, C.E.; Kim, E.S.; Nissen, S.E.; et al. Bariatric surgery versus intensive medical therapy for diabetes-3-year outcomes. *N. Engl. J. Med.* **2014**, *370*, 2002–2013. [CrossRef]
15. Choi, Y.Y.; Noh, S.H.; An, J.Y. A randomized controlled trial of roux-en-y gastrojejunostomy vs. Gastroduodenostomy with respect to the improvement of type 2 diabetes mellitus after distal gastrectomy in gastric cancer patients. *PLoS ONE* **2017**, *12*, e0188904. [CrossRef] [PubMed]
16. Kim, J.H.; Huh, Y.J.; Park, S.; Park, Y.S.; Park, D.J.; Kwon, J.W.; Lee, J.H.; Heo, Y.S.; Choi, S.H. Multicenter results of long-limb bypass reconstruction after gastrectomy in patients with gastric cancer and type ii diabetes. *Asian J. Surg.* **2020**, *43*, 297–303. [CrossRef]
17. Kim, J.W.; Cheong, J.H.; Hyung, W.J.; Choi, S.H.; Noh, S.H. Outcome after gastrectomy in gastric cancer patients with type 2 diabetes. *World J. Gastroenterol.* **2012**, *18*, 49–54. [CrossRef] [PubMed]

18. Lee, E.K.; Kim, S.Y.; Lee, Y.J.; Kwak, M.H.; Kim, H.J.; Choi, I.J.; Cho, S.J.; Kim, Y.W.; Lee, J.Y.; Kim, C.G.; et al. Improvement of diabetes and hypertension after gastrectomy: A nationwide cohort study. *World J. Gastroenterol.* **2015**, *21*, 1173–1181. [CrossRef]
19. American Diabetes Association. Standards of medical care in diabetes—2011. *Diabetes Care* **2011**, *34* (Suppl. 1), S11–S61.
20. Khorgami, Z.; Shoar, S.; Saber, A.A.; Howard, C.A.; Danaei, G.; Sclabas, G.M. Outcomes of bariatric surgery versus medical management for type 2 diabetes mellitus: A meta-analysis of randomized controlled trials. *Obes. Surg.* **2019**, *29*, 964–974. [CrossRef]
21. Park, C.H.; Nam, S.J.; Choi, H.S.; Kim, K.O.; Kim, D.H.; Kim, J.W.; Sohn, W.; Yoon, J.H.; Jung, S.H.; Hyun, Y.S.; et al. Comparative efficacy of bariatric surgery in the treatment of morbid obesity and diabetes mellitus: A systematic review and network meta-analysis. *Obes. Surg.* **2019**, *29*, 2180–2190. [CrossRef]
22. Sheng, B.; Truong, K.; Spitler, H.; Zhang, L.; Tong, X.; Chen, L. The long-term effects of bariatric surgery on type 2 diabetes remission, microvascular and macrovascular complications, and mortality: A systematic review and meta-analysis. *Obes. Surg.* **2017**, *27*, 2724–2732. [CrossRef]
23. Yan, G.; Wang, J.; Zhang, J.; Gao, K.; Zhao, Q.; Xu, X. Long-term outcomes of macrovascular diseases and metabolic indicators of bariatric surgery for severe obesity type 2 diabetes patients with a meta-analysis. *PLoS ONE* **2019**, *14*, e0224828. [CrossRef] [PubMed]
24. Billeter, A.T.; Scheurlen, K.M.; Probst, P.; Eichel, S.; Nickel, F.; Kopf, S.; Fischer, L.; Diener, M.K.; Nawroth, P.P.; Müller-Stich, B.P. Meta-analysis of metabolic surgery versus medical treatment for microvascular complications in patients with type 2 diabetes mellitus. *Br. J. Surg.* **2018**, *105*, 168–181. [CrossRef] [PubMed]
25. Cummings, D.E.; Cohen, R.V. Bariatric/metabolic surgery to treat type 2 diabetes in patients with a bmi < 35 kg/m^2. *Diabetes Care* **2016**, *39*, 924–933. [CrossRef] [PubMed]
26. Rubio-Almanza, M.; Hervás-Marín, D.; Cámara-Gómez, R.; Caudet-Esteban, J.; Merino-Torres, J.F. Does metabolic surgery lead to diabetes remission in patients with bmi < 30 kg/m^2?: A meta-analysis. *Obes. Surg.* **2019**, *29*, 1105–1116. [CrossRef]
27. Ji, G.; Li, P.; Li, W.; Sun, X.; Yu, Z.; Li, R.; Zhu, L.; Zhu, S. The effect of bariatric surgery on asian patients with type 2 diabetes mellitus and body mass index < 30 kg/m^2: A systematic review and meta-analysis. *Obes. Surg.* **2019**, *29*, 2492–2502. [CrossRef]
28. Xiong, S.W.; Zhang, D.Y.; Liu, X.M.; Liu, Z.; Zhang, F.T. Comparison of different gastric bypass procedures in gastric carcinoma patients with type 2 diabetes mellitus. *World J. Gastroenterol.* **2014**, *20*, 18427–18431. [CrossRef]
29. Hayashi, S.Y.; Faintuch, J.; Yagi, O.K.; Yamaguchi, C.M.; Faintuch, J.J.; Cecconello, I. Does roux-en-y gastrectomy for gastric cancer influence glucose homeostasis in lean patients? *Surg. Endosc.* **2013**, *27*, 2829–2835. [CrossRef]
30. Askarpour, M.; Alizadeh, S.; Hadi, A.; Symonds, M.E.; Miraghajani, M.; Sheikhi, A.; Ghaedi, E. Effect of bariatric surgery on the circulating level of adiponectin, chemerin, plasminogen activator inhibitor-1, leptin, resistin, and visfatin: A systematic review and meta-analysis. *Horm. Metab. Res.* **2020**, *52*, 207–215. [CrossRef]
31. Kelesidis, T.; Kelesidis, I.; Chou, S.; Mantzoros, C.S. Narrative review: The role of leptin in human physiology: Emerging clinical applications. *Ann. Intern. Med.* **2010**, *152*, 93–100. [CrossRef]
32. Katsiki, N.; Mikhailidis, D.P.; Banach, M. Leptin, cardiovascular diseases and type 2 diabetes mellitus. *Acta Pharmacol. Sin.* **2018**, *39*, 1176–1188. [CrossRef] [PubMed]
33. Simonds, S.E.; Pryor, J.T.; Ravussin, E.; Greenway, F.L.; Dileone, R.; Allen, A.M.; Bassi, J.; Elmquist, J.K.; Keogh, J.M.; Henning, E.; et al. Leptin mediates the increase in blood pressure associated with obesity. *Cell* **2014**, *159*, 1404–1416. [CrossRef]
34. Boutari, C.; Perakakis, N.; Mantzoros, C.S. Association of adipokines with development and progression of nonalcoholic fatty liver disease. *Endocrinol. Metab.* **2018**, *33*, 33–43. [CrossRef] [PubMed]
35. Goldberg, R.B. Cytokine and cytokine-like inflammation markers, endothelial dysfunction, and imbalanced coagulation in development of diabetes and its complications. *J. Clin. Endocrinol. Metab.* **2009**, *94*, 3171–3182. [CrossRef]
36. Jung, R.G.; Motazedian, P.; Ramirez, F.D.; Simard, T.; Di Santo, P.; Visintini, S.; Faraz, M.A.; Labinaz, A.; Jung, Y.; Hibbert, B. Association between plasminogen activator inhibitor-1 and cardiovascular events: A systematic review and meta-analysis. *Thromb. J.* **2018**, *16*, 12. [CrossRef] [PubMed]
37. Cabrera, L.O.; Trindade, E.N.; Leite, C.; Abegg, E.H.; Trindade, M.R.M. Preoperative level of leptin can be a predictor of glycemic control for patients with diabetes undergoing bariatric surgery. *Obes. Surg.* **2020**, *30*, 4829–4833. [CrossRef]

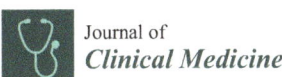

Article

Prevalence and Clinical Implications of Ascites in Gastric Cancer Patients after Curative Surgery

Ju-Hee Lee [1,*], Sung-Joon Kwon [1], Mimi Kim [2] and Bo-Kyeong Kang [2]

[1] Department of Surgery, Hanyang University College of Medicine, 222 Wangsimri-ro, Seongdong-gu, Seoul 04763, Korea; sjkwon@hanyang.ac.kr
[2] Department of Radiology, Hanyang University College of Medicine, 222 Wangsimri-ro, Seongdong-gu, Seoul 04763, Korea; bluefish010@naver.com (M.K.); msbbogri@naver.com (B.-K.K.)
* Correspondence: leejuhee79@gmail.com; Tel.: +82-2-2290-8451

Abstract: We aimed to determine the frequency and clinical significance of ascites that developed during the follow-up period in patients who underwent curative resection for gastric cancer. The study included 577 patients with gastric cancer who underwent curative gastrectomy. Among them, 184 showed ascites in postoperative follow-up images. Benign ascites was observed in 131 of 490 patients without recurrence, 48 patients (of 87) with recurrence had malignancy-related ascites, and the remaining 5 patients had ascites only prior to recurrence. In most patients without recurrence (97.7%) and in 50% of patients with malignancy-related ascites, the ascites was small in volume and located in the pelvic cavity at the time that it was first identified. However, with the exception of nine patients, malignancy-related pelvic ascites occurred simultaneously or after obvious recurrence. Of those nine patients who had minimal pelvic ascites before obvious recurrence, only one had a clear association with a malignancy-related ascites. In the multivariate analysis, an age of ≤45 was the only independent risk factor for the occurrence of benign ascites. A small volume of pelvic ascites fluid is common in young gastric cancer patients who do not have recurrence after gastrectomy, regardless of sex. It is rare for ascites to be the first manifestation of recurrence.

Keywords: gastric cancer; ascites; postoperative follow-up

1. Introduction

Gastric cancer is one of the leading causes of cancer-related deaths worldwide [1] and most gastric cancer-related deaths are due to recurrence [2]. The peritoneal region is the most common site of gastric cancer recurrence and is associated with a poor prognosis [3–5]. Diagnosis of peritoneal metastasis is typically determined by a computed tomography [CT] scan. Ascites is one of the most common findings suggestive of peritoneal carcinomatosis; others include peritoneal thickening, nodularity, and contrast enhancement in CT [6–9]. Although there is little convincing evidence that intense surveillance improves survival, routine follow-up after curative resection for the early detection of recurrence in gastric cancer is considered general practice, as some research findings indicate that asymptomatic patients had longer post-recurrence and overall survival than symptomatic patients [10–12]. Physicians often encounter ascites in abdominal imaging during the post-gastrectomy follow-up period and there are concerns that this finding may indicate early peritoneal recurrence, especially in men, despite a lack of evidence otherwise. Preoperatively detected ascites in CT strongly suggests the presence of peritoneal metastasis and free cancer cells in patients with advanced gastric cancer [13,14]. However, the clinical significance of ascites detected by postoperative CT or other abdominal imaging during the follow-up period is not well-studied. In this study, we evaluated the frequency and clinical implications of ascites in patients who underwent curative surgery for gastric cancer.

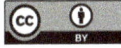

2. Materials and Methods

A total of 634 patients with gastric cancer who underwent curative gastrectomy at the Hanyang University Seoul Hospital between January 2008 and December 2015 were selected from a prospective gastric cancer database. Fifty-seven patients were excluded for the following reasons: (1) mortality after surgery ($n = 3$); (2) synchronous or metachronous cancers ($n = 14$); (3) recurrent ascites due to liver cirrhosis or chronic kidney disease ($n = 3$); (4) ascites due to ileus ($n = 1$); and (5) follow-up loss or a short follow-up time of <12 months due to unknown causes (in patients without recurrence) after surgery ($n = 35$). A postoperative follow-up was conducted every 3–6 months for up to 5 years and annually thereafter. Standard clinical practice included evaluation by physical examination, laboratory tests including the measurement of tumor markers, radiologic imaging, and endoscopy. Imaging was conducted alternatively by abdominopelvic and chest CT and abdominal sonography. Medical records of the remaining 577 patients were retrospectively reviewed. The median period of follow-up was 61.0 months (range of 4.0–146.0 months).

Ascites was primarily detected in CT imaging, having been initially identified by abdominal sonography in only one patient. Images were reviewed by at least two experienced radiologists and ascites was considered present when a low radiologic density of ≤10 Hounsfield units was found within the abdominal cavity outside the intra-abdominal or pelvic organs. Intraperitoneal fluid collection that occurred within 3 months after surgery was excluded to distinguish from postoperative changes in benign ascites. The volume of ascites fluid was estimated using ruler grids applied to CT images using the method described by Chang et al. [15]. A small degree of ascites was defined as a volume of <50 mL, moderate as 50–500 mL, and large as >500 mL (Figure 1).

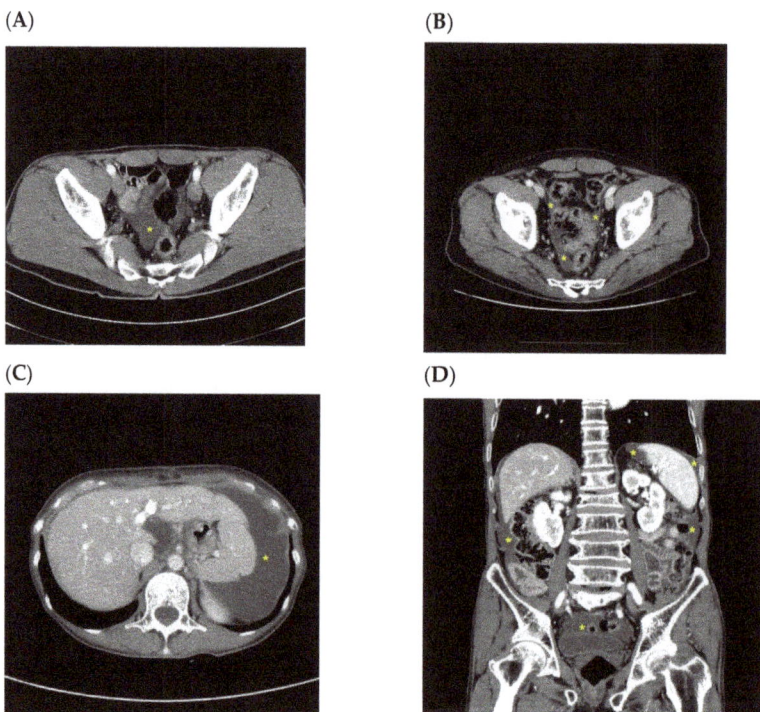

Figure 1. *Cont.*

(E) 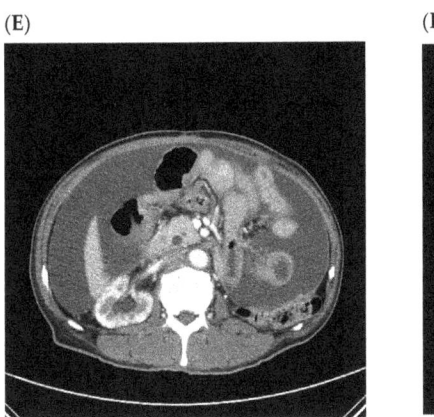 (F)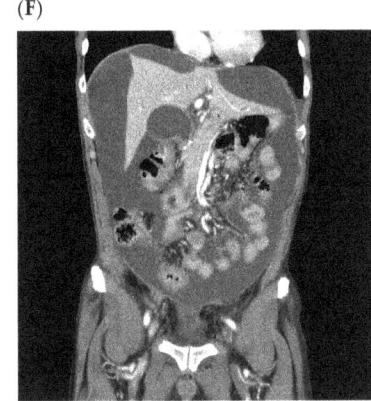

Figure 1. Typical ascites imaging in CT: (**A**) benign small pelvic ascites; (**B**) malignant small pelvic ascites with peritoneal thickening; (**C**) benign moderate ascites in perisplenic area (left abdomen); (**D**) malignant moderate ascites; and (**E**,**F**) alignant large ascites. Yellow stars indicate ascites.

Cases of benign ascites were those in which patients developed ascites without recurrence during the follow-up period. None of the patients had an interval of <12 months from identification of ascites to the follow-up conclusion, excluding eight patients whose follow-up period exceeded to 5 years without recurrence. If only ascites was present without symptoms or other findings suggesting intra-abdominal recurrence, the ascites was considered benign at that time and routine radiologic follow-up was performed according to the gastric cancer follow-up protocol of our hospital. Short-term radiologic tests including positron emission tomography and/or abdominopelvic CT were performed within 3 months in 40 patients with benign ascites for the following reasons: (1) an advanced-stage disease with newly detected ascites ($n = 13$); (2) a remaining or increased infiltration around the surgical site ($n = 11$); (3) combined intra-abdominal lymphadenopathy, ultimately confirmed as reactive lymph node enlargement by repeat tests ($n = 7$); (4) combined abnormal laboratory findings ($n = 2$) or levels of tumor markers ($n = 1$); (5) complaints of abdominal symptoms ($n = 1$); (6) the presence of portal vein thrombosis; (7) moderate volume of ascites fluid ($n = 1$); (8) an increased volume of ascites fluid compared to the findings immediately after surgery ($n = 2$); and (9) a liver cyst of increasing size ($n = 1$). The phrase "malignancy-related ascites" is used as a more appropriate descriptor than "malignant ascites" considering malignant cells were confirmed by ascites cytology in only some patients with recurrence. Intra-abdominal recurrence or peritoneal metastasis was diagnosed by serial changes in the CT and/or positron emission tomography performed when recurrence was suspected based on the CT. A histological examination of biopsy specimens or ascites cytology for patients with recurrence was performed whenever possible. Death due to disease progression was confirmed in all patients classified as having recurrence.

Statistical analyses were performed using SPSS version 22.0 (SPSS Inc., Chicago, IL, USA). Chi-squared tests and independent Student's t-tests were used for comparisons between groups. A binary logistic regression model was used for multivariate analysis. The threshold for statistical significance was set at $p \leq 0.05$.

3. Results

Of the 577 eligible patients, ascites was identified in 184 patients during the follow-up period. Among them, 131 patients had benign ascites, accounting for 26.7% of the 490 patients without recurrence. Of the 131 patients with benign ascites, 78 were male (78/328; 23.8% of all males without recurrence) and 53 were female (53/162; 32.7% of all females without recurrence). Ascites was observed in 53 (60.7%) of the 87 patients with recurrence. Patients fell into three groups: (1) 40 patients with malignancy-related ascites at the same time as the findings of peritoneal seeding or intra-abdominal recurrence, including one patient who on initial recurrence had ascites only; (2) eight patients with ascites presumed to be benign before obvious recurrence and considered to have malignancy-related ascites after the obvious recurrence; and (3) five patients with ascites before recurrence but no evidence of malignancy-related ascites upon recurrence. Groups (1) and (2) were classified as patients with malignancy-related ascites. Among 48 patients with malignancy-related ascites, ascites appeared prior to recurrence in eight patients (16.7%, Group (2)), simultaneous with the recurrence detection in 25 (48.1%) and following recurrence in 15 (31.3%) (Figure 2).

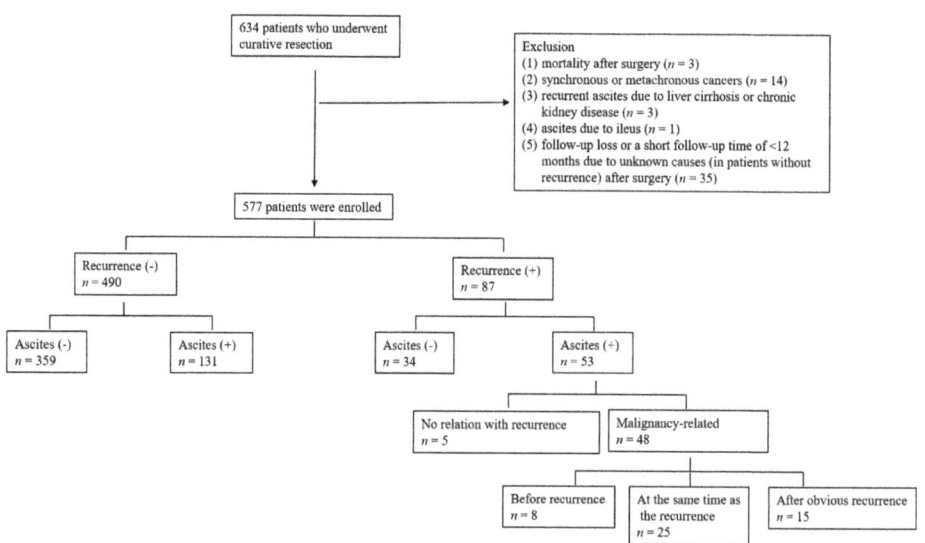

Figure 2. Study population.: +, presence; −, absence.

Comparisons between patients with and without recurrence are shown in Table 1. The T and N stages, type of resection, mean albumin and hemoglobin level, and history of adjuvant chemotherapy were significantly different between patients with and without recurrence. The most common location of ascites at first appearance was the pelvic cavity both in patients with (29/53, 54.7%) and without (128/131, 97.7%) recurrence, followed by the whole abdominal region (16/53, 30.2%), perihepatic area (6/53, 11.3%), and paracolic gutter (2/53, 3.8%) in patients with recurrence. In the remaining patients without recurrence, ascites was located in the perihepatic area (2/131, 1.5%) and the left abdominal cavity (1/131, 0.8%). Ascites fluid was small in volume and located in the pelvic cavity in most patients without recurrence (128/131, 97.7%). In the majority of patients with malignancy-related ascites, the volume of ascites fluid at first detection was small (33/48, 68.8%). Among 131 patients with benign ascites, repeatability was observed in 79 (60.3%). With the exception of one case, there was no difference in the amount and location of ascites after the initial detection in patients with recurrent benign ascites. The one exceptional case had a moderate amount of benign ascites in the perisplenic area (Figure 1C) and a small volume of pelvic ascites fluid on later examination. Median time for the first appearance of ascites was 10.5 months post-surgery (range of 3.0–108.0) in all patients with ascites, 9.0 months (range of 3.0–108.0) in those with benign ascites, and 11.5 months (range of 3.0–71.0) in those with recurrence. There was a significant difference in the mean age of males and females at the detection of benign ascites (58.8 ± 11.5 vs. 51.6 ± 12.4, $p = 0.001$). Repeatability (45 (57.0%) vs. 34 (65.4%), $p = 0.366$) and the history of adjuvant chemotherapy (32 (41.8%) vs. 18 (34.6%), $p = 0.466$) were not significantly different between males and females with benign ascites.

Table 1. Clinicopathologic features.

	Ascites without Recurrence	Ascites with Recurrence	p
	n (%)	n (%)	
Sex			0.869
Male	78 (60.3)	31 (58.5)	
Female	53 (39.7)	22 (41.5)	
Age (years ± SD)	55.9 ± 12.3	60.0 ± 12.1	0.046
Type of resection			<0.001
Partial gastrectomy	105 (80.2)	26 (49.1)	
Total gastrectomy	26 (19.8)	27 (50.9)	
Surgical approach			<0.001
Open	89 (67.9)	52 (98.1)	
Laparoscopy	42 (32.1)	1 (1.9)	
pT stage			<0.001
T1	80 (61.1)	4 (7.5)	
T2	12 (9.2)	4 (7.5)	
T3	18 (13.7)	24 (45.3)	
T4	21 (16.0)	21 (39.6)	
pN stage			<0.001
N0	80 (61.1)	8 (15.1)	
N1	23 (17.6)	5 (9.4)	
N2	19 (14.5)	7 (13.2)	
N3	9 (6.9)	33 (62.3)	
Nutritional parameters			
Albumin (g/dL ± SD)	4.2 ± 0.4	4.0 ± 0.6	<0.001
Hemoglobin (g/dL ± SD)	12.3 ± 1.4	11.4 ± 1.4	<0.001
Adjuvant chemotherapy			<0.001
No	80 (61.1)	8 (15.1)	
Yes	51 (38.9)	45 (84.9)	
Location of ascites at first appearance			<0.001
Pelvic cavity only	128 (97.7)	29 (54.7)	
Whole abdomen	0 (0)	16 (30.2)	
Other	3 (2.3)	8 (15.1)	
Volume of ascites at first appearance			<0.001
Small	130 (99.2)	38 (71.7)	
Moderate	1 (0.8)	10 (18.9)	
Large	0 (0)	5 (9.4)	
Repeatability [†]			
No	52 (39.7)		
Yes	79 (60.3)		
Timing of first appearance (months after surgery)	9.0 (range of 3.0–108.0)	11.5 (range of 3.0–71.0)	

"Ascites with recurrence" includes patients with malignancy-related ascites (n = 40), patients in whom ascites before recurrence were reclassified as malignancy-related ascites at a later stage (n = 8), and patients with benign ascites before recurrence but with no evidence of malignancy-related ascites after recurrence (n = 5). Abbreviations: SD, standard deviation. [†] In the case of ascites without recurrence.

According to the presence or absence of ascites, sensitivity, specificity, accuracy, and positive and negative predictive values for intra-abdominal recurrence were 60.9%, 73.3%, 71.4%, 28.8%, and 91.3%, respectively. Positive and negative likelihood ratios were 2.28 and 0.53, respectively. Values for intra-abdominal recurrence were then calculated according to location of ascites (pelvic vs. other). Sensitivity, specificity, and positive and negative predictive values for the pelvic location were 54.7%, 2.3%, 18.5%, and 1.1%, respectively, and for other locations, 45.3%, 97.7%, 88.9%, and 81.5%, respectively. The positive and negative likelihood ratios for the pelvic location were 0.56 and 19.7, respectively, and 19.7 and 0.56 for other locations, respectively.

Risk factors for the occurrence of benign ascites were evaluated in recurrence-free patients (Table 2). Univariate analyses showed that younger age (≤45), a pN2–3 stage, and a history of adjuvant chemotherapy were associated with the occurrence of benign ascites. Patient sex (p = 0.065) and pT stage (p = 0.054), significant at the 0.1 level, were included with these factors in a multivariate analysis to evaluate the risk for benign ascites. Younger age (≤45) was the only independent risk factor associated with the occurrence of benign ascites post-surgery.

Table 2. Risk factors related to the occurrence of benign ascites in disease-free patients.

	Univariate Analysis			Multivariate Analysis		
	Ascites (−), n (%)	Ascites (+), n (%)	p-Value	Hazard Ratio	95% CI	p-Value
Sex			0.065			
Male	249 (75.9)	79 (24.1)		1		
Female	110 (67.9)	52 (32.1)		1.436	0.926–2.227	0.106
Age (years)			<0.001			
≤45	9 (32.1)	19 (67.9)		6.465	2.803–14.915	<0.001
>45	350 (75.8)	112 (24.2)		1		
Type of surgery			0.211			
Total gastrectomy	306 (74.5)	105 (25.5)				
Partial gastrectomy	53 (67.1)	26 (32.9)				
Surgical approach			0.581			
Open	252 (74.0)	89 (26.0)				
Laparoscopy	106 (71.6)	42 (28.4)				
Depth of invasion			0.054			
pT1–2	283 (75.5)	92 (24.5)		1		
pT3–4	76 (66.1)	39 (33.9)		0.889	0.435–1.819	0.748
Lymph node metastasis						
pN0–1	310 (75.1)	103 (24.9)	0.049	1		
pN2–3	49 (63.6)	28 (36.4)		1.088	0.553–2.140	0.806
Adjuvant chemotherapy			0.003			
No	268 (77)	80 (23.0)		1		
Yes	91 (64.1)	51 (35.9)		2.098	0.985–4.470	0.055

+, presence; −, absence. Abbreviation: CI, confidence interval.

Table 3 shows the characteristics of the nine patients with undefined ascites at the first discovery. This group includes eight patients with ascites presumed to be benign before definitive recurrence and one patient with eventual recurrence who developed ascites without other evidence of peritoneal and/or intra-abdominal recurrence. Short-term follow-up abdominopelvic CT and ascites cytology examinations were conducted one month later due to increased ascites, and peritoneal recurrence was eventually confirmed in the latter patient mentioned previously (Figure 3). All of these patients were in an advanced stage of pathology and the ascites fluid was small in volume and located in the pelvic cavity at first appearance.

(A) 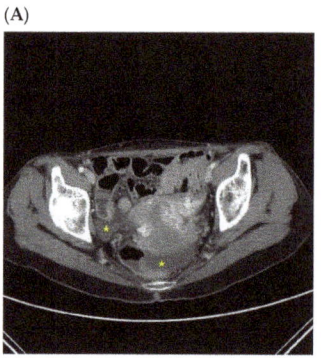 (B)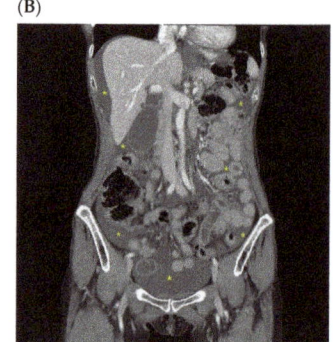

Figure 3. CT images of a patient on initial recurrence of malignant ascites without other CT findings related to peritoneal seeding, later confirmed by cytology. A small volume of pelvic ascites fluid was observed at first appearance (A). Follow-up CT (B) showed an increased volume of ascites fluid. Yellow stars indicate ascites.

Table 3. Characteristics of patients with temporarily undefined ascites.

	Age/Sex	Type of Operation	TN Stage	Characteristic of Ascites	Timing of Malignant Ascites	Site of First Recurrence	Interval between Surgery and Recurrence (Month)	Interval between First Appearance of Benign Ascites and Recurrence (Month)
				Patients with ascites presumed to be benign before confirmation of recurrence (n = 8)				
Pt 1	65/M	PG	T3N3a	small pelvic cavity	Simultaneous with recurrence	T colon (increased ascites in the pelvic cavity)	44.4	8.1
Pt 2	53/F	TG	T4bN3b	small pelvic cavity	Simultaneous with recurrence	Peritoneum (increased ascites, peritoneal thickening, bowel obstruction, and Krukenberg tumors)	18.2	13.2
Pt 3	40/F	TG	T4aN3a	small pelvic cavity	Simultaneous with recurrence	Peritoneum (nodularity and increased ascites)	73.2	70.3
Pt 4	59/F	TG	T4aN3a	small pelvic cavity	Simultaneous with recurrence	Peritoneum (increased ascites and peritoneal thickening)	25.2	21.7
Pt 5	39/F	TG	T3N3b	small pelvic cavity	Simultaneous with recurrence	Peritoneum (Krukenberg tumors, nodularity, and increased ascites)	12.1	9
Pt 6	57/F	TG	T3N3a	small pelvic cavity	Simultaneous with recurrence	Peritoneum (bowel obstruction and increased ascites)	9.8	4.4
Pt 7	61/F	TG	T3N1	small pelvic cavity	Simultaneous with recurrence	Peritoneum (increased ascites, T colon, and mesentery LNs)	29.6	26
Pt 8	68/F	PG	T4aN2	small pelvic cavity	Simultaneous with recurrence	Peritoneum (increased ascites and peritoneal thickening)	11.7	5.3
	A patient who first recurred with malignant ascites without other CT findings related to peritoneal seeding (later confirmed by cytology) (n = 1)							
Pt 9	49/F	TG	T3N3a	small pelvic cavity				

Abbreviations: PG, partial gastrectomy; TG, total gastrectomy; and CT, computed tomography.

4. Discussion

In gastric cancer patients, the most common cause of ascites after surgery is thought to be intra-abdominal recurrence but this is not supported by our study. In this study, a small volume of pelvic ascites fluid that had no identified pathological cause was noted in a substantial number of patients, notably an incidental finding during regular follow-ups. Malignancy-related ascites was observed in only 28.8% of patients with a history of ascites.

Normal peritoneal fluid that keeps the peritoneum moist and smooth may accumulate in the deep region of the pelvis in both males and females [16]. It is more frequently observed in premenopausal females than in males or postmenopausal females. In premenopausal females, the fluid that accumulates in the pelvis is thought to originate from ovarian exudation and decreased absorption of peritoneal fluid due to adhesions caused by various factors including endometriosis [17,18]. In a board sense, this fluid is called "physiologic ascites". The precise incidence of physiologic ascites has rarely been studied. According to Yoshikawa et al., a small amount of physiologic pelvic ascites was observed in 3.8% of healthy males and 16.8% of healthy postmenopausal females in pelvic magnetic resonance imaging conducted during health screenings [17]. In our study, benign ascites was identified in 23.8% of all male patients and 32.7% of all female patients without recurrence. There was no statistically significant difference in ascites detection between the sexes on either univariate or multivariate analyses. Peritoneal fluid accumulation seems to occur more often after gastric cancer surgery regardless of sex. A possible explanation for this is that the absorption capacity of the peritoneum decreases when it is infected or injured [19]. It is assumed that ascites accumulation increases after surgery due to peritoneal injury and adhesion. This reaction may be stronger in younger patients because an age of ≤45 was the only independent factor significantly linked to the occurrence of benign ascites in our study. In addition, young female patients are more likely to have ascites due to gynecological causes but those were not investigated in this study because of insufficient medical records. Therefore, the level of concern regarding recurrence is lower if the patient's ascites has a gynecological cause.

Cheon et al. reported that a small amount of pelvic fluid was detected in follow-up CT after curative surgery for gastric cancer in 3.9% of male patients [20]. This incidence is quite low when compared with our study. The authors obtained data only from radiology reports without a review of all CT images, whereas in our study, all images were independently reviewed by two radiologists. In addition, their definition of a "small" volume of ascites fluid was less than 20 mL, while in our study, it was defined as less than 50 mL. These reasons may explain the discrepancy between the results of the two studies. Further prospective observation is required for clarification.

According to reports from South Korea as well as western countries, malignant tumors are the second most common pathologic cause of ascites, following portal hypertension due to cirrhosis [21,22]. Malignancy-related ascites typically develops in the setting of recurrent and/or advanced cancer. The primary pathophysiological mechanism of malignancy-related ascites is peritoneal carcinomatosis, which blocks the drainage of lymphatic channels and increases vascular permeability [23]. Along with peritoneal carcinomatosis, some tumors may metastasize in the liver, which can cause ascites because of the obstruction/compression of the portal veins, further leading to portal hypertension or liver failure. Other types of tumors such as lymphomas can cause lymph node obstruction with accumulation of chylous ascites [24]. In gastric cancer, multiple pathophysiological mechanisms of ascites formation can occur but the primary mechanism is peritoneal carcinomatosis. There are few reports considering ascites as the first manifestation of gastric cancer despite its being the first detected sign of intra-abdominal malignancy in 50% of patients with peritoneal carcinomatosis [23,25]. To date, there are no reports considering ascites as the first manifestation of recurrence in postgastrectomy gastric cancer patients. In our study, most cases of malignancy-related ascites were accompanied by other findings of recurrence or were discovered during disease progression. Malignancy-related ascites is indicated as a late manifestation of intra-abdominal metastasis after gastrectomy for gastric cancer, as in the first diagnosis of gastric cancer [26]. Therefore, a small amount of pelvic ascites cannot be excluded from consideration as an early indicator of peritoneal carcinomatosis. This judgment requires caution. In our study, ascites was the only initially detected sign of intra-abdominal recurrence in one patient (Table 3; Figure 3). Furthermore, among patients with ascites presumed to be benign before obvious recurrence, the possibility of malignancy-related ascites due to peritoneal recurrence cannot be excluded because of the relatively short time between the first occurrence of ascites and the recurrence in some cases (Pt. 1, 5, 6, and 8 in Table 3). All patients mentioned above were in far-advanced stages of the disease (Table 3). The possibility of recurrence should be suspected in all gastric cancer patients with advanced disease who develop ascites even when the characteristics of the ascites are similar to those of benign ascites and there are no definitive findings suggesting peritoneal metastasis.

CT is frequently used for the postoperative surveillance of patients with gastric carcinoma. CT allows for the detection of even small amounts of ascites and provides information that is difficult to obtain in ultrasonography [16]. It would be desirable if intra-abdominal recurrence could be predicted with CT-detected ascites; however, this does not seem to be possible. The likelihood ratios were not at appropriate levels in our study. According to previous reports, malignancy-related ascites is often loculated or septated, or may be absent in typical or dependent areas such as the pelvis [8,27]. Similarly, in our study, the specificity and positive and negative predictive values for intra-abdominal recurrence were improved when calculated for ascites at locations other than the pelvis. In terms of the volume of the ascites fluid, that of >50 mL in a preoperative CT was found to be related to peritoneal metastasis in gastric cancer patients in a recently published study [13]. Additionally, in our study, malignancy-related ascites fluid volumes were larger (>50 mL are considered moderate and large amounts) than benign ascites at the time of initial detection. However, except for some patients with undefined ascites, all patients with malignancy-related ascites exhibited definitive peritoneal metastasis or intra-abdominal recurrence in the CT when ascites was first detected. Ascites alone therefore seems to be inappropriate as a diagnostic marker for intra-abdominal or peritoneal recurrence in postgastrectomy gastric cancer patients.

5. Conclusions

The presence of small-volume pelvic ascites fluid in follow-up images has minimal clinical significance in the majority of patients who undergo gastrectomy for gastric cancer. This phenomenon is more common in younger patients, regardless of sex. Although the presence of malignant ascites alone in the pelvic cavity can precede obvious intra-abdominal recurrence involving peritoneal seeding, ascites is more likely to be an indicator of disease progression in patients with recurrent gastric cancer.

Author Contributions: Conceptualization, J.-H.L. and S.-J.K.; methodology, M.K., J.-H.L. and S.-J.K.; software, J.-H.L.; validation, J.-H.L., S.-J.K., M.K. and B.-K.K.; formal analysis, J.-H.L.; investigation, J.-H.L., M.K. and B.-K.K.; resources, S.-J.K. and B.-K.K.; data curation, J.-H.L.; writing—original draft preparation, J.-H.L.; writing—review and editing, J.-H.L., S.-J.K., M.K. and B.-K.K.; visualization, J.-H.L.; supervision, S.-J.K.; project administration, J.-H.L.; funding acquisition, J.-H.L. All authors have read and agreed to the published version of the manuscript.

Funding: This work was supported by the research fund of Hanyang University (HY-202100000000767).

Institutional Review Board Statement: The study was conducted according to the guidelines of the Declaration of Helsinki and was approved by the Institutional Review Board (or Ethics Committee) of the Hanyang University hospital (protocol code 2021-03-050-004 and date of approval 23 April 2021).

Informed Consent Statement: Patient consent was waived due to the minimal risk of a retrospective study.

Data Availability Statement: The data presented in this study are available on request from the corresponding author.

Conflicts of Interest: The authors declare no conflict of interest.

References

1. Jemal, A.; Bray, F.; Center, M.M.; Ferlay, J.; Ward, E.; Forman, D. Global cancer statistics. *CA Cancer J. Clin.* **2011**, *61*, 69–90. [CrossRef]
2. Kim, C.D.; Chang, M.C.; Roh, H.R.; Chae, G.B.; Yang, D.H.; Choi, W.J. Factors influencing recurrence after curative resection for advanced gastric cancer. *J. Korean Surg. Soc.* **2003**, *65*, 301–308.
3. Yoo, C.H.; Noh, S.H.; Shin, D.W.; Choi, S.H.; Min, J.S. Recurrence following curative resection for gastric carcinoma. *Br. J. Surg.* **2000**, *87*, 236–242. [CrossRef] [PubMed]
4. Chu, D.Z.; Lang, N.P.; Thompson, C.; Osteen, P.K.; Westbrook, K.C. Peritoneal carcinomatosis in nongynecologic malignancy. A prospective study of prognostic factors. *Cancer* **1989**, *63*, 364–367.
5. Sadeghi, B.; Arvieux, C.; Glehen, O.; Beaujard, A.C.; Rivoire, M.; Baulieux, J.; Fontaumard, E.; Brachet, A.; Caillot, J.L.; Faure, J.L.; et al. Peritoneal carcinomatosis from non-gynecologic malignancies: Results of the EVOCAPE 1 multicentric prospective study. *Cancer* **2000**, *88*, 358–363. [CrossRef]
6. Raptopoulos, V.; Gourtsoyiannis, N. Peritoneal carcinomatosis. *Eur. Radiol.* **2001**, *11*, 2195–2206. [CrossRef]
7. Kim, S.J.; Kim, H.H.; Kim, Y.H.; Hwang, S.H.; Lee, H.S.; Park, D.J.; Kim, S.Y.; Lee, K.H. Peritoneal metastasis: Detection with 16-or 64-detector row CT in patients undergoing surgery for gastric cancer. *Radiology* **2009**, *253*, 407–415. [CrossRef] [PubMed]
8. Friedman, A.C.; Sohotra, P.; Radecki, P.D. CT manifestations of peritoneal carcinomatosis. *Am. J. Roentgenol.* **1988**, *150*, 1035–1041.
9. Lee, H.J.; Kim, M.J.; Lim, J.S.; Kim, K.W. Follow up CT findings of various types of recurrence after curative gastric surgery. *J. Korean Radiol. Soc.* **2007**, *57*, 553–562. [CrossRef]
10. Bennett, J.J.; Gonen, M.; D'Angelica, M.; Jaques, D.P.; Brennan, M.F.; Coit, D.G. Is detection of asymptomatic recurrence after curative resection associated with improved survival in patients with gastric cancer? *J. Am. Coll Surg.* **2005**, *201*, 503–510. [CrossRef]
11. Kim, J.H.; Jang, Y.J.; Park, S.S.; Park, S.H.; Mok, Y.J. Benefit of post-operative surveillance for recurrence after curative resection for gastric cancer. *J. Gastrointest. Surg.* **2010**, *14*, 969–976. [CrossRef] [PubMed]
12. Lee, J.H.; Lim, J.K.; Kim, M.G.; Kwon, S.J. The influence of post-operative surveillance on the prognosis after curative surgery for gastric cancer. *Hepatogastroenterology* **2014**, *61*, 2123–2132. [PubMed]
13. Kim, S.H.; Choi, Y.H.; Kim, J.W.; Oh, S.; Lee, S.; Kim, B.G.; Lee, K.L. Clinical significance of computed tomography-detected ascites in gastric cancer patients with peritoneal metastases. *Medicine* **2018**, *97*, e9343. [CrossRef] [PubMed]
14. Yajima, K.; Kanda, T.; Ohashi, M.; Wakai, T.; Nakagawa, S.; Sasamoto, R.; Hatakeyama, K. Clinical and diagnostic significance of preoperative computed tomography findings of ascites in patients with advanced gastric cancer. *Am. J. Surg.* **2006**, *192*, 185–190. [CrossRef]
15. Chang, D.K.; Kim, J.W.; Kim, B.K.; Lee, K.L.; Song, C.S.; Han, J.K.; Song, I.S. Clinical significance of CT-defined minimal ascites in patients with gastric cancer. *World J. Gastroenterol.* **2005**, *11*, 6587–6592. [CrossRef]
16. Healy, J.C.; Reznek, R.H. The peritoneum, mesenteries and omenta: Normal anatomy and pathological processes. *Eur. Radiol.* **1998**, *8*, 886–900. [CrossRef] [PubMed]
17. Yoshikawa, T.; Hayashi, N.; Maeda, E.; Matsuda, I.; Sasaki, H.; Ohtsu, H.; Ohtomo, K. Peritoneal fluid accumulation in healthy men and postmenopausal women: Evaluation on pelvic MRI. *Am. J. Roentgenol.* **2013**, *200*, 1181–1185. [CrossRef]
18. Koninckx, P.R.; Renaer, M.; Brosens, I.A. Origin of peritoneal fluid in women: An ovarian exudation product. *Br. J. Obstet. Gynaecol.* **1980**, *87*, 177–183. [CrossRef]
19. Verger, C.; Luger, A.; Moore, H.L.; Nolph, K.D. Acute changes in peritoneal morphology and transport properties with infectious peritonitis and mechanical injury. *Kidney Int.* **1983**, *23*, 823–831. [CrossRef]
20. Cheon, H.J.; Ryeom, H.K.; Bae, J.H.; Jang, Y.J.; Kim, G.C.; Kim, J.H.; Shin, K.M.; Chung, H.Y. Clinical significance of a small amount of isolated pelvic free fluid at multidetector CT in male patients after curative surgery for gastric carcinoma. *J. Korean Soc. Radiol.* **2014**, *71*, 69–74. [CrossRef]
21. Hwangbo, Y.; Jung, J.H.; Shim, J.; Kim, B.H.; Jung, S.H.; Lee, C.K.; Jang, J.Y.; Dong, S.H.; Kim, H.J.; Chang, Y.W.; et al. Etiologic and laboratory analyses of ascites in patients who underwent diagnostic paracentesis. *Korean J. Hepatol.* **2007**, *13*, 185–195. [PubMed]
22. Runyon, B.A. Management of adult patients with ascites caused by cirrhosis. *Hepatology* **1998**, *27*, 264. [CrossRef]
23. Sangisetty, S.L.; Miner, T.J. Malignant ascites: A review of prognostic factors, pathophysiology and therapeutic measures. *World J. Gastrointest. Surg.* **2012**, *4*, 87–95. [CrossRef]
24. Press, O.W.; Press, N.O.; Kaufman, S.D. Evaluation and management of chylous ascites. *Ann. Intern. Med.* **1982**, *96*, 358. [CrossRef] [PubMed]
25. Duarte, I.; Outerelo, C. Gastric cancer presenting as isolated ascites: A diagnostic challenge. *Eur. J. Case Rep. Intern. Med.* **2019**, *6*, 001141. [PubMed]
26. Maeda, H.; Kobayashi, M.; Sakamoto, J. Evaluation and treatment of malignant ascites secondary to gastric cancer. *World J. Gastroenterol.* **2015**, *21*, 10936–10947. [CrossRef]
27. Kim, K.W.; Choi, B.I.; Han, J.K.; Kim, T.K.; Kim, A.Y.; Lee, H.J.; Kim, Y.H.; Choi, J.; Do, K.; Kim, H.C.; et al. Postoperative anatomic and pathologic findings at CT following gastrectomy. *Radiographics* **2002**, *22*, 323–336. [CrossRef] [PubMed]

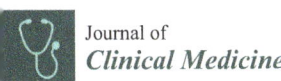

Article

Colorectal Cancer Risk in Women with Gynecologic Cancers—A Population Retrospective Cohort Study

Szu-Chia Liao [1,2], Hong-Zen Yeh [1,3], Chi-Sen Chang [1], Wei-Chih Chen [4], Chih-Hsin Muo [5] and Fung-Chang Sung [5,6,7,*]

[1] Division of Gastroenterology, Department of Internal Medicine, Taichung Veterans General Hospital, Taichung 407, Taiwan; b8401084@gmail.com (S.-C.L.); hzen.yeh@gmail.com (H.-Z.Y.); changcs@vghtc.gov.tw (C.-S.C.)
[2] Department of Public Health, China Medical University, Taichung 404, Taiwan
[3] Department of Internal Medicine, National Yang-Ming University, Taipei 112, Taiwan
[4] Department of Obstetrics and Gynecology, Taichung Veterans General Hospital, Taichung 407, Taiwan; awe@vghtc.gov.tw
[5] Management Office for Health Data, China Medical University Hospital, Taichung 404, Taiwan; b8507006@gmail.com
[6] Department of Health Services Administration, China Medical University, Taichung 404, Taiwan
[7] Department of Food Nutrition and Health Biotechnology, Asia University, Taichung 413, Taiwan
* Correspondence: fcsung1008@yahoo.com; Tel.: +886-4-2296-7979 (ext. 6220)

Abstract: We conducted a retrospective cohort study to evaluate the subsequent colorectal cancer (CRC) risk for women with gynecologic malignancy using insurance claims data of Taiwan. We identified patients who survived cervical cancer (N = 25,370), endometrial cancer (N = 8149) and ovarian cancer (N = 7933) newly diagnosed from 1998 to 2010, and randomly selected comparisons (N = 165,808) without cancer, matched by age and diagnosis date. By the end of 2011, the incidence and hazard ratio (HR) of CRC were estimated. We found that CRC incidence rates were 1.26-, 2.20-, and 1.61-fold higher in women with cervical, endometrial and ovarian cancers, respectively, than in comparisons (1.09/1000 person–years). The CRC incidence increased with age. Higher adjusted HRs of CRC appeared within 3 years for women with endometrial and ovarian cancers, but not until the 4th to 7th years of follow up for cervical cancer survivals. Cancer treatments could reduce CRC risks, but not significantly. However, ovarian cancer patients receiving surgery alone had an incidence of 3.33/1000 person–years for CRC with an adjusted HR of 3.79 (95% CI 1.11–12.9) compared to patients without any treatment. In conclusion, gynecologic cancer patients are at an increased risk of developing CRC, sooner for those with endometrial or ovarian cancer than those with cervical cancer.

Keywords: colorectal cancer; gynecologic cancer; retrospective cohort study; colonoscopy screening

1. Introduction

Cervical, endometrial and ovarian cancers are gynecologic (GYN) cancers among the ten leading causes of deaths from cancer for women. Cervical cancer is the most common female cancer in developing countries and the eighth most common in the US women [1–3]. The prevalence of endometrial cancer is on the rise in developed countries, with the incidence higher than that of cervical cancer. Ovarian cancer is the second-most common cancer in women, with a higher incidence in developed countries. The 5-year survival rates of GYN cancers have improved over the past few decades due to the improved treatments [1]. GYN cancer survivors are at risk for a second cancer [4–10]. Human papillomavirus infection, smoking, obesity, hormone replacement therapy, radiotherapy and hereditary nonpolyposis colorectal cancer (HNPCC) are associated with a secondary malignancy [6,10,11]. A meta-analysis found that the standardized incidence ratios (SIRs) on all types of second cancer risk ranged from 1.0 to 1.4 for women with primary breast

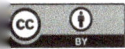

cancer, with the risk greater for women of less than 50 years than those who were older (SIR 1.51 vs. 1.11) [11].

Colorectal cancer (CRC) has become the second or third leading cause in cancer-related deaths in women [12–15]. GYN cancers and CRC share some common risk factors, such as obesity, lifestyle and socioeconomic status [10–12,14,16]. Thus, the risk of CRC development is an important concern for women with GYN cancer. Previous epidemiologic studies have shown conflicting results about the CRC risk in women with prior cervical or endometrial cancers [4,17–22]. Studies on the risk of subsequent CRC after radiotherapy for cervical cancer have conflicting results. Women with previous endometrial or ovarian cancer with or without radiotherapy have been found to be at increased risk for CRC [14,22].

Using cancer registries in European countries and the United States, Chaturvedi et al. followed 104,760 one-year survivors of cervical cancer for 40 years [19]. Patients treated with heavy radiotherapy have a higher SIR for second cancers, including colorectal cancer and other GYN cancers. Limited data are available on the risk of CRC for Asian women with GYN. A retrospective study followed 52,972 women with cervical cancer for 9 years using the Taiwan Cancer Registry and found the second cancer risk was greater for rectal cancer than for colon cancer (SIR = 1.31 vs. 1.13) [5]. The effects of treatment for cervical cancer on the risk of CRC have not been clarified in the study.

No study has compared the CRC risk for women with GYN cancers by treatment modality other than with or without radiotherapy. In the present study, we established cohorts of survivors with major GYN cancers, including cervical, endometrial and ovarian cancers, to evaluate the risk of subsequent CRC. Risks of the second CRC cancers were also assessed for patients with GYN treatment methods.

2. Methods and Materials

2.1. Study Design, Data Source and Study Subjects

We performed a population-based retrospective cohort study using data obtained from Taiwan National Health Insurance, which is a universal health insurance system with over 99% of the population covered. We used 1998–2011 claims data, which included inpatient and outpatient records for cancer care and a registry for catastrophic illnesses. The International Classification of Diseases, 9th Revision, Clinical Modification (ICD-9-CM) and A-code was applied to retrieve information on diagnosis.

From the registry for catastrophic illnesses, we identified 41,452 cases of GYN cancers with at least one-year survival from 1998 to 2010, for the study cohorts. Patients with the history of CRC at the baseline were excluded. The GYN cancer cohort included 25,370 cases of cervical cancer (ICD-9-CM code 180), 8149 cases of endometrial cancer (ICD-9-CM code 182) and 7933 cases of ovarian cancer (ICD-9-CM code 183). The diagnosis date was designated as index date. Using a ratio of 1:4, 165,808 women free from any cancer were randomly selected as the reference cohort, and frequency matched with all GYN cases by age and index date. Follow up began 1 year after the subject was included in the cohort until the date of CRC diagnosis or the end of 2011, whichever occurred first. Subjects lost to follow up were censored. Subsequent CRC cases were identified by linkage within the respective cancer registry files and confirmed by the registry for catastrophic illnesses.

2.2. Statistical Analysis

Data analysis first displayed sociodemographic characteristics (age and occupation) and comorbidities among cohorts. Comorbidities included diabetes mellitus (ICD-9-CM 250), hypertension (ICD-9-CM 401–405,997.91), hyperlipidemia (ICD-9-CM 272), non-infectious enteritis and colitis (ICD-9-CM 555–558), anal and rectal polyp (ICD-9-CM 560.9), benign neoplasm of the colon (ICD-9-CM 211.3), and cholecystectomy (ICD-9-CM 51.22–51.23) [23]. Distributions of age (30–39, 40–49, 50–64, and >60 years), occupation and comorbidities were compared between the GYN cohorts and reference cohort and examined using a Chi-square test for categorical variables and a t-test for continuous variables. We calculated the incidence rates of subsequent CRC for each cohort during the follow-up period. The Cox proportional hazards regression analysis was used to estimate the hazard ratios (HRs) and 95% confidence intervals (CIs) of CRC associated with GYN cancers and treatment modalities. The multivariable Cox model was used to calculate adjusted HR (aHR) controlling for demographic factors and comorbidities. To assess the effect of cancer therapy, GYN cohorts were stratified into five groups by therapeutic modalities: radiation therapy (RT) only, chemotherapy (CT) only, combination of RT and CT (RT/CT), surgery only and no treatment (non-RT/CT/surgery). We used the no treatment group as a reference to examine whether RT, CT, surgery, and RT/CT were associated the CRC risk. We also calculated the HRs of CRC by the follow-up duration, <1, 2–3, 4–5, 6–7, 8–9 and ≥10 years for the GYN cohorts. In order to evaluate the competing risk of death, we also used the sub-distribution model to estimate the overall sub-hazard ratio (SHR) of CRC cancer associated with each of the 3 GYN cancers. All data analyses were performed using the SAS 9.3 statistical package (SAS Institute Inc., Cary, NC, USA). The study was approved by Research Ethics Committee at China Medical University and Hospital (CMUH104-REC2-115).

3. Results

All GYN cancer cases and the reference cohort were similar in distributions of age, with the mean age of 54.9 years (Table 1). Patients with cervical cancer were older than patients with endometrial and ovarian cancers (means 56.2, 53.2 and 52.0 years, respectively). Women with endometrial cancer and ovarian cancer were more likely to work in white collar jobs. Overall, GYN cancer patients were more prevalent than the reference cohort with diabetes mellitus, hypertension, non-infectious enteritis and colitis, anal and rectal polyps, and benign neoplasm of the colon. The prevalence rates of hyperlipidemia and cholecystectomy were similar.

Table 1. Distributions of gender, age, and comorbidity among gynecologic cancer cohorts and reference cohort identified from 1998 to 2010.

	Cancer Cohorts				Reference	p Value
	Cervical	Endometrial	Ovarian	Total		
Total population, n (%)	25,370 (61.2)	8149 (19.7)	7933 (19.1)	41,452 (100)	165,808 (100)	
Age, n (%)						
30–39	2905 (11.5)	770 (9.45)	1284 (16.2)	4959 (12.0)	19,836 (12.0)	
40–49	6727 (26.5)	2293 (28.1)	2514 (31.7)	11,534 (27.8)	46,136 (27.8)	0.95
50–64	8513 (33.6)	3914 (48.0)	2845 (35.9)	15,272 (36.8)	61,088 (36.8)	
≥65	7225 (28.5)	1172 (14.4)	1290 (16.3)	9687 (23.4)	38,748 (23.4)	
Mean (SD)	56.2 (13.5)	53.6 (10.7)	52.0 (12.1)	54.9 (12.8)	54.8 (12.9)	0.36
Occupation n, (%)						
White collar	11,034 (43.5)	4495 (55.2)	4421 (55.7)	19,950 (48.1)	81,365 (49.1)	
Blue collar	11,902 (46.9)	2963 (36.4)	2805 (35.4)	17,670 (42.6)	71,622 (43.2)	<0.0001
Others	2405 (9.48)	651 (8.36)	693 (8.74)	3779 (9.12)	12,634 (7.62)	
Missing	29 (0.11)	10 (0.12)	14 (0.18)	53 (0.13)	187 (0.11)	
Comorbidity, n (%)						
Diabetes	3139 (12.4)	1325 (16.3)	794 (10.0)	5258 (12.7)	18,894 (11.4)	<0.0001
Hypertension	2938 (11.6)	1180 (14.5)	848 (10.7)	4966 (12.0)	12,275 (7.40)	<0.0001
Hyperlipidemia	520 (2.05)	187 (2.29)	143 (1.80)	850 (2.05)	3366 (2.03)	0.79
Non-infectious enteritis and colitis	419 (1.65)	70 (0.86)	86 (1.08)	575 (1.39)	1944 (1.17)	0.0004
Anal and rectal polyp	25 (0.10)	0 (0.00)	6 (0.08)	31 (0.07)	56 (0.03)	0.0003
Benign neoplasm of colon	94 (0.37)	18 (0.22)	42 (0.53)	154 (0.37)	153 (0.09)	<0.0001
Cholecystectomy	267 (1.05)	104 (1.28)	104 (1.31)	475 (1.15)	1911 (1.15)	0.91

p value: reference vs. total cases.

The overall CRC incidence rate was the highest in the endometrial cohort, followed by the ovarian cohort and cervical cohort (2.20, 1.76 and 1.37 per 1000 person–years, respectively) with aHRs of 2.26 (95% confidence interval (CI): 1.77–2.90), 2.09 (95% CI: 1.59–2.76) and 1.20 (95% CI: 1.03–1.40), compared to the reference cohort (1.09 per 10,000 person–years) (Table 2). The age-specific CRC cancer incidence increased with age in each cohort.

However, the age-specific HR of CRC, relative to the reference cohort, decreased with age, particularly for patients with endometrial and ovarian cancer. We further used the sub-distribution model to estimate the adjusted hazard ratio (aSHR) of CRC associated with the competing risk of death in women with these GYN cancers. The overall aSHRs of developing CRC were 1.04 (95% CI: 0.89–1.21), 1.97 (95% CI: 1.54–2.52) and 1.53 (95% CI: 1.16–2.01), respectively, in women with cervical, endometrial and ovarian cancers.

Table 2. Incidence of colorectal cancer and gynecologic cancer cohorts to reference cohort adjusted hazard ratio by age.

	Reference	Cervical Cancer		Endometrial Cancer		Ovarian Cancer	
Age	Rate	Rate	aHR (95% CI)	Rate	aHR (95% CI)	Rate	aHR (95% CI)
	CRC						
All	1.09	1.37	1.20 (1.03–1.40) *	2.20	2.26 (1.77–2.90) ***	1.76	2.09 (1.59–2.76) ***
30–39	0.19	0.22	1.14 (0.40–3.31)	1.11	6.18 (2.11–18.1) ***	1.18	6.37 (2.71–15.0) ***
40–49	0.46	0.78	1.67 (1.13–2.48) *	1.54	3.46 (2.05–5.84) ***	1.25	2.83 (1.59–5.01) ***
50–64	1.13	1.51	1.32 (1.02–1.70) *	2.34	2.19 (1.55–3.09) ***	1.48	1.41 (0.84–2.36)
≥65	2.40	2.46	1.02 (0.81–1.29)	2.84	1.23 (0.69–2.18)	4.52	1.94 (1.23–3.08) **

Incidence rate: per 1000 person–years, aHR: adjusted for age, diabetes, hypertension, benign neoplasm of colon, anal and rectal polyp and cholecystectomy. CRC, colorectal cancer. * $p < 0.05$; ** $p < 0.01$; *** $p < 0.001$.

Table 3 shows the CRC risk associated with treatment modalities. The incidence rates were higher in patients with cervical cancer and endometrial cancer receiving no treatment (1.90 and 3.84 per 1000 person–years, respectively) than those with treatment. The aHR was significant for those with endometrial cancer (aHR = 3.38, 95% CI: 1.61–7.11), compared to the reference cohort, but not significant for those with cervical cancer. Treatments reduced the CRC incidence rates in both cohorts, with significant aHRs in the endometrial cancer cohort but not significant in the cervical cancer cohort. However, all reduced aHRs were not significant for patients with treatments, compared to those with no treatment. On the other hand, the CRC incidence rate in ovarian cancer patients was 4.6-fold greater in those undergoing surgery than those receiving no treatment (3.33 vs. 0.73 per 1000 person–years), with an aHR of 3.56 (95% CI: 2.23–5.68) compared with controls. Most ovarian cancer patients received chemotherapy (5069/7933) and had an adjusted HR of 1.95 (95% CI: 1.35–2.80).

Table 3. Incidence and adjusted hazard ratio of colorectal cancer by type of treatment for patients with gynecologic cancers and reference cohort.

Treatment	N	Event	Person-Years	Incidence Rate ++	aHR (95% CI)	aHR (95% CI)
Control	165,808	1033	945,889	1.09	1.00	
Cervical cancer						
Non-RT/CT/surgery	3369	43	22,573	1.90	1.32 (0.97–1.79)	1.00
RT	4250	40	21,555	1.86	1.11 (0.81–1.52)	0.90 (0.59–1.40)
CT	1544	8	8904	0.90	1.08 (0.54–2.16)	0.74 (0.34–1.59)
RT/CT	7558	39	29,471	1.32	1.24 (0.90–1.71)	0.97 (0.62–1.50)
Only surgery	8649	62	57,181	1.08	1.19 (0.92–1.54)	0.83 (0.56–1.25)
Endometrial cancer						
Non-RT/CT/surgery	350	7	1823	3.84	3.38 (1.61–7.11) **	1.00
RT	1376	12	5466	2.20	2.19 (1.24–3.87) **	0.61 (0.24–1.56)
CT	826	8	2872	2.79	3.39 (1.69–6.80) ***	0.83 (0.30–2.32)
RT/CT	1055	7	3325	2.11	2.38 (1.13–5.01) *	0.61 (0.21–1.76)
Only surgery	4542	34	20,132	1.69	1.97 (1.40–2.78) ***	0.50 (0.22–1.14)
Ovarian cancer						
Non-RT/CT/surgery	84	3	4121	0.73	0.98 (0.32–3.04)	1.00
RT	51	0	261	0.00		
CT	5069	30	18,368	1.63	1.95 (1.35–2.80) ***	1.88 (0.57–6.18)
RT/CT	785	3	2545	1.18	1.45 (0.47–4.49)	1.33 (0.27–6.60)
Only surgery	1184	18	5402	3.33	3.56 (2.23–5.68) ***	3.79 (1.11–12.9) *

aHR: Adjusted for age, diabetes, hypertension, benign neoplasm of colon, anal and rectal polyp and cholecystectomy. RT, radiation therapy; CT, chemotherapy. Incidence rate ++: per 1000 person–years. * $p < 0.05$; ** $p < 0.01$; *** $p < 0.001$.

Figure 1 shows the Cox model-estimated aHRs of CRC for GYN cohorts in a 10-year follow-up period, compared with the reference cohort. The incident CRC developed earlier in women with the endometrial cohort and the ovarian cohort than in women with cervical cancer. Elevated aHRs were significant within the first 3 years of follow up for women with endometrial cancer and ovarian cancer, but not until 4th to 7th years for women with cervical cancer.

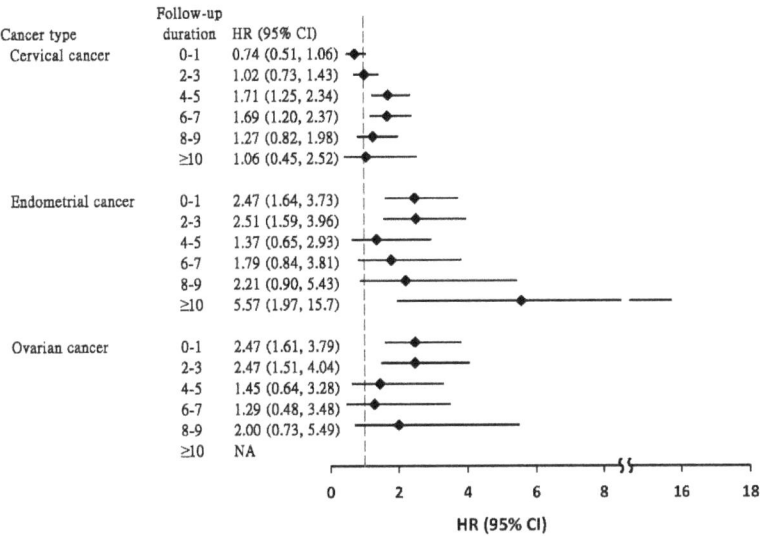

Figure 1. Cox proportional hazards regression analysis estimated adjusted hazard ratio of colorectal cancer for patients with gynecologic cancers compared to reference cohort by follow-up year.

Figure 2 shows the Cox model estimated age-specific aHRs of CRC during the follow-up period. The hazards of developing CRC were all greater for younger GYN patients, particularly during the first 3 years of follow up for women <50 years old with endometrial cancer and ovarian cancer.

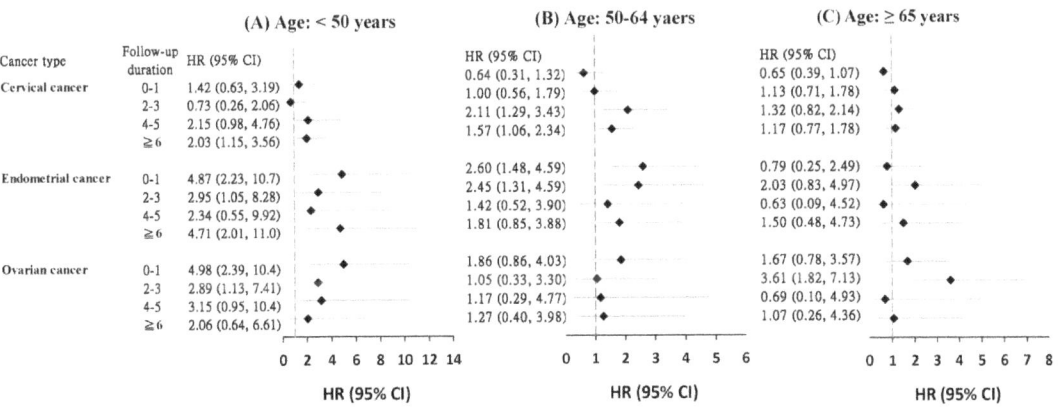

Figure 2. Cox proportional hazards regression analysis estimated adjusted hazard ratios of colorectal cancer for patients with gynecologic cancers relative to comparison cohort by follow-up year and age group. (**A**) Age: <50 years, (**B**) Age: 50–64 years, (**C**) Age: ≥65 years.

4. Discussion

This population-based retrospective cohort study showed that women with major GYN cancers are at an elevated risk of developing CRC. The CRC risk is the highest for women with endometrial cancer, followed by ovarian cancer and cervical cancer. The CRC risk varied not only by GYN cancer type, but also by the follow-up period, cancer treatment modality and age. Previous studies on relationships between a second CRC and GYN cancers are inconsistent [4,17–22]. In general, the CRC risks found were stronger for patients with ovarian cancer and endometrial cancer than for patients with cervical cancer. Weaker relationships between CRC and cervical cancer in these studies are consistent with our findings. We failed to identify the CRC risk in association with treatment modality in cervical cancer.

A retrospective cohort study using the US cancer registry data of the Surveillance, Epidemiology, and End Results (SEER) program found women with GYN cancer tended to have a higher CRC incidence in the first 6 months after the diagnosis of the cancer; the estimated SIR of subsequent CRC is significant for those with ovarian cancer (SIR: 2.20, 95% CI: 1.06–2.58), but not for endometrial cancer [22]. Another study using SEER data found the risk of CRC was the highest in 12–24 months after the diagnosis of endometrial cancer [14]. The Swedish record-linkage study also found a significant SIR of 1.64 (95% CI: 1.24–2.11) for CRC within 2 years for women with ovarian cancer [4].

The exact mechanisms associated with CRC risk among women with GYN cancers remain unclear. GYN cancers shared the same risk factors with CRC, including hormone modulation, lifestyle and hereditary diseases. Decreased exposure to estrogen may protect against colorectal, endometrial, and ovarian cancer [24]. Nulliparous women and women using hormone replacement therapy are at a high risk [16]. Dietary factors and obesity are the shared risk factors in colorectal and ovarian or endometrial cancer [14]. Estrogen levels are elevated in obese persons [25]. In addition, the familial CRC syndrome of HNPCC can appear in the early development of colorectal, endometrial and ovarian cancer [26]. However, HNPCC is not prevalent in our population. HNPCC may do little to explain the association between GYN cancers and CRC.

GYN cancer detection and treatment may in part explain the CRC risk variations among GYN cancers. The latent periods of subsequent CRC for women with cervical cancer is longer than that for women with endometrial cancer and ovarian cancer. The pap test helps to detect cervical cancer in the early stages. The detection and treatment of carcinoma in situ of the cervix may prevent not only the development of an invasive carcinoma of the cervix but also other cancer. On the other hand, ovarian cancer and endometrial cancer are more likely not detected until they are in more advanced stages. This may also explain in part why the incidence of CRC in cervical cancer patients was lower than that in ovarian cancer and endometrial cancer patients.

Some women may have developed CRC by the time they are diagnosed with ovarian cancer and endometrial cancer. In our study, the CRC incidence was the highest in women receiving surgery alone for ovarian cancer treatment. These patients might have received more screening modalities. A higher CRC incidence is thus identified in a shorter follow-up time for ovarian cancer patients than for cervical cancer patients. Most patients with endometrial cancer received surgery alone, but they had the lowest CRC incidence. These patients might have the disease diagnosed at an advanced stage. This is probably why CRC incidence was the highest in endometrial cancer patients receiving no treatment. On the other hand, the incidence among ovarian cancer patients was the lowest for those receiving no treatment. However, there were few ovarian cases receiving no treatment. A further investigation with a more ovarian cases is needed to address the finding.

Evidence from previous studies has shown the risk of CRC is elevated for cervical cancer patients after receiving RT [18,19]. Brown et al. found the RT treatment increased colon cancer risk after endometrial cancer [18]. In the present study, the CRC risk increased after RT for endometrial cancer and ovarian cancer, but not for cervical cancer. The relationship between CRC risk and endometrial cancers treated with RT in our study is compatible with findings in two studies using the US Survival, Epidemiology, and End Results database [18,20].

In our study, 70.7% patients with ovarian cancer, 10.1% patients with endometrial cancer and 6.09% patients with cervical cancer received CT. The subsequent CRC risk after CT was significant for those with endometrial cancer and ovarian cancer. No previous study has observed the CRC risk for GYN cancers after CT. Further data analysis showed that the age-specific GYN cancer cohort to the reference cohort risk of CRC was greater for younger patients than older patients after CT. As for 30–49 years old patients, the adjusted HRs of CRC were 5.44 (95% CI: 2.23–13.3) for those with endometrial cancer and 3.29 (95% CI: 1.86–5.84) for those with ovarian cancer. In general, younger women might have these cancers diagnosed at an earlier stage and have longer survival than older women have. Longer survival increases the detection of CRC cancer. The greater impact of CT for young GYN patients than older patients could be true, because of low CRC incidence in younger general population [27]. A further investigation for the impact of CT regimens needs to be addressed. Routine gynecologic examination and cancer screening are also recommended for these younger women.

Boice et al. found the risk of secondary cancer was greater for young GYN patients after RT [28]. A previous study on testicular cancer patients noted that platinum-based chemotherapy had induced leukemia and solid organ tumors, including colon cancer [15,29–31]. Travis et al. found a higher risk of leukemia in ovarian cancer patients after receiving CT [32], but no report on the risk of CRC. No other report has addressed the carcinogenic effect after CT for endometrial and ovarian cancers. We suspect that harder follow-up checks for GYN cancer patients may also explain in part the increased identification of CRC.

Our study results should be interpreted with caution because of limitations. First, data on patient lifestyles and family history of diseases were not adjusted in data analyses because the information is not available from the NHRI records. Second, the NHRI records also provide no information on cancer stage and dosages of CT and RT, and we are unable to measure the dose–response association between treatment and CRC risk. Third, cancer patients covered in the insurance system are registered in the catastrophic illnesses group eligible for treatment benefit with discounted treatment costs. The insurance system provides no guides on which treatment modalities are usually used on treatment by the cancer stage. Our study could not differentiate whether the health insurance policies affect the development of CRC. However, further study is needed to investigate factors associated with increased CRC risk in women receiving surgery for ovarian cancer. Information on images of colonoscopy screening is also unavailable, and we are unable to prove whether hard follow-up checkups increase the diagnosis of CRC for GYN patients. However, all cancer patients have been registered as catastrophic illnesses, and the misdiagnosis of GYN cancer and CRC is unlikely in this study.

5. Conclusions

In this study, the number of patients with cervical cancer was much greater than that of endometrial and ovarian cancers. The risk of developing a second CRC was higher for patients with endometrial and ovarian cancers than for those with cervical cancer. The younger patients were at a higher impact after treatment. The risk of developing CRC after GYN cancer therapy is an important concern, because the CRC risk varied by the cancer treatment method among GYN cancers. The elevated incidence of CRC associated with surgery in patients with endometrial and ovarian cancers, but not cervical cancer should prompt the mechanism investigation. Colonoscopy screening for the subsequent development of CRC in these GYN cancer patients should be performed as soon as possible, especially for patients below 50 years old, in the early years after cancer diagnosis and after ever receiving chemotherapy or radiotherapy.

Author Contributions: Conceived and designed the study: S.-C.L., H.-Z.Y., C.-S.C., W.-C.C., C.-H.M. and F.-C.S. Data analysis and interpretation: C.-H.M., S.-C.L., F.-C.S. Data evaluation: H.-Z.Y., C.-S.C.,

W.-C.C., F.-C.S. Manuscript preparation: S.-C.L. and F.-C.S. Manuscript editing: F.-C.S. Manuscript review: All authors. All authors have read and agreed to the published version of the manuscript.

Funding: This study was supported in part by the Ministry of Health and Welfare, Taiwan (MOHW109-TDU-B-212-114004), MOST Clinical Trial Consortium for Stroke (MOST 109-2321-B-039-002), the Ministry of Science and Technology, Taiwan (Grant no. MOST108-2410-H-039-001 and MOST109-2410-H-039-001), the China Medical University, Taiwan (Grant no. CMU109-MF-119), and Tseng-Lien Lin Foundation, Taichung, Taiwan.

Institutional Review Board Statement: This study was approved by the Research Ethics Committee of China Medical University and Hospital (CMUH104-REC2-115). Surrogate identification numbers were used for data linkage to protect the privacy. No consents are required.

Data Availability Statement: Data are available from the Ministry of Health and Welfare of Taiwan by request after IRB approval. Authors are not allowed to duplicate data files.

Conflicts of Interest: The authors declare no conflict of interest.

References

1. Gray, H.J. Primary management of early stage cervical cancer (IA1-IB) and appropriate selection of adjuvant therapy. *J. Natl. Compr. Cancer Netw.* **2008**, *6*, 47–52. [CrossRef]
2. Wild, C. *World Cancer Report 2014*; Christopher, P.W., Bernard, W., Eds.; WHO Press: Geneva, Switzerland, 2014; pp. 465–482. ISBN 109283204298.
3. Howlader November 10. SEER Stat Fact Sheets: Cervix Uteri. National Cancer Institute. Available online: https://seer.cancer.gov/statfacts/ (accessed on 7 February 2012).
4. Bergfeldt, K.; Einhorn, S.; Rosendahl, I.; Hall, P. Increased risk of second primary malignancies in patients with gynecological cancer: A Swedish record-linkage study. *Acta Oncol.* **1995**, *34*, 771–777. [CrossRef] [PubMed]
5. Boice, J.D., Jr.; Day, N.E.; Andersen, A.; Brinton, L.A.; Brown, R.; Choi, N.W.; Clarke, E.A.; Coleman, M.P.; Curtis, R.E.; Flannery, J.T.; et al. Second cancers following radiation treatment for cervical cancer. An international collaboration among cancer registries. *J. Natl. Cancer Inst.* **1985**, *74*, 955–975. [CrossRef]
6. Chen, C.Y.; Lai, C.H.; Lee, K.D.; Huang, S.H.; Dai, Y.M.; Chen, M.C. Risk of second primary malignancies in women with cervical cancer: A population-based study in Taiwan over a 30-year period. *Gynecol. Oncol.* **2012**, *127*, 625–630. [CrossRef] [PubMed]
7. Hemminki, K.; Dong, C.; Vaittinen, P. Second primary cancer after in situ and invasive cervical cancer. *Epidemiology* **2000**, *11*, 457–461. [CrossRef] [PubMed]
8. Kaldor, J.M.; Day, N.E.; Band, P.; Choi, N.W.; Clarke, E.A.; Coleman, M.P.; Hakama, M.; Koch, M.; Langmark, F.; Neal, F.E.; et al. Second malignancies following testicular cancer, ovarian cancer and Hodgkin's disease: An international collaborative study among cancer registries. *Int. J. Cancer* **1987**, *39*, 571–585. [CrossRef] [PubMed]
9. Kleinerman, R.A.; Boice, J.D., Jr.; Storm, H.H.; Sparen, P.; Andersen, A.; Pukkala, E.; Lynch, C.F.; Hankey, B.F.; Flannery, J.T. Second primary cancer after treatment for cervical cancer. An international cancer registries study. *Cancer* **1995**, *76*, 442–452. [CrossRef]
10. Rabkin, C.S.; Biggar, R.J.; Melbye, M.; Curtis, R.E. Second primary cancers following anal and cervical carcinoma: Evidence of shared etiologic factors. *Am. J. Epidemiol.* **1992**, *136*, 54–58. [CrossRef]
11. Molina-Montes, E.; Requena, M.; Sanchez-Cantalejo, E.; Fernandez, M.F.; Arroyo-Morales, M.; Espin, J.; Arrebola, J.P.; Sanchez, M.J. Risk of second cancers cancer after a first primary breast cancer: A systematic review and meta-analysis. *Gynecol. Oncol.* **2015**, *136*, 158–171. [CrossRef]
12. Curtis, R.E.; Hoover, R.N.; Kleinerman, R.A.; Harvey, E.B. Second cancer following cancer of the female genital system in Connecticut, 1935–1982. *Natl. Cancer Inst. Monogr.* **1985**, *68*, 113–137.
13. Jemal, A.; Murray, T.; Samuels, A.; Ghafoor, A.; Ward, E.; Thun, M.J. Cancer statistics, 2003. *CA Cancer J. Clin.* **2003**, *53*, 5–26. [CrossRef] [PubMed]
14. Terry, P.D.; Miller, A.B.; Rohan, T.E. Obesity and colorectal cancer risk in women. *Gut* **2002**, *51*, 191–194. [CrossRef] [PubMed]
15. Travis, L.B.; Rabkin, C.S.; Brown, L.M.; Allan, J.M.; Alter, B.P.; Ambrosone, C.B.; Begg, C.B.; Caporaso, N.; Chanock, S.; DeMichele, A.; et al. Cancer survivorship–genetic susceptibility and second primary cancers: Research strategies and recommendations. *J. Natl. Cancer Inst.* **2006**, *98*, 15–25. [CrossRef] [PubMed]
16. Newcomb, P.A.; Taylor, J.O.; Trentham-Dietz, A. Interactions of familial and hormonal risk factors for large bowel cancer in women. *Int. J. Epidemiol.* **1999**, *28*, 603–608. [CrossRef] [PubMed]
17. Bergfeldt, K.; Silfversward, C.; Einhorn, S.; Hall, P. Overestimated risk of second primary malignancies in ovarian cancer patients. *Eur. J. Cancer* **2000**, *36*, 100–105. [CrossRef]
18. Brown, A.P.; Neeley, E.S.; Werner, T.; Soisson, A.P.; Burt, R.W.; Gaffney, D.K. A population-based study of subsequent primary malignancies after endometrial cancer: Genetic, environmental, and treatment-related associations. *Int. J. Radiat. Oncol. Biol. Phys.* **2010**, *78*, 127–135. [CrossRef]

19. Chaturvedi, A.K.; Engels, E.A.; Gilbert, E.S.; Chen, B.E.; Storm, H.; Lynch, C.F.; Hall, P.; Langmark, F.; Pukkala, E.; Kaijser, M.; et al. Second cancers among 104,760 survivors of cervical cancer: Evaluation of long-term risk. *J. Natl. Cancer Inst.* **2007**, *99*, 1634–1643. [CrossRef]
20. Kumar, S.; Shah, J.P.; Bryant, C.S.; Awonuga, A.O.; Imudia, A.N.; Ruterbusch, J.J.; Cote, M.L.; Ali-Fehmi, R.; Morris, R.T.; Malone, J.M., Jr. Second neoplasms in survivors of endometrial cancer: Impact of radiation therapy. *Gynecol. Oncol.* **2009**, *113*, 233–239. [CrossRef]
21. Travis, L.B.; Curtis, R.E.; Boice, J.D., Jr.; Platz, C.E.; Hankey, B.F.; Fraumeni, J.F., Jr. Second malignant neoplasms among long-term survivors of ovarian cancer. *Cancer Res.* **1996**, *56*, 1564–1570.
22. Weinberg, D.S.; Newschaffer, C.J.; Topham, A. Risk for colorectal cancer after gynecologic cancer. *Ann. Intern. Med.* **1999**, *131*, 189–193. [CrossRef]
23. Chen, C.H.; Lin, C.L.; Kao, C.H. The Effect of Cholecystectomy on the Risk of Colorectal Cancer in Patients with Gallbladder Stones. *Cancers* **2020**, *12*, 550. [CrossRef]
24. Calle, E.E.; Miracle-McMahill, H.L.; Thun, M.J.; Heath, C.W., Jr. Estrogen replacement therapy and risk of fatal colon cancer in a prospective cohort of postmenopausal women. *J. Natl. Cancer Inst.* **1995**, *87*, 517–523. [CrossRef] [PubMed]
25. Hardcastle, J.D.; Chamberlain, J.O.; Robinson, M.H.; Moss, S.M.; Amar, S.S.; Balfour, T.W.; James, P.D.; Mangham, C.M. Randomised controlled trial of faecal-occult-blood screening for colorectal cancer. *Lancet* **1996**, *348*, 1472–1477. [CrossRef]
26. Watson, P.; Lynch, H.T. Extracolonic cancer in hereditary nonpolyposis colorectal cancer. *Cancer* **1993**, *71*, 677–685. [CrossRef]
27. Imperiale, T.F.; Wagner, D.R.; Lin, C.Y.; Larkin, G.N.; Rogge, J.D.; Ransohoff, D.F. Results of screening colonoscopy among persons 40 to 49 years of age. *N. Engl. J. Med.* **2002**, *346*, 1781–1785. [CrossRef] [PubMed]
28. Boice, J.D., Jr.; Engholm, G.; Kleinerman, R.A.; Blettner, M.; Stovall, M.; Lisco, H.; Moloney, W.C.; Austin, D.F.; Bosch, A.; Cookfair, D.L.; et al. Radiation dose and second cancer risk in patients treated for cancer of the cervix. *Radiat. Res.* **1988**, *116*, 3–55. [CrossRef]
29. Fung, C.; Fossa, S.D.; Milano, M.T.; Oldenburg, J.; Travis, L.B. Solid tumors after chemotherapy or surgery for testicular nonseminoma: A population-based study. *J. Clin. Oncol.* **2013**, *31*, 3807–3814. [CrossRef]
30. Travis, L.B.; Curtis, R.E.; Storm, H.; Hall, P.; Holowaty, E.; Van Leeuwen, F.E.; Kohler, B.A.; Pukkala, E.; Lynch, C.F.; Andersson, M.; et al. Risk of second malignant neoplasms among long-term survivors of testicular cancer. *J. Natl. Cancer Inst.* **1997**, *89*, 1429–1439. [CrossRef] [PubMed]
31. Travis, L.B.; Fossa, S.D.; Schonfeld, S.J.; McMaster, M.L.; Lynch, C.F.; Storm, H.; Hall, P.; Holowaty, E.; Andersen, A.; Pukkala, E.; et al. Second cancers among 40,576 testicular cancer patients: Focus on long-term survivors. *J. Natl. Cancer Inst.* **2005**, *97*, 1354–1365. [CrossRef] [PubMed]
32. Travis, L.B.; Holowaty, E.J.; Bergfeldt, K.; Lynch, C.F.; Kohler, B.A.; Wiklund, T.; Curtis, R.E.; Hall, P.; Andersson, M.; Pukkala, E.; et al. Risk of leukemia after platinum-based chemotherapy for ovarian cancer. *N. Engl. J. Med.* **1999**, *340*, 351–357. [CrossRef]

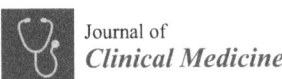

Article

Association between Hepatitis C Virus Infection and Esophageal Cancer: An Asian Nationwide Population-Based Cohort Study

Yin-Yi Chu [1,2,3], Jur-Shan Cheng [4,5], Ting-Shu Wu [3,6], Chun-Wei Chen [1,3], Ming-Yu Chang [3,7,8], Hsin-Ping Ku [2], Rong-Nan Chien [3,9] and Ming-Ling Chang [3,9,*]

[1] Division of Gastroenterology, Department of Gastroenterology and Hepatology, Chang Gung Memorial Hospital, Taoyuan 333423, Taiwan; chu2235@yahoo.com (Y.-Y.C.); 8902088@cgmh.org.tw (C.-W.C.)
[2] Department of Gastroenterology and Hepatology, New Taipei Municipal Tu Cheng Hospital, New Taipei City 236, Taiwan; find94132@yahoo.com
[3] Department of Medicine, College of Medicine, Chang Gung University, Taoyuan 333323, Taiwan; tingshu.wu@gmail.com (T.-S.W.); p123073@gmail.com (M.-Y.C.); ronald@adm.cgmh.org.tw (R.-N.C.)
[4] Clinical Informatics and Medical Statistics Research Center, College of Medicine, Chang Gung University, Taoyuan 333423, Taiwan; jscheng@mail.cgu.edu.tw
[5] Department of Emergency Medicine, Chang Gung Memorial Hospital, Keelung 20401, Taiwan
[6] Division of Infectious Diseases, Department of Internal Medicine, Linkou 333423, Taiwan
[7] Division of Pediatric Neurologic Medicine, Chang Gung Children's Hospital, Taoyuan 333423, Taiwan
[8] Division of Pediatrics, Chang Gung Memorial Hospital, Keelung 20401, Taiwan
[9] Division of Hepatology, Department of Gastroenterology and Hepatology, Chang Gung Memorial Hospital, Taoyuan 333423, Taiwan
* Correspondence: mlchang8210@gmail.com; Tel.: +886-3-3281200 (ext. 8102); Fax: +886-3-3272236

Abstract: Background: Hepatitis C virus (HCV) infection causes many extrahepatic cancers, and whether HCV infection is associated with esophageal cancer development remains inconclusive. **Methods:** A nationwide population-based cohort study of the Taiwan National Health Insurance Research Database (TNHIRD) was conducted. **Results:** From 2003 to 2012, of 11,895,993 patients, three 1:1:1 propensity score-matched cohorts, including HCV-treated (interferon-based therapy ≧6 months, n = 9047), HCV-untreated (n = 9047), and HCV-uninfected cohorts (n = 9047), were enrolled. The HCV-untreated cohort had the highest 9-year cumulative incidence of esophageal cancer among the three cohorts (0.174%; 95% confidence interval (CI): 0.068–0.395) (p = 0.0292). However, no difference in cumulative incidences was identified between the HCV-treated (0.019%; 0.002–0.109%) and HCV-uninfected cohorts (0.035%; 0.007–0.133%) (p = 0.5964). The multivariate analysis showed that HCV positivity (hazard ratio (HR): 5.1, 95% CI HR: 1.39–18.51) and male sex (HR: 8.897; 95% CI HR: 1.194–66.323) were independently associated with the development of esophageal cancer. Of the three cohorts, the HCV-untreated cohort had the highest cumulative incidence of overall mortality at 9 years (21.459%, 95% CI: 18.599–24.460) (p < 0.0001), and the HCV-treated (12.422%, 95% CI: 8.653–16.905%) and HCV-uninfected cohorts (5.545%, 95% CI: 4.225–7.108%) yielded indifferent cumulative mortality incidences (p = 0.1234). **Conclusions:** Although HCV positivity and male sex were independent factors associated with esophageal cancer development, whether HCV infection is the true culprit or a bystander for developing esophageal cancer remains to be further investigated. Interferon-based anti-HCV therapy might attenuate esophageal risk and decrease overall mortality in HCV-infected patients.

Keywords: HCV; esophageal cancer; male; interferon; mortality

Citation: Chu, Y.-Y.; Cheng, J.-S.; Wu, T.-S.; Chen, C.-W.; Chang, M.-Y.; Ku, H.-P.; Chien, R.-N.; Chang, M.-L. Association between Hepatitis C Virus Infection and Esophageal Cancer: An Asian Nationwide Population-Based Cohort Study. *J. Clin. Med.* **2021**, *10*, 2395. https://doi.org/10.3390/jcm10112395

Academic Editor: Gian Paolo Caviglia

Received: 3 April 2021
Accepted: 27 May 2021
Published: 28 May 2021

Publisher's Note: MDPI stays neutral with regard to jurisdictional claims in published maps and institutional affiliations.

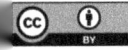

Copyright: © 2021 by the authors. Licensee MDPI, Basel, Switzerland. This article is an open access article distributed under the terms and conditions of the Creative Commons Attribution (CC BY) license (https://creativecommons.org/licenses/by/4.0/).

1. Introduction

Esophageal cancer is the sixth leading cause of cancer death in males, with an estimated >500,000 new cases and >500,000 deaths annually, accounting for 3.2% of cancer cases and 5.37% of cancer deaths worldwide [1]. China, South Africa, and North Central Asia are considered to have the highest incidence of esophageal cancer [2]. The 5-year survival rate among patients with esophageal cancer is 19%, decreasing to 0.9% in patients with advanced esophageal cancer [3]. There are two main histological types of esophageal cancer: esophageal squamous cell carcinoma (ESCC) and esophageal adenocarcinoma (EAC). The risk factors for esophageal SCC include alcohol, smoking, betel nut chewing [4], and hypertension [5]. Metabolic syndrome (MetS) [6] and body mass index (BMI)/obesity [5,7] are related to a higher risk of EAC. In contrast, a high BMI significantly decreases the risk of ESCC [5].

Hepatitis C virus (HCV) is a human pathogen responsible for acute and chronic liver disease that infects an estimated 150 million individuals worldwide [8]. In addition to hepatic complications such as steatosis, cirrhosis, and hepatocellular carcinoma (HCC), HCV causes extrahepatic complications, including mixed cryoglobulinemia [9], dyslipidemia, diabetes [10], obesity, cardiovascular events [11], and neurological manifestations [12]. Moreover, HCV infection is associated with many extrahepatic malignancies, including lymphoid [13], head and heck [14], thyroid [15], lung, pancreas, kidney [13], and gastric cancers [16], B-cell non-Hodgkin's lymphomas, and intrahepatic cholangiocarcinoma [17]. However, the link between HCV infection and esophageal cancer has been elucidated but remains inconclusive. An Asian study showed that compared with HCV seronegative patients, HCV seropositive patients had a higher multivariate-adjusted hazard ratio (HR) for esophageal cancer [15], while another study of a U.S. population showed that esophageal cancers were not more frequent among HCV-infected patients compared with the general population [13]. Combination therapy with pegylated interferon (Peg-IFN) and ribavirin has provided a "cure" for a considerable proportion of HCV-infected patients, particularly in those with the favorable interferon λ 3 (IFNL3) genotype [8]. The cure rates were further improved by replacing interferon-based therapy with direct-acting antiviral agents (DAAs) [8], which led to a sustained virological response (SVR) rate as high as 100% [18]. However, HCV-associated malignancies are not eradicable, especially among patients with baseline diabetes and cirrhosis [19,20]. Whether HCV infection accelerates the risk of esophageal cancer is still a crucial issue in the era of using DAA to eliminate HCV infection.

Accordingly, we aimed to examine the impacts of HCV infection on the development of esophageal cancer in Taiwan, an Asian country where HCV infection is rampant [21], by conducting a nationwide population-based cohort study using the Taiwan National Health Insurance Research Database (TNHIRD). The cumulative incidences of esophageal cancer and esophageal cancer-associated mortalities among HCV-infected subjects with and without anti-HCV therapy and HCV-uninfected subjects were compared to explore the impacts of HCV infection and anti-HCV therapy.

2. Methods

2.1. Samples and Measurements

National-level data, including the National Health Insurance (NHI) administrative database, the Cancer Registry Database, and the Death Registry Database, were used to retrieve data for this population-based retrospective cohort study. The NHI program is a mandatory, single-payer system that covers >99% of the population and offers comprehensive coverage, ranging from laboratory tests and prescription drugs to ambulatory care and hospital services. The HCV-treated cohort consisted of patients who had an HCV RNA test and received Peg-IFN and ribavirin (RBV) for more than 6 months between 1 January 2003 and 31 December 2012. The date of their first HCV test was the index date. The baseline was defined as the date of six months after completing the combination therapy, which was the time to ensure SVR. Patients with cirrhosis-related complications, including hepatoencephalopathy, esophageal or gastric varices, ascites or hepatorenal syndrome, were excluded to avoid interference from these complications or from the associated treatment on the development of esophageal cancer. Those diagnosed with esophageal cancer and those who died before baseline were also excluded. The HCV-untreated subjects included patients who met all the following criteria: (1) received HCV tests (HCV antibody or HCV RNA test); (2) had a diagnosis of HCV infection (International Classification of Diseases, Ninth Revision, Clinical Modification (ICD-9-CM) codes: 070.41, 070.44, 070.51, 070.54, 070.70, 070.71, V02.62)); (3) received hepatoprotective agent therapy, including silymarin, liver hydrolysate, choline bitartrate, and ursodeoxycholic acid; and (4) did not have any history of anti-HCV therapy (Peg-IFN or RBV). Their index date was the date of their first HCV test. The HCV-uninfected individuals consisted of those without any HCV diagnosis, HCV tests, and hepatoprotective agent therapy or anti-HCV treatment. Their index date was the date of one of their physician visits randomly selected from their claims database. The HCV-treated cohort was 1:1:1 matched with the HCV-untreated cohort and with the HCV-uninfected cohort using a propensity score-matched method to assure comparable observed characteristics among the three cohorts. The probability of receiving the combination therapy was estimated by adopting a logistic model with the following covariates: age, NHI registration location, Charlson Comorbidity Index (CCI) score [22], and year of the index date. In the HCV-untreated and HCV-uninfected cohorts, the baseline was determined based on the time elapsed from the index date to the baseline of their matched HCV-treated counterparts. The same exclusion criteria were applied to the HCV-untreated and HCV-uninfected cohorts. The matching processes of the three cohorts are demonstrated in Supplementary Figure S1.

Development of esophageal cancer (ICD-9-CM:150) was identified from the Cancer Registry data that provides types of cancers and dates of diagnosis. Esophageal cancer-related mortality (ICD-9-CM code: C15) was retrieved from the Death Registry data that contains information on causes and dates of death. Subjects were followed from baseline until the date of event (esophageal cancer or esophageal cancer-related mortality), death, or the end of follow-up (31 December 2013), whichever occurred first.

2.2. Statistical Analysis

Statistical Package for Statistical Analysis System (SAS version 9.4, SAS Institute Inc., Cary, NC, USA) software was used to perform the analyses. The modified Kaplan–Meier method and the Gray method that took into account death as a competing risk event [23] were used to estimate and compare cumulative incidences. A subdistribution hazards model [24], which is a modified Cox proportional hazards model that considers competing mortality, was used to estimate the adjusted HR of esophageal cancer development. Covariates of the models included age, sex, NHI registration location, CCI score, year of the index date, baseline liver cirrhosis, end-stage renal disease (ESRD), chronic obstructive pulmonary disease (COPD), diabetes mellitus (DM), hypertension, dyslipidemia, cardiovascular events, and stroke. Cardiovascular events consisted of percutaneous coronary intervention, myocardial infarction, cardiogenic heart failure, shock, coronary artery bypass graft, and peripheral vascular disease. Statistical significance level was defined at 5%.

2.3. Informed Consent

The study protocol conformed to the ethical guidelines of the 1975 Declaration of Helsinki and was approved by the Chang Gung Medical Foundation Institutional Review Board. The need for consent was waived because the national-level data used in this study were deidentified by encrypting personal identification information.

3. Results

3.1. Baseline Characteristics

From a total of 19,298,735 individuals assessed between 1 January 2003 and 31 December 2012, 11,895,993 patients without baseline esophageal cancer were identified; 114,304 patients with HCV infection and 11,781,689 patients without HCV infection were eligible for the study. In total, three cohorts, including HCV-treated (n = 9047), HCV-untreated (n = 9047) and HCV-uninfected (n = 9047) cohorts, were enrolled (Figure 1). The three cohorts were matched with the propensity scores and did not differ in demographic factors, residency, CCI score or index year, which were the covariates in the models to calculate propensity scores, although baseline comorbidities were not similar (Table 1). Compared with HCV-untreated cohorts, the HCV-treated cohort had higher rates of baseline cirrhosis but comparable rates of COPD and lower rates of other comorbidities. Compared with the HCV-uninfected cohort, the HCV-treated cohort had higher rates of baseline cirrhosis, COPD, ESRD, and hypertension but lower rates of dyslipidemia and stroke. Compared with the HCV-uninfected cohort, the HCV-untreated cohort had higher rates of all baseline comorbidities except dyslipidemia and stroke. To determine the HCV-associated complications, we compared the baseline factors between the HCV-infected cohort (which was a combination of the HCV-treated and HCV-untreated cohorts) and HCV-uninfected cohort. The HCV-infected cohort had higher rates of all baseline comorbidities except dyslipidemia and stroke for which there were lower rates than that of the HCV-uninfected cohort (Supplementary Table S1).

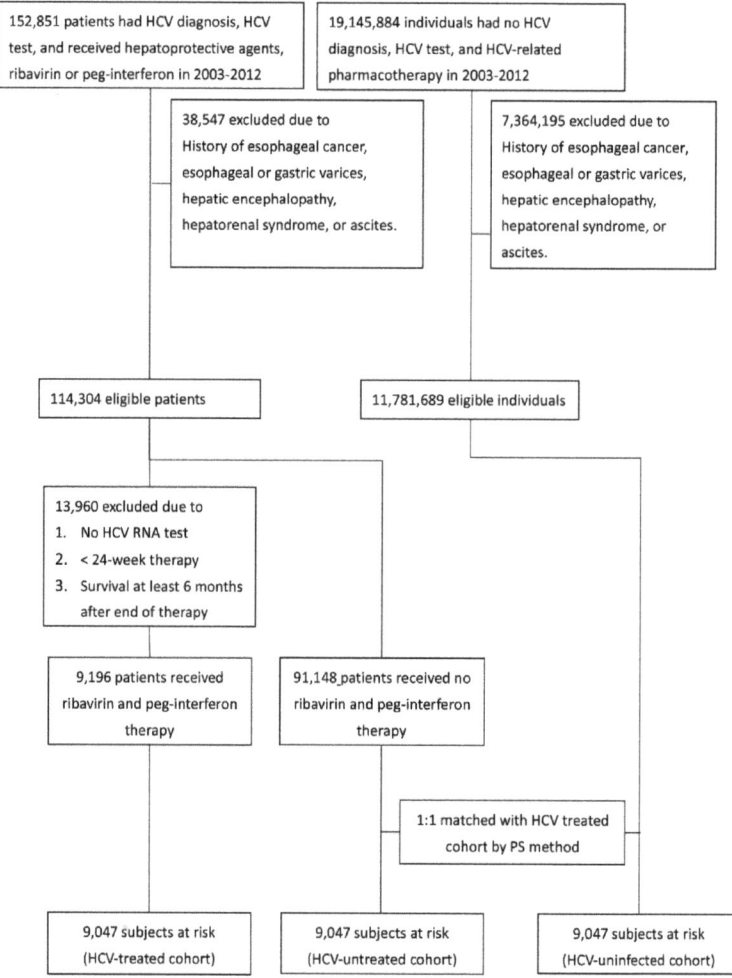

Figure 1. Flow chart of TNHIRD study subjects' selection. TNHIRD: Taiwan National Health Insurance Research Database; HCV: hepatitis C virus; Peg-IFN: pegylated interferon; PS: propensity score.

Table 1. Baseline characteristics of the 3 HCV cohorts of TNHIRD.

	(1)	(2)	(3)	p-Values		
	HCV-Treated	HCV-Untreated	HCV-Uninfected	(1),(2)	(1),(3)	(2),(3)
n	9047	9047	9047			
Gender						
Female, n, (%)	4182 (46.23)	4182 (46.23)	4182 (46.23)	1	1	1
Age range (years), n, (%)						
20–39	1569 (17.34)	1569 (17.34)	1569 (17.34)	1	1	1
40–49	2515 (27.80)	2515 (27.80)	2515 (27.80)			
50–59	3260 (36.03)	3260 (36.03)	3260 (36.03)			
≥60	1703 (18.82)	1703 (18.82)	1703 (18.82)			
Area, n, (%)						
city	2205 (24.37)	2205 (24.37)	2205 (24.37)	1	1	1
township	2785 (30.78)	2785 (30.78)	2785 (30.78)			
rural area	4057 (44.84)	4057 (44.84)	4057 (44.84)			
CCI score, n, (%)						
0	4292 (47.44)	4292 (47.44)	4292 (47.44)	1	1	1
1	3029 (33.48)	3029 (33.48)	3029 (33.48)			
≥2	1726 (19.08)	1726 (19.08)	1726 (19.08)			
Index year, n, (%)						
2003–2006	4400 (48.63)	4400 (48.63)	4400 (48.63)	1	1	1
2007–2009	2805 (31.00)	2805 (31.00)	2805 (31.00)			
2010–2012	1842 (20.36)	1842 (20.36)	1842 (20.36)			
Baseline factor, n, (%)						
Liver cirrhosis	969 (10.71)	546 (6.04)	6 (0.07)	<0.0001	<0.0001	<0.0001
COPD	1050 (11.61)	1017 (11.24)	892 (9.86)	0.4406	0.0001	0.0025
ESRD	61 (0.67)	253 (2.80)	23 (0.25)	<0.0001	<0.0001	<0.0001
DM	1702 (18.81)	2051 (22.67)	1677 (18.54)	<0.0001	0.6334	<0.0001
Hypertension	2668 (29.49)	3154 (34.86)	2498 (27.61)	<0.0001	0.0051	<0.0001
Dyslipidemia	1107 (12.24)	1781 (19.69)	1686 (18.64)	<0.0001	<0.0001	0.0727
Cardiovascular events	234 (2.59)	360 (3.98)	255 (2.82)	<0.0001	0.3357	<0.0001
Stroke	298 (3.29)	441 (4.87)	466 (5.15)	<0.0001	<0.0001	0.3944

(1): HCV-treated cohort; (2): HCV-untreated cohort; (3): HCV-untreated cohort; HCV: hepatitis C virus; TNHIRD: Taiwan National Health Insurance Research Database; CCI: Charlson Comorbidity Index; COPD: Chronic obstructive pulmonary disease; ESRD: end stage renal disease; DM: diabetes.

3.2. Cumulative Incidences and Associated Factors of Esophageal Cancer

The HCV-treated, untreated, and uninfected cohorts were followed up until death for a duration of up to 9 years. The HCV-untreated cohort had the highest cumulative incidence of esophageal cancer among the three cohorts (Figure 2, Table 2). However, no difference in cumulative incidences of esophageal cancer was identified between the HCV-treated and HCV-uninfected cohorts ($p = 0.5965$). The multivariate analysis of the three cohorts showed that male patients had a higher hazard ratio (HR: 8.894, 95% confidence interval (CI) of HR: 1.194–66.227) than female patients; compared with the HCV-untreated cohort, the HCV-treated cohort had a borderline lower HR ($p = 0.054$) (Supplementary Figure S2). Because the HCV-treated and HCV-uninfected cohorts yielded similar cumulative incidences of esophageal cancer, we combined the HCV-treated and HCV-uninfected cohorts to form an HCV-negative cohort to determine the impact of the presence of HCV on the development of esophageal cancer. Compared with the HCV-negative cohort, the HCV-positive (i.e., HCV-untreated) cohort had a higher risk of incident esophageal cancer ($p < 0.0001$). The multivariate analyses of these two cohorts showed that HCV positivity (HR: 5.1, 95% CI HR: 1.39–18.51) and male sex were independently associated with the development of esophageal cancer (Figure 3).

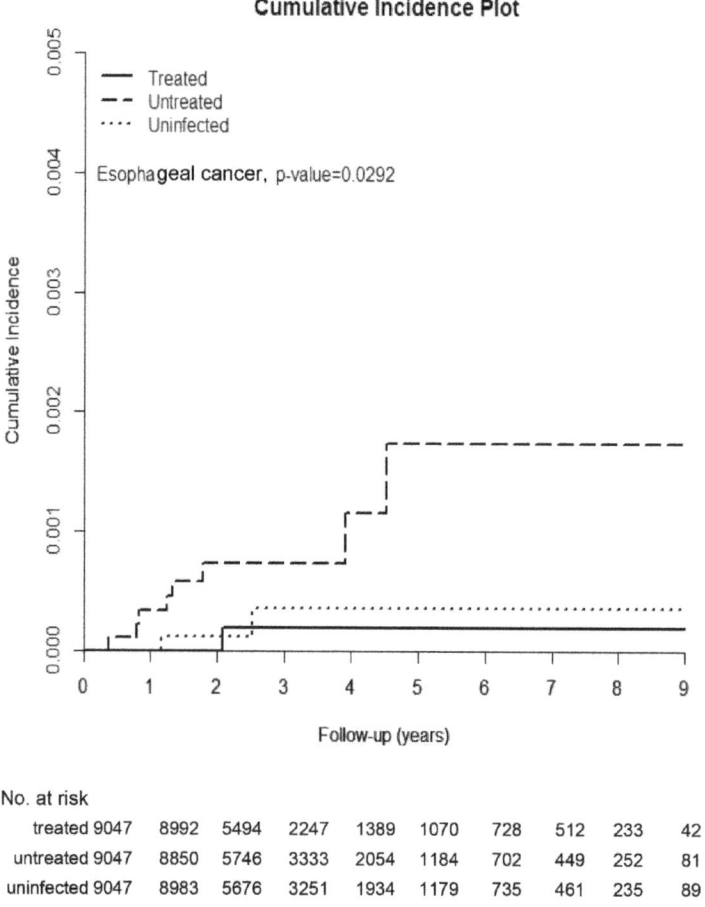

Figure 2. Cumulative incidence of esophageal cancers among the three TNHIRD cohorts, including HCV-treated, HCV-untreated, and HCV-uninfected cohorts.

Table 2. Comparison of the cumulative incidences of esophageal cancers among (1) HCV-treated, (2) HCV-untreated, and (3) HCV-uninfected cohorts.

	HCV-Treated	HCV-Untreated	HCV-Uninfected	*p*-Value
	n = 9047	*n* = 9047	*n* = 9047	
Follow-up years, mean ± SD	2.76 ± 1.75	2.97 ± 1.83	2.96 ± 1.81	
Event number, *n* (%)	1 (0.01)	86 (0.56)	40 (0.26)	
Competing mortality, *n* (%)	209 (2.31)	762 (4.95)	272 (1.77)	
CI, % (95% CI)	0.019 (0.002–0.109)	0.174 (0.068–0.395)	0.035 (0.007–0.133)	0.0292

HCV: hepatitis C virus; SD: standard deviation; CI: cumulative incidence; 95% CI: 95% confidence interval of cumulative incidence 0.007–0.133.

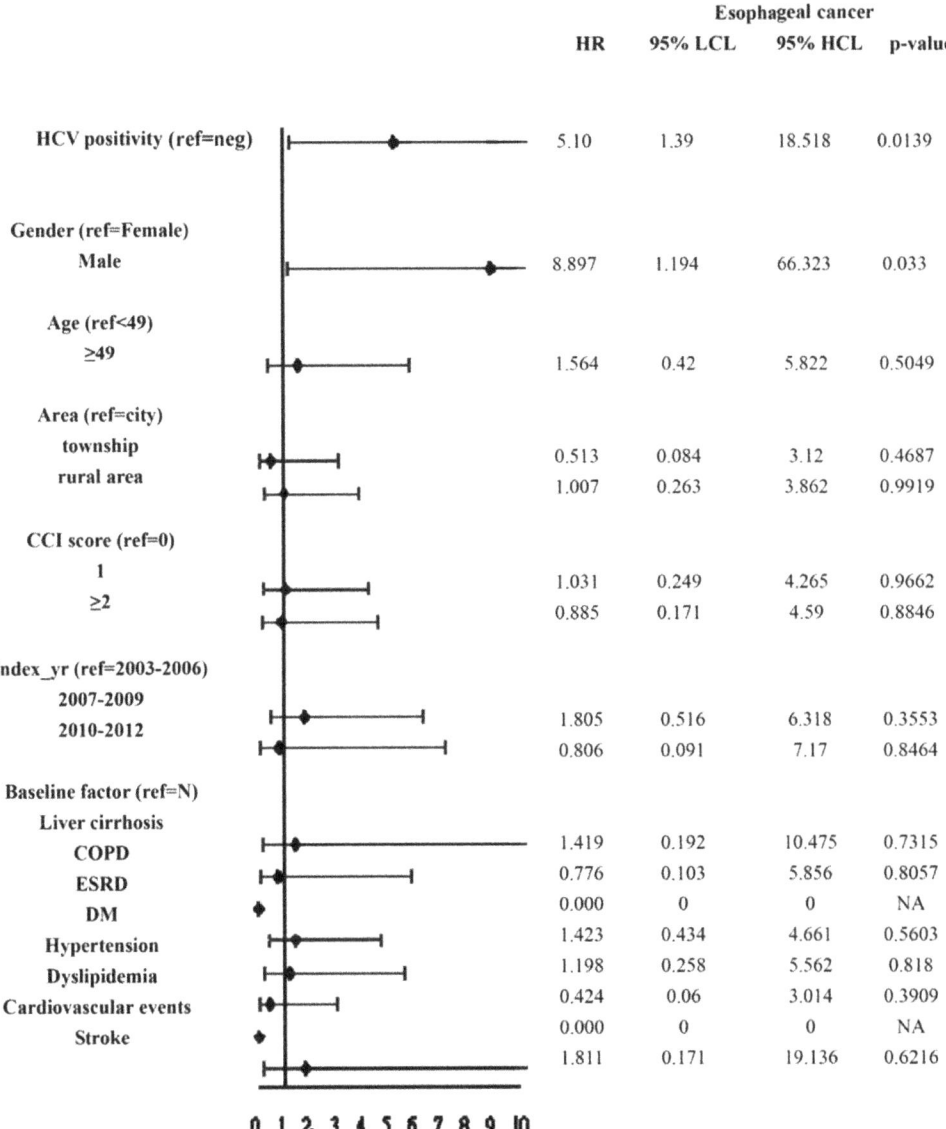

Figure 3. Forest plot of factors associated with incident esophageal cancers in the two TNHIRD cohorts, including HCV-positive and HCV-negative cohorts. neg: Negative; HR: hazards ratio; CI: confidence interval; LCL: lower confidence limit; HCL: higher confidence limit; HCV: hepatitis C virus; COPD: Chronic obstructive pulmonary disease; ESRD: end stage renal disease; DM: diabetes.

3.3. Mortality

Of the three cohorts, the HCV-untreated cohort had the highest cumulative incidence of overall mortality at 9 years (21.459%, 95% CI: 18.599–24.460) ($p < 0.0001$), and the HCV-treated (12.422%, 95% CI: 8.653–16.905%) and HCV-uninfected (5.545%, 95% CI: 4.225–7.108%) cohorts yielded nonsignificant mortality rates ($p = 0.1234$). No differences in esophageal cancer-associated mortality were noted among the three cohorts ($p = 0.1966$).

4. Discussion

The most compelling results of the current study were as follows: (1) The HCV-untreated cohort had the highest 9-year cumulative incidence of esophageal cancer among the three cohorts, while no difference in cumulative incidences was identified between the HCV-treated and HCV-uninfected cohorts; (2) HCV positivity and male sex were independent factors associated with esophageal cancer development; and (3) The HCV-untreated cohort had the highest cumulative incidence of overall mortality, while the HCV-treated and HCV-uninfected cohorts yielded nonsignificant mortality incidences.

At baseline, the findings that the HCV-treated cohort had a higher cirrhosis rate than the untreated cohort and that the HCV-infected cohort had higher cirrhosis and cardiometabolic complication rates but lower dyslipidemia rates than the HCV-uninfected cohorts were consistent with the ideas that only patients with significant fibrosis were reimbursed for interferon-based anti-HCV therapy by NHI, Taiwan [25], and HCV infection causes cirrhosis, cardiometabolic events, and hypolipidemia [8]. These different baseline comorbidities thus supported the reliability of the results based on TNHIRD.

The fact that the HCV-untreated cohort had the highest esophageal cancer cumulative incidence, and that HCV positivity was independently associated with esophageal cancer development suggests that HCV infection might increase the risk of esophageal cancer, although the reported data are conflicting, as mentioned above [13,15], and different ethnicities might account for the discrepancy. More than 90% of patients with esophageal cancer in Asian countries suffer from ESCC [26]. In contrast, in Western countries, most esophageal cancers are EACs [5]. Interestingly, both current and other cohort studies observing the positive link between HCV infection and esophageal cancer were conducted in Taiwan, an Asian country endemic for the practice of Areca nut and betel quid chewing [27], and a negligible association between HCV infection and esophageal cancers was noted in the U.S. population [13]. In particular, in Taiwan, there is an increasing trend of the incidence of ESCC but not that of EAC [26]. Moreover, betel nut chewing has been regarded as a risk factor for HCV infection in Taiwan [28]. Although MetS was associated with poor prognosis in ESCC patients [29], as mentioned, MetS, including increased BMI, decreases the risks of ESCC [5]. Together, the connection between HCV infection and esophageal cancer might accelerate ESCC through a betel liquid chewing habit in HCV-infected patients rather than through metabolic alteration subsequent to HCV infection to accelerate EAC, based on the unique pathology trend of esophageal cancer and the betel liquid chewing practices of Taiwan [27]. Of note, the fact that the cumulative incidences of esophageal cancer were similar between the HCV-treated and HCV-uninfected cohorts suggests that the HCV-associated esophageal cancer risk might be reversed by interferon-based anti-HCV therapy. Future studies are needed to verify the reversibility of esophageal cancer risk in HCV-infected patients with viral clearance following DAA therapy [8].

In addition to HCV positivity, male sex was independently associated with the cumulative incidence of esophageal cancer among the three TNHIRD cohorts. Consistently, the risks of developing esophageal cancer among men have increased worldwide [30]. It is possible that the risk factors for the development of ESCC [4,5] are more common among men, which potentially, at least partly, explains the higher cumulative incidence of esophageal cancer among men. Thus, male HCV-infected patients have a higher risk of esophageal cancer, regardless of anti-HCV therapy.

Although the esophageal cancer-associated mortality was similar among the three cohorts, the HCV-untreated cohort yielded the highest overall mortality, which might be caused by HCV-associated events, such as cirrhosis, HCC or cardiometabolic events [8] other than esophageal cancer-associated complications, as no difference in esophageal cancer-associated mortality was noted among the three cohorts. This phenomenon indicates the importance of prescribing anti-HCV therapy in HCV-infected patients to decrease overall mortality.

There are limitations in the current study. First, because linking the results from TNHIRD to the laboratory results of individual patients was forbidden, the correlation of SVR with esophageal cancer could not be identified. Regardless, we are confident of the antiviral efficacy in the HCV-treated cohort because interferon-based therapy for HCV infection generally achieves an SVR rate ranging from 70% to 90% in Taiwan [31], where favorable genetic variation in IFNL3is prevalent [32]. Second, HCV testing is not universally performed in Taiwan, and HCV-uninfected individuals were the patients who did not receive any HCV diagnosis, HCV tests, hepatoprotective agent therapy, or anti-HCV treatment. There might be undiagnosed HCV-infected patients in the HCV-uninfected cohort. However, because the reimbursement of anti-HCV therapy in Taiwan is nationwide and only up to 2.7% of the Taiwanese were HCV-positive [33,34], the undiagnosed HCV infection rate of the HCV-uninfected cohort might be negligible. Third, the case numbers of patients who developed esophageal cancer were low in the TNHIRD cohort, which might lead to some statistical biases. In particular, the difference between HCV-untreated and HCV-uninfected cohorts could be due to random variation. Fourth, the precise mechanism of the increased risk of esophageal cancer in HCV-infected patients was undetermined, and some documented risks for esophageal cancer, such as alcohol, smoking, betel nut chewing [4], MetS [6,29], hypertension [35], and obesity [7] cannot be identified from the TNHIRD. Fifth, the ICD-9 CM code cannot differentiate ESCC and EAC. The trend of specific histology of esophageal cancer in HCV-infected patients thus cannot be identified. Lastly, as mentioned above, what we found in the current study that adopted interferon-based therapy demands further verification by using DAAs as anti-HCV therapy. Future prospective studies in other independent cohorts with a large number of esophageal cancer cases, definite HCV-uninfected diagnosis confirmed by negative HCV serological tests, identifiable SVR following DAAs with comprehensive risk and histology surveys, and sophisticated molecular investigations are required to elucidate the fundamental mechanisms underlying the findings described here.

Taken together, both HCV positivity and male sex were associated with the development of esophageal cancer. However, whether HCV infection is the true culprit or only a bystander for developing esophageal cancer remains to be further investigated. Interferon-based anti-HCV therapy might attenuate the risk of esophageal cancer development and decrease the mortality of HCV-infected patients.

Supplementary Materials: The following are available online at https://www.mdpi.com/article/10.3390/jcm10112395/s1, Figure S1: Matching process of the 3 TNHIRD cohorts, including HCV-treated, HCV-untreated, and HCV-uninfected cohorts, Figure S2: Forest plot of factors associated with esophageal cancers in the 3 TNHIRD cohorts, including HCV-treated, HCV-untreated, and HCV-uninfected cohorts. esoph.: esophageal. Table S1. Baseline characteristics of the 2 HCV cohorts of TNHIRD.

Author Contributions: Data curation, Y.-Y.C., T.-S.W., C.-W.C., M.-Y.C., R.-N.C., and M.-L.C.; Formal analysis, Y.-Y.C., J.-S.C., C.-W.C., H.-P.K., and M.-L.C.; Funding acquisition, M.-L.C.; Supervision, M.-L.C. All authors have read and agreed to the published version of the manuscript.

Funding: This study was supported by grants from the Chang Gung Medical Research Program (CMRPG3I0413, CMRPG3K0721, and CMRPG1K0111) and the National Science Council (MOST 109-2314-B-182-024- and MOST 109-2629-B-182-002-). The funders had no role in study design, data collection and analysis, decision to publish, or preparation of the manuscript. The opinions expressed in this paper are those of the authors and do not necessarily represent those of Chang Gung Medical Hospital and National Science Council, Taiwan.

Institutional Review Board Statement: The study protocol conformed to the ethical guidelines of the 1975 Declaration of Helsinki and was approved by the local Institutional Review Board.

Informed Consent Statement: The need for consent was waived because the national-level data used in this study were de-identified by encrypting personal identification information.

Data Availability Statement: The datasets generated during and/or analysed during the current study are available from the corresponding author on reasonable request.

Acknowledgments: The authors thank Shu-Chun Chen, Chia-Hui Tsai, Chun-Kai Liang, and Shuen-Shian Shiau from the Liver Research Center, Chang Gung Memorial Hospital, Taiwan for their assistance with data mining.

Conflicts of Interest: The authors declare no conflict of interest.

References

1. Bray, F.; Me, J.F.; Soerjomataram, I.; Siegel, R.L.; Torre, L.A.; Jemal, A. Global cancer statistics 2018: GLOBOCAN estimates of incidence and mortality worldwide for 36 cancers in 185 countries. *CA Cancer J. Clin.* **2018**, *68*, 394–424. [CrossRef]
2. Siegel, R.L.; Mph, K.D.M.; Jemal, A. Cancer statistics, 2018. *CA Cancer J. Clin.* **2018**, *68*, 7–30. [CrossRef]
3. Testa, U.; Castelli, G.; Pelosi, E. Esophageal Cancer: Genomic and Molecular Characterization, Stem Cell Compartment and Clonal Evolution. *Medicines* **2017**, *4*, 67. [CrossRef] [PubMed]
4. Lee, C.-H.; Lee, J.-M.; Wu, D.-C.; Hsu, H.-K.; Kao, E.-L.; Huang, H.-L.; Wang, T.-N.; Huang, M.-C.; Wu, M.-T. Independent and combined effects of alcohol intake, tobacco smoking and betel quid chewing on the risk of esophageal cancer in Taiwan. *Int. J. Cancer* **2004**, *113*, 475–482. [CrossRef]
5. Huang, F.-L.; Yu, S.-J. Esophageal cancer: Risk factors, genetic association, and treatment. *Asian J. Surg.* **2018**, *41*, 210–215. [CrossRef]
6. Zhang, J.; Wu, H.; Wang, R. Metabolic syndrome and esophageal cancer risk: A systematic review and meta-analysis. *Diabetol. Metab. Syndr.* **2021**, *13*, 8. [CrossRef] [PubMed]
7. Chang, M.-L.; Yang, Z.; Yang, S.-S. Roles of Adipokines in Digestive Diseases: Markers of Inflammation, Metabolic Alteration and Disease Progression. *Int. J. Mol. Sci.* **2020**, *21*, 8308. [CrossRef] [PubMed]
8. Chang, M.-L. Metabolic alterations and hepatitis C: From bench to bedside. *World J. Gastroenterol.* **2016**, *22*, 1461–1476. [CrossRef] [PubMed]
9. Cheng, Y.T.; Cheng, J.S.; Lin, C.H.; Chen, T.-H.; Lee, K.-C.; Chang, M.-L. Rheumatoid factor and immunoglobulin M mark hepatitis C-associated mixed cryo-globulinaemia: An 8-year prospective study. *Clin. Microbiol. Infect.* **2020**, *26*, 366–372. [CrossRef] [PubMed]
10. Chang, M.-L.; Chen, W.-T.; Hu, J.-H.; Chen, S.-C.; Gu, P.-W.; Chien, R.-N. Altering retinol binding protein 4 levels in hepatitis C: Inflammation and steatosis matter. *Virulence* **2020**, *11*, 1501–1511. [CrossRef] [PubMed]
11. Chang, M.-L.; Lin, Y.-S.; Hsu, C.-L.; Chien, R.-N.; Fann, C.S. Accelerated cardiovascular risk after viral clearance in hepatitis C patients with the NAMPT-rs61330082 TT genotype: An 8-year prospective cohort study. *Virulence* **2021**, *12*, 270–280. [CrossRef] [PubMed]
12. Negro, F.; Forton, D.; Craxì, A.; Sulkowski, M.S.; Feld, J.J.; Manns, M.P. Extrahepatic Morbidity and Mortality of Chronic Hepatitis C. *Gastroenterology* **2015**, *149*, 1345–1360. [CrossRef] [PubMed]
13. Allison, R.D.; Tong, X.; Moorman, A.C.; Ly, K.N.; Rupp, L.; Xu, F.; Gordon, S.C.; Holmberg, S.D. Increased incidence of cancer and cancer-related mortality among persons with chronic hepatitis C infection, 2006–2010. *J. Hepatol.* **2015**, *63*, 822–828. [CrossRef]
14. Mahale, P.; Sturgis, E.M.; Tweardy, D.J.; Ariza-Heredia, E.J.; Torres, H.A. Association Between Hepatitis C Virus and Head and Neck Cancers. *J. Natl. Cancer Inst.* **2016**, *108*. [CrossRef] [PubMed]
15. Lee, M.-H.; Yang, H.-I.; Lu, S.-N.; Jen, C.-L.; You, S.-L.; Wang, L.-Y.; Wang, C.-H.; Chen, W.J.; Chen, C.-J.; Reveal-HCV Study Group. Chronic Hepatitis C Virus Infection Increases Mortality from Hepatic and Extrahepatic Diseases: A Community-Based Long-Term Prospective Study. *J. Infect. Dis.* **2012**, *206*, 469–477. [CrossRef]
16. Chen, C.-W.; Cheng, J.-S.; Chen, T.-D.; Le, P.-H.; Ku, H.-P.; Chang, M.-L. The irreversible HCV-associated risk of gastric cancer following interferon-based therapy: A joint study of hospital-based cases and nationwide population-based cohorts. *Ther. Adv. Gastroenterol.* **2019**, *12*. [CrossRef]
17. Fiorino, S.; Bacchi-Reggiani, L.; De Biase, D.; Fornelli, A.; Masetti, M.; Tura, A.; Grizzi, F.; Zanello, M.; Mastrangelo, L.; Lombardi, R.; et al. Possible association between hepatitis C virus and malignancies different from hepatocellular carcinoma: A systematic review. *World J. Gastroenterol.* **2015**, *21*, 12896–12953. [CrossRef]
18. Vermehren, J.; Park, J.; Jacobson, I.M.; Zeuzem, S. Challenges and perspectives of direct antivirals for the treatment of hepatitis C virus infection. *J. Hepatol.* **2018**, *69*, 1178–1187. [CrossRef]
19. Toyoda, H.; Kumada, T.; Tada, T.; Kiriyama, S.; Tanikawa, M.; Hisanaga, Y.; Kanamori, A.; Kitabatake, S.; Ito, T. Risk factors of hepatocellular carcinoma development in non-cirrhotic patients with sustained virologic response for chronic hepatitis C virus infection. *J. Gastroenterol. Hepatol.* **2015**, *30*, 1183–1189. [CrossRef]
20. Kalaitzakis, E.; Gunnarsdottir, S.A.; Josefsson, A.; Björnsson, E. Increased Risk for Malignant Neoplasms Among Patients with Cirrhosis. *Clin. Gastroenterol. Hepatol.* **2011**, *9*, 168–174. [CrossRef]
21. Hu, J.-H.; Chen, M.-Y.; Yeh, C.-T.; Lin, S.-H.; Lin, M.-S.; Huang, T.-J.; Chang, M.-L. Sexual Dimorphic Metabolic Alterations in Hepatitis C Virus-infected Patients: A Community-Based Study in a Hepatitis B/Hepatitis C Virus Hyperendemic Area. *Medicine* **2016**, *95*, e3546. [CrossRef]
22. Deyo, R.A.; Cherkin, D.C.; Ciol, M.A. Adapting a clinical comorbidity index for use with ICD-9-CM administrative databases. *J. Clin. Epidemiol.* **1992**, *45*, 613–619. [CrossRef]
23. Gray, R.J. A Class of K-Sample Tests for Comparing the Cumulative Incidence of a Competing Risk. *Ann. Stat.* **1988**, *16*, 1141–1154. [CrossRef]

24. Fine, J.P.; Gray, R.J. A Proportional Hazards Model for the Subdistribution of a Competing Risk. *J. Am. Stat. Assoc.* **1999**, *94*, 496–509. [CrossRef]
25. Available online: https://www.nhi.gov.tw/Content_List.aspx?n=A4EFF6CD1C4891CA&topn=3FC7D09599D25979 (accessed on 3 April 2021).
26. Lu, C.-L.; Lang, H.-C.; Luo, J.-C.; Liu, C.-C.; Lin, H.-C.; Chang, F.-Y.; Lee, S.-D. Increasing trend of the incidence of esophageal squamous cell carcinoma, but not adenocarcinoma, in Taiwan. *Cancer Causes Control* **2009**, *21*, 269–274. [CrossRef] [PubMed]
27. Gunjal, S.; Pateel, D.G.S.; Yang, Y.-H.; Doss, J.G.; Bilal, S.; Maling, T.H.; Mehrotra, R.; Cheong, S.C.; Zain, R.B.M. An Overview on Betel Quid and Areca Nut Practice and Control in Selected Asian and South East Asian Countries. *Subst. Use Misuse* **2020**, *55*, 1533–1544. [CrossRef]
28. Lin, C.H.; Lin, C.C.; Liu, C.S. Betel nut chewing as a risk factor for hepatitis C infection in Taiwan—A community-based study. *Ann. Saudi Med.* **2011**, *31*, 204–205. [CrossRef] [PubMed]
29. Peng, F.; Hu, D.; Lin, X.; Chen, G.; Liang, B.; Zhang, H.; Dong, X.; Lin, J.; Zheng, X.; Niu, W. Analysis of Preoperative Metabolic Risk Factors Affecting the Prognosis of Patients with Esophageal Squamous Cell Carcinoma: The Fujian Prospective Investigation of Cancer (FIESTA) Study. *EBioMedicine* **2017**, *16*, 115–123. [CrossRef]
30. Dix, O.; Thakur, M.; Genova, A. Increased Risk of Esophageal Cancers Among Men in Taiwan. *Cureus* **2020**, *12*, e6990. [CrossRef] [PubMed]
31. Yu, M.-L.; Dai, C.-Y.; Huang, J.-F.; Hou, N.-J.; Lee, L.-P.; Hsieh, M.-Y.; Chiu, C.-F.; Lin, Z.-Y.; Chen, S.-C.; Wang, L.-Y.; et al. A randomised study of peginterferon and ribavirin for 16 versus 24 weeks in patients with genotype 2 chronic hepatitis C. *Gut* **2007**, *56*, 553–559. [CrossRef] [PubMed]
32. Yu, M.-L.; Huang, C.-F.; Huang, J.-F.; Chang, N.-C.; Yang, J.-F.; Lin, Z.-Y.; Chen, S.-C.; Hsieh, M.-Y.; Wang, L.-Y.; Chang, W.-Y.; et al. Role of interleukin-28B polymorphisms in the treatment of hepatitis C virus genotype 2 infection in Asian patients. *Hepatology* **2010**, *53*, 7–13. [CrossRef] [PubMed]
33. Cheng, Y.L.; Wang, Y.C.; Lan, K.H.; Huo, T.-L.; Huang, Y.-H.; Su, C.-W.; Lin, H.-C.; Lee, F.-Y.; Wu, J.-C.; Lee, S.-D. Anti-hepatitis C virus seropositivity is not associated with metabolic syndrome irrespective of age, gender and fibrosis. *Ann. Hepatol.* **2015**, *14*, 181–189. [CrossRef]
34. Polaris Observatory HCV Collaborators. Global prevalence and genotype distribution of hepatitis C virus infection in 2015: A modelling study. *Lancet Gastroenterol. Hepatol.* **2017**, *2*, 161–176. [CrossRef]
35. Seo, J.H.; Kim, Y.D.; Park, C.S.; Han, K.-D.; Joo, Y.-H. Hypertension is associated with oral, laryngeal, and esophageal cancer: A nationwide population-based study. *Sci. Rep.* **2020**, *10*, 10291. [CrossRef] [PubMed]

MDPI
St. Alban-Anlage 66
4052 Basel
Switzerland
www.mdpi.com

Journal of Clinical Medicine Editorial Office
E-mail: jcm@mdpi.com
www.mdpi.com/journal/jcm

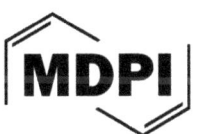

Disclaimer/Publisher's Note: The statements, opinions and data contained in all publications are solely those of the individual author(s) and contributor(s) and not of MDPI and/or the editor(s). MDPI and/or the editor(s) disclaim responsibility for any injury to people or property resulting from any ideas, methods, instructions or products referred to in the content.

www.ingramcontent.com/pod-product-compliance
Lightning Source LLC
LaVergne TN
LVHW070614100526
838202LV00012B/649